1 MONTH OF
FREE
READING

at

www.ForgottenBooks.com

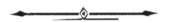

By purchasing this book you are eligible for one month membership to ForgottenBooks.com, giving you unlimited access to our entire collection of over 1,000,000 titles via our web site and mobile apps.

To claim your free month visit:

www.forgottenbooks.com/free439017

ISBN 978-0-483-42817-1
PIBN 10439017

SAINT LOUIS

Medical and Surgical

JOURNAL.

1873.

PUBLISHED MONTHLY.

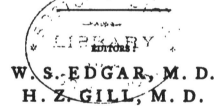

EDITORS:

W. S. EDGAR, M. D.
H. Z. GILL, M. D.

NEW SERIES. VOL X.

ST. LOUIS:
E. F. HOBART & CO., PUBLISHERS.
1873.

Table of Contents.

VOLUME X.

Original Communications.

Hospital Reports.

Reviews and Bibliographical Notices.

Extracts from Current Medical Literature.

Proceedings.

Editorial.

Miscellaneous.

PAGE.

Obituary. 292, 511
Specialties 570
Linton District Medical Society 570
Medical Schools 624

Books and Pamphlets.

Books and Pamphlets received 41, 165, 214, 336, 458, 494, 561, 621

Meteorological.

Thermometric 55, 113, 167, 291, 347, 403, 459, 515, 571, 625, 687

Official Report of Deaths, Diseases, etc.

Mortality Reports 56, 114, 168, 232, 292, 348, 404, 460, 516, 572, 626, 688

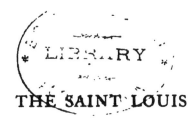

THE SAINT LOUIS
Medical and Surgical Journal.

JANUARY, 1873.

Original Communications.

ON THE TREATMENT OF FEVER.

By Prof. C. LIEBERMEISTER, of Tübingen.

(*Volkman's Clinical Lectures.*)

(Translated from the German, by HENRY KIRCHNER, M. D., St. Louis, Mo)

(Continued from page 740, vol. IX.)

In the fever patient the conditions above mentioned, exist in the same manner, only with this difference, that with him the remedies do not reach so far, and that accordingly the boundary at which the cooling of the internal parts of the body begins is passed somewhat sooner. Besides, the fever patient has the same tendency to retain his temperature; he maintains his abnormally high temperature by the same means as the healthy does his normal temperature. In the fever patient the existing high temperature is increased in an extraordinary manner, by the cold bath, as direct observations on the production of heat show, and are corroborated by investigation on the production of carbonic acid by exhalation.

In this constancy of the regulatory power of temperature is to be found the impediment to a sufficient artificial lowering of it.   This explains why many observers, who with high hopes took up the cold water treatment, but did not go far enough in the abstraction of heat, were much disappointed.   There is no doubt, that by abstraction of heat, at least during its continuance, the consumption of the tissues is increased, the increase in the production of heat and carbonic acid during both is a proof thereof.   This circumstance must not be lost sight of, and it may, in particular cases, furnish a contra-indication against the energetic use of the cold bath.   But for the majority of cases of acute fever, in spite of the danger that lies in a temporary increase of temperature *per se*, can this increase in consumption of bodily material, hardly be taken into account.   And furthermore, as observations show, is the increase in consumption during the abstraction of heat compensated by this : that in a little while the production of heat falls below the usual degree.

But is the first object, the cooling of the body, really affected by the abstraction of heat?   And when it is affected, how does it agree with the fact that in fever this regulation of heat still exists ?   You will notice in the fever patient, as the first and immediate effect of abstraction of heat, that the inner temperature does not fall, but rises.   But it is remarkable, that this only happens in moderate abstractions of heat, and, on the other hand, follows after its cessation in all cases, a considerable falling of the temperature and the sinking in this "after effect," similar as in the healthy, is much greater than the preceding rise.   According to this, the desired effect that often is missed during the process, constantly takes place after the discontinuing of it. While in an abstraction of heat of moderate intensity, the favorable result depends exclusively upon this "after effect," is another important circumstance to be taken into consideration in the more intense abstraction of heat. In the healthy we are only able, in spite of the complete regulatory power to lower the temperature after persevering application of somewhat intense cold. In the fever patient the same may be accomplished, and a degree of cold suffices there, and of less duration than in the healthy would be quite sufficient.

From the above, then, we draw the conclusion that, although during fever any external cooling of the body is followed by an increased production of heat, that we are nevertheless able, by abstraction of heat, to diminish the temperature in a fever patient. We sometimes succeed by this "after effect," and sometimes by a forcible conquering of the regulatory power. In spite of all impediment, and the effective resistance of the organism, we gain our object by an abstraction of heat of sufficient intensity—a cold bath or cold effusions—it cools the body of our patient externally and internally. But it takes a considerable effort to lower the inner temperature for one or two degrees.

Finally, remains one difficulty to be observed, and this, perhaps, chiefly it was that impeded so long the introduction of an effective cold water treatment. If you pour cold water upon a person in fever heat, he is evidently benefitted by this violent procedure, he will be something better. But the fever heat is not overcome permanently, or for a longer time, as some observers expected. Mostly after the lapse of a few hours his condition is the same as before; and even if they had concluded to apply this unpleasant procedure daily it could have had no perceptible influence upon the course of the disease.

Up to a few years ago, the few physicians who employed the cold water treatment to a later period fell into the error (and I have to count myself among these), of believing that it was already a very serious affair to subject a fever patient daily to this rather violent procedure ; only in exceptional cases have we dared to give a cold bath twice a day, and these baths were mostly not as cold as they should have been.

A great merit is due to Bartels and Jürgensen of Kiel, as pioneers in this direction. These observers have shown that in the majority of cases, cold baths can be employed without any danger, as often as may be necessary, that is, as often as the inner temperature transgresses a certain boundary. Since the publication of their experience (1866), dates the great success of cold water treatment. It was everywhere experienced that great successes are then only gained, when day and night the temperature of the patient is controlled, and the cold bath employed as often as the temperature requires.

There are generally necessary from four or six to eight cold baths in twenty-four hours. In severe cases it may become necessary to bathe twelve times in twenty-four hours. I have treated some cases of typhus where the number of baths exceeded two hundred during their illness. They were extraordinarily obstinate cases, that in consequence of the fever, surely would have been fatal, if a less energetic treatment had been instituted.

The most frequent employment of cold water, has, up to this time, been in abdominal typhus, and wherever the treatment was carried through with the necessary perseverance, the result has been surprisingly favorable.

At the hospital in Kiel, there died during the years from 1850 to 1861, of 330 patients with typhus, 51, consequently 15.4 per cent. with an indifferent treatment. During the years 1863 to 1866, died, of 160 treated perseveringly with cold water, only five; consequently 3.1 per cent.; and in later times the result of this treatment appears still more favorable. Also at the hospital in Basel, where abdominal typhus occurred in remarkable frequency and malignity, the antipyretic method had a surprising success. I give a statistical list of mortality, by the different plans of treatment.

Up to 1865, the treatment had been the usual expectant, symptomatic, yet they had commenced in latter years to give a cold or lukewarm bath. When I took the management of the division, in August, 1865, the baths were given regularly only once a day, in exceptional cases twice. In connection with it there was employed, for the purpose of antipyresis, quinine, or digitalis, but not in so energetic a manner, and not according to the fixed indications of a later period. Finally, since September, 1866, after having seen the convincing communication of Jürgensen, on the results they had at Kiel, the baths were employed, gradually increasing in frequency, and gradually somewhat colder, until since the beginning of the year 1868, this method of treatment became a more fixed one.

I.　WITH INDIFFERENT TREATMENT.

	Typhus patients.	Died.	Mortality. Per cent.
1843–1853	444	135	30.4
1854–1859	643	172	26.7
1860–1864	631	16a	25.7

II.　WITH IMPERFECT ANTIPYRETIC TREATMENT.

	Typhus patients received.	Died.	Mortality. Per cent.
Beginning 1865 to Sept. 1866	982	159	16.2

III.　WITH PERSEVERING ANTIPYRETIC TREATMENT.

	Typhus patients received.	Of which died.	Mortality. Per cent.
Sept.　1866, to end of 1867,	339	33	9.7
1868,	181	11	6.1
1869,	186	10	5.4
1870,	139	10	7.2
	845	64	7.6

The figures as shown in these statistics are in so far not properly comparable, as formerly the name typhus was applied somewhat closer, so that it excludes many light cases. We are perfectly able however, to determine the boundaries of this error and conclude that it does not count much. Upon carefully weighing all evidences, we come to the conclusion, that in the last years, with the antipyretic treatment, the number of deaths is hardly one-third of those occurring with an indifferent treatment. The results reported from various other hospitals were, almost without an exception, very favorable especially from Munich, Enlargen, Würzburg, Nüremberg, Greifswell, Jena, Halle, etc. Only in Vienna it appears that up to the present time, they were not able to succeed. On the battle field and in military hospitals, numerous physicians approved of the antipyretic treatment, and in private practice it was employed with a great deal of success. But this method is not only useful in abdominal typhus, but in every febrile ailment in which the temperature, by its height and duration brings danger. The number of diseases is much larger than formerly was supposed; it comprises all diseases in which the danger lies especially in the fever and very little depends on the local disturbance, as for instance abdominal and exanthemetic typhus, scarlatina, etc. In those diseases in which exist severe and dangerous local alterations, is gained a great deal when we succeed to conquer the danger solely dependent upon the fever. So for instance are the results very favorable in treating the severe cases of pneumonia designated as typhous, bilious, or asthenic, perseveringly with cold water; we diminish by it the mortality considerable, if even not in the same proportion as in typhus, as I can state from my own experience, after having treated more than two hundred cases of pneumonia in this manner.

The temperature of the baths as I employ them in hospital and private practice is generally 20° C. = 16° R. = 68° F. or less. For the same patient I use the same water for many baths, the tub remains in the sick room, the water assumes nearly the temperature of the room and I generally leave it so. In the heat of summer only, or when for various reasons a lower temperature is necessary I lower it with pieces of ice. The duration of a bath, as a rule, is ten minutes, a much longer time is for the patient mostly very unpleasant and might possibly lead to bad consequences. When feeble patients are much exausted by the bath, feeling very chilly, or collapse, it will be well to shorten the same to five or

seven minutes. Such a short cold bath always performs
more than a lukewarm of longer duration. Immediately
after the bath the patient requires rest, he is therefore
dried, wrapped in a dry sheet and put to bed (which,
especially at the foot, may be warmed), lightly covered,
he receives, according to circumstances, a glass of wine,
and is dressed after a lapse of some time. Very feeble
patients may have the bath in the beginning at 24° C.
=20° R. =77° F. Such baths are to be of a longer
duration.

Cold effusions have, as the calorimetric investigation
shows, a far inferior effect than cold baths of equal temperature and duration and are for the patient much more
unpleasant. They would suggest themselves, when it
is impossible to apply any other mode of lowering the
temperature, or when you desire less the cooling effect,
than a forcible excitement of the psychical or respiratory
function.

Wrapping in the cold sheets are mostly well borne,
even by the most feeble patients, especially when you
leave the feet and legs free. A series of successive cold
wrappings of ten to twenty minutes each, has about the
same cooling effect as a cold bath of ten minutes duration. Especially in children, where on account of the
relative extent of bodily surface, the abstraction of heat
acts by far more intensely, and where the bath needs to
be less cold and shorter, cold envelopments may be substituted for the bath.

Cold ablutions, even with ice water, appear to have a
slight cooling effect, but by frequent repetition may be
raised to some significance. As substitutes for the bath
they cannot be used.

Local abstraction of heat by cold applications, bladders

of ice, etc., appear to have no decided influence on the temperature of distant parts. Only when the patient is laid on a large india rubber bed, filled with a cooling mixture, a general antipyretic effect may be gained.

By cold drinks, by swallowing ice, by using cold enemata, etc., is the temperature of the body lowered in the healthy person and to such a degree as is necessary to warm what may have been introduced. A regulatory increase in the production of heat, as in the cooling of the external surface, does not take place.

This circumstance is of some importance, and if even the general effect of such internal methods of lowering the temperature is not very great, they have the preference, for you need not conquer a resistance and the organism is not excited to greater expenditure. If it was possible, without serious inconveniences to abstract great quantities of heat from internal organs, this would be the most commendable mode. A suggestion made by a *collegue* with such a view appears to me worth a trial; namely, to bring the mucous membrane of the rectum in contact with cold water during a longer space of time, by introducing into the rectum a stomach tube à *double courant* and connect one of the tubes with a current of water.

The extraordinary obstinacy of fever in many cases, that sometimes is not subdued by the most persevering employment of baths, and the circumstance that many patients cannot bear a sufficiently frequent employment of them, necessitates the employment of other remedies for the purpose of lowering the temperature. The most suitable medicines are chiefly quinine, digitalis and veratria [in this country *veratrum viride*]. Quinine has, aside from malarial fevers, a plain anti-

pyretic effect only then, when it is given in large
doses; for the adult I use as a rule 1½ to 2½ grammes
=23 to 40 grains sulphate or muriate (I find no
difference between the two salts), but it is of importance
that the whole dose be given within the space of half to
one hour at most. If you were to use that quantity
divided during a longer space of time, the effect would
be so much the less, even a much larger quantity taken
in a half or whole day, has often a hardly perceptible
influence upon the temperature. But I do not generally
repeat the dose before the lapse of forty-eight hours.
I would call attention to this: that in cases where the fever
spontaneously remits or intermits the quinine, contrary to a formerly very common notion is much less
indicated than in a febris continua or sub-continua.
Its favorable effect consists in the latter case only in
effecting if ever a transitory intermission. Where such
intermissions occur spontaneously, this indication is
not to be fulfilled, that is to say quinine is not necessary. The known fact that a violent fever, which at
times completely intermits, is much less dangerous
than a less severe fever, that is continued or intermits
very lightly and the experience that this rule holds
good in the artificial depression of fever, has brought
me to the conclusion in the employment of antipyretic
medicines, to look to complete intermission. I estimate therefore the effect of a dose of quinine as sufficient only then, when by it the temperature becomes
normal, or is depressed to nearly 38° C. = 100.5° F. If
we do not succeed with the first dose, we give the next
time a larger one. Should the temperature have fallen
to 37° C. upon the first dose, what not unfrequently occurs,
then you can give a somewhat smaller dose the next

time. This is the most simple way to individualize and to suit the requirements of each single case.

In this way I employed quinine in abdominal typhus, further in pneumonia, in simple as well as in the typhoid or asthenic forms; in variola, scarlatina, erysipelas, acute articular rheumatism, pleurisy, in the symptomatic fevers accompanying profuse discharge of pus; in phthisis florida, with strong continued' fever, in meningitis cerebro-spinalis epidemica. An antipyretic effect is always observed if the quantity is sufficient and used in a short time, yet it appears, there are isolated cases, where the effect of quinine is difficult to gain. I can name as such the suppurative fever in variola and acute articular rheumatism. But also in all other febrile diseases there occur not unfrequently severe and obstinate cases, where even a dose of 37½ grs. is not sufficient to reduce the temperature to its normal standard. In such cases the purpose may be gained by other antipyretic remedies or by their combination with quinine.

Digitalis, I employ for the purpose of antipyresis only in powder. It is thus, when such effect is desired, by far the most reliable, while the commonly used infusion deserves the preference where you chiefly want its action on the heart. The total dose, when taken in powder is considerably less than the less effective infusion. I generally give from 12 to 24 grains divided through thirty-six hours. Digitalis, however, in severe febrile diseases is so much the less indicated, the more excessive the frequency of the pulse is; in dreaded paralysis of the heart it appears rather to aid that event. In typhus abdominalis it may also be employed with great advantage, as the action of the heart is not

excessive, and is somewhat strong.   In especially severe
and obstinate cases, when quinine alone does not sufficiently lower the temperature, the desired effect may be
gained by a combination of both quinine and digitalis.
¾ to 1½ grammes digitalis in powder is to be used in
the course of twenty-four or thirty-six hours, and immediately thereafter a full dose of quinine (2 to 2½
grammes).   If we once succeed in this way to reach
a complete intermission we will be enabled after this to
produce it by quinine alone.

Veratria is a very reliable antipyretic, it causes a complete intermission in cases in which the same could not
be reached by quinine.   I generally give it in pills each
containing five milligrammes of Veratria (about 1.15
grain), one every hour, until sickness of the stomach or
emesis follows.   The collapse which follows upon the
emesis, together with a sudden decline of temperature is,
even in typhus patients, not dangerous, and is treated
with wine and other analeptics.

To say anything definite on the effect of other strong
antipyretic remedies, I must confess that I have not
sufficient experience with them.

Cold water treatment, as well as the employment of
the above named remedies in the large doses mentioned,
is a very thorough, and we may say powerful one, which,
when favorable results are to be obtained, has to be
carried out with great perseverance and circumspection,
that, however, like every other harsh treatment must be
modified according to the peculiarities of each individual
case, and for which reason the very careful managment
of an experienced physician is required.   But the experience of thousands of years has shown that in this
line of small remedies no great effects can be expected

and that as everywhere else great effects require great causes. And finally, the knife of the surgeon is no plaything either, and must not be delivered into the hands of the inexperienced.

The extraordinary practical success, that a perseveringly executed antipyresis shows, tells more than all theoretical deductions that we find ourselves in the right way. The continued experience and with it the correct explanation of its theory will add to secure the way, which we hope to be somewhat more even and comfortable hereafter.

As a paradigma I will make a short sketch of the antipyretic treatment of typhus abdominalis, as it has become fixed in the course of time in Basel.

When a patient comes in before the ninth day of the disease, we give him calomel two to four doses of ½ gramme each (7 grs.) in the course of a few hours; any existing diarrhœa is only momentarily increased by it, on the whole rather diminished. In the majority of cases upon this administration of calomel follows a considerable decrease in temperature. From the time of his admission the temperature of the axilla is examined and as often as the thermometer shows 39° C. (102°F.) or more, a bath of 20° C. or even less, and of ten minutes duration is given. Somewhat severe cases, who get six to twelve baths in twenty-four hours, get the second evening 1½ to 2 grammes quinine; the examination of the temperature and the baths are not suspended. If a decrease of temperature follows toward morning to less than 38° C., and if it continues long enough, so that for the next twelve hours another bath is not required, then we give, forty-eight hours after the first dose of quinine, an equal one, or if admissible a smaller one, but if the decline in temperature was not sufficient, a large dose is given.   If this one appears sufficient, we repeat the same every second day, or a smaller one, as long as the continuity of the fever requires.   In very severe cases, in which even a dose of quinine of 2½ grammes is not sufficient, we give the digitalis in the course of the next thirty-six hours, under constant attention to the temperature and the pulse, until gradatim, ¾ to 1½ grammes in powder are used. Immediately after this, that is, forty-eight hours after the last quinine dose we repeat the quinine again. The temperature goes down almost constantly to below 38°C. and sometimes to 36°C., and the obstinacy of the fever for the whole course of the disease is so broken that you need but to continue the baths and a dose of quinine every two days, but if necessary, we may try the combination of digitalis and quinine again.   Should we not be able to procure a sufficient remission by digitalis and quinine, which occurs very rarely, though sometimes then we must have recourse to veratria, which sometimes suffices to diminish the obstinacy of the fever for the rest of its course.   When, on account of hemorrhage from the bowels, or for other reasons, the employment of the baths has to be interrupted, we can yet give the quinine from time to time, when hemorrhage of the bowels does occur, we give it (the quinine), in solution, with the addition of Tinct. Opii, or else it may be used in the same form as an injection.

The severe asthenic, typhous or bilious pneumonias, so frequent in Basel, are treated on the whole in the same manner, especially the cold baths and the quinine are used according to the same indications ; only in very high fever, 41° C. and over (106° F.), a full dose of quinine is given on entering the hospital and at the same time powdered digitalis.

In pneumonia also, quinine has the preference over digitalis in order to gain a remission sooner.

In all other severe fevers, the same procedure is proper, yet it is necessary to act according to circumstances in each case and also carefully individualize according to the nature of the disease and the presumed course of the fever.

So, for instance, it is not needed in a common case of intermittent fever or a simple febrile angina, even when there appear the highest degrees of temperature to set in motion the whole antipyretic therapeutic apparatus while the excessive temperature has not a long duration and for that reason is not dangerous.

And therefore you will not interfere antipyretically with typhus in the later stage, when spontaneously in the morning sufficient remission occurs, even when the evening temperature rises very high.

In chronic fevers, especially in phthisis pulmonalis, I do not employ the more decided abstraction of heat. The increase in its production, and in consequence the waste of tissue occuring during this abstraction of heat appears to contra-indicate such procedure in a disease in which the chief danger lies in the consumption. But I allow that direct experience finally will decide it, as possibly a complete compensation, or even more than this may occur as an after effect. Quinine, in large doses, in phthisis is so much the more indicated the more the fever assumes the character of a continued fever (for instance in many cases of phthisis florida).

We may sometimes succeed by one or more large doses of quinine, given within the space of two days,

to not only diminish the fever at once, but to break it for
a longer time, we must consider that in such patients
exists a very fatal circle, inasmuch as the local disease
feeds the fever, and on the other hand by the elevation
of temperature the progress of the local disease is
favored.   For cases of phthisis with strong remittent
or intermittent fever is to be recommended the continued use of digitalis and quinine in smaller doses
combined.   For a day is to be given 1½ grs. digitalis
and from 5 to 7½ grs. quinine in pills and to be continued until we have the effect, or until disturbing consequences of the effect of digitalis are observed, for
instance, loss of appetite, sickness of the stomach, or
even emesis.

I will not enter upon dietetic measures that are so
important in the treatment of fevers, the lecture being
already somewhat extended.   Physicians generally agree
upon the necessity of bodily and mental rest, *suitable*
bedding, the importance of pure, not too hot air, plenty
of cooling drinks, etc.   Only a short remark upon the
choice of nutriment for fever patients might be in place.
With regard to the consuming febrile diseases, I will
remind of the widely-known experience of the effects of
the so-called Banting diet, which give a sufficient explanation of the fact that beefsteak and eggs are not the
nourishment by which you can sustain and invigorate
patients affected with phthisis, that rather show that the
nourishment proven by experience as effective, in which
the hydro-carbons, and especially the fats (cod liver oil),
are abundantly represented, for such cases are also theoretically justified.   And as in acute fevers, the fats in
larger quantities are not digested and resorbed, there
remain as suitable nutriments only those that especially

contain hydra-carbons, and we therefore arrive at such fever diet as has been employed since the time of Hippocrates, by experienced physicians.

We may look upon the knowledge as a special progress that alcoholic drinks do not increase the fever, but of late, rather tend to diminish it.

PROGRESS OF THE SCIENCES.

By CHAS. L. CARTER, M. D., Holden, Mo.

Our habitat is a world of wonders. The universe is a vast laboratory in which our brief lives afford us scarcely ample time to investigate our surroundings, to examine and admire the handiwork of the Creator, and to reverence Him for His power, wisdom and beneficence. Here, by the way, we have a theology that cannot be counterfeited by the errors of repeated translations, nor by the superstitions of Grecian mythology.

But it is a lamentable fact that most of the human family pass through life totally unconscious of the beauties and wonders ever present in and around them. These crude minds, without others to think for them, would never have aspired above Patagonian darkness, and the orgies of barbarism. Many noble brains have dwindled—atrophied—for want of proper stimulus to thought and culture. I am inclined to paraphrase the sacred old text, thus : He that has a brain to think, let him think.

Fortunately for humanity, some splendid minds are continually engaged in investigating the phenomena, and utilizing researches in the natural sciences. These sciences have been cultivated by slow degrees. Each has been developed from occult mysteries; each has had its stage of incipiency, and withstood the anathemas of the ignorant, who are always largely in the majority. With profound pleasure do we retrospect the culture and growth of some of these sciences for only a few years—of others, for centuries. We do rejoice that those researches have illumined this day with the light of science, and astounded us with the strides of art.

The wild Arabs gave us the rudiments of Algebra, and six centuries ago these Ishmaelites and the Chinese devised the mariner's compass and the astrolobe, which were, in navigation, vast improvements on the night-sailing of ancient Tyria. The Y Zeddies—devil. worshippers—once held their carnivals on the ground afterwards consecrated by Babylon in her pride, and finally in her ruins.

Physical science has been developed from the falling of an apple to the correlation of forces. Franklin caught the electric spark that now goes on our swiftest errands, traverses the furious ocean, binds two continents together, and makes of antipodes door neighbors. The accidental heating of a flask containing some fluid, has brought enterprise, convenience and wealth to cover all the land and waters of our earth.

Geology, though a young science presents an attractive field for thought. It has heightened our conceptions and expanded our knowledge much in every way. Beyond doubt our earth is many thousands of years older than the Mosaic account had led us to suppose.

Whether our globe was formed of nothing by Omnipotent power, or resulted from the condensation of gases, or was originally a molten liquid thrown from the burning sun, its ten strata mark as many thousands of years.

Fossils of animals have been exhumed from the solid rock five miles deep, under the very spot where Eden bloomed. Even our coal beds are the fossils of trees that grew before Moses' Adam had an existence. What then of the Silurian, Cambrian, and Laurentian eras? What of the fossil infusoria that are continually sifting down from near the watery surface till they have in many places filled up the ocean bed, and their calcareous mausoleum is now covered with deep soil and stately trees? It is interesting to know that naturalists have classified and named about 200 varieties of these diminutive beings.

The microscope, as well as the telescope, has opened new worlds to our astonished gaze. How boundless the wisdom, the works and the empire of the Deity. Let man who stands midway between God and nothing, for a moment look with a telescope in one hand and a microscope in the other. Here, he beholds a vast system of infinitely ponderous worlds. There, he sees a world of animalculæ,—creatures so small that a drop of water would make an ocean for millions of them— so diminutive that a batallion of them could drill on the point of a cambric needle. And yet, these animalculæ are as various in their forms and characters as are the huge beasts that roam our forests and plains— each has a complex system of organs, and the adaptations and functions for digestion, nutrition and reproduction.

Now we have confined life to the smallest possible compass, still it is a mystery that baffles all science. What is life? What the origin of living matter? Faleopius, of England, called it "vital force." Beale called it "germinal matter." Prof Nelson of Chicago, calls it "Bioplasm,"* and Huxley calls it "Protoplasm" and maintains, if I understand him, that life inheres in "Protoplasm" which is spontaneously generated by accidental combinations of hydrogen, oxygen, carbon, and nitrogen, but in equivalents yet incognito. I believe that life can not originate spontaneously, and that its origin will ever remain a mystery to all but the Creator. Whatever of life's origin we find in every drop of water, grain of sand, and in the petal of every flower, there may be lives enough to populate a continent.

Now, looking again upward, and we muse; strange, our mighty earth is not more than a grain of sand compared with the systems of worlds we behold. By the use of the spectroscope the sun is found to be surrounded by a gaseous envelope more than 4,000 miles thick. This is called its chromosphere, and consists mainly of glowing hydrogen, but in its deeper strata are found the vapors of sodium and magnesium. The moon has been really photographed, and in different lunations. Her surface has been thus accurately mapped out, showing her mountains, valleys and rocks, but not her rivers, for she has no water. The highest lunar mountain has an altitude of more than 26,000 feet. Another of her

---

* Of "Bioplasm" Beale says (Disease Germs, 2d edition, page 12): "The term I propose to apply to the *living* or *germinal self-propagating* matter of living beings, and to restrict to this, is '*Bioplasm*' (Βιος, life; πλασνα, plasma)." "Bioplasm involves no theory as regards the nature or origin of the matter. It simply distinguishes it as living."   H. Z. G.

mountains received the name "Tycho," and has a perpendicular height of 17,000 feet.

It has been ascertained that centrifugal force is stronger than the centripetal, and that all the planets are therefore extending their orbits further from the sun, and it is probable that eventually as they become less dense because less attracted, the present system of planets will disappear or dissolve into gases. Meantime other will be thrown off from the sun and "cool down" to take their places. There is also reason to believe that such chemical changes are being wrought spontaneously on our earth that it will at long intervals be alternately enveloped in floods and flames.

Chemistry reveals volumes of startling wonders, and is a boon to the world of arts and sciences In photogrophy and photogeny light has been chemicalized, but it is in the department of medicine that it has worked the greatest wonders and the greatest good. Especially has organic chemistry promoted and given positive character to physiology and histology.

But medicine, though progressing slowly, has made the grandest march, and achieved for mankind countless blessings, most sacred to mortals. Dark was its day, and puerile its claims, when the mythic god "Apollo," through his son Esculapius, was the "healer" and the superstitious invalids would visit the Grecian temple of Coos and Cuidos, prostrate their bodies on the skins of sacrificed animals for the priest to diagnose their cases and heal them through power derived from the "gods" In after times the barbers were the doctors ;—next the preachers ;—then empirical prescriptions handed down through family traditions. Finally, some attention began to be given to anatomy and physiology, and medicine came to be cultivated as a science.

From Galen down to the present, a retinue of wise men and illustrious names have been associated with medicine. Certainly more bright and intellectual minds have been devoted to medical science than to any other department of thought. It is true, however, that most young men who embark in medicine, do so without properly estimating the vast depth of these sciences, and without considering whether they have the requisite and natural adaptations. The result is, that while all may make the practice the means of a livelihood, but few are capable of understanding the sciences and giving strength to the profession. The indispensable adaptations are, a good intellect, large perception, reason, eventuality, and caution. Then a good literary education, with good and industrious habits. These characteristics strongly indicate success. Those without them had better follow something else.

But is phrenology a science? It is. It is physiology pertaining to the brain and its functions. The brain does not act as an unit. Certain definite regions of the brain do control certain definite faculties of the mind. These facts are demonstrably true. There are no facts in the whole domain of physiology more positive than those which support the cardinal principles of phrenology. They are as much physiological facts as they are phrenological facts. They are phrenological facts because they are physiological facts. Physiology and pathology have ever been my darling sciences, and I have long since found that phrenology is so nearly related as to make a harmonious trio.

Years ago I stood almost alone in the medical profession as a friend to, and student of phrenology. For then most medical men rejected it through the bias of traditional but ill-founded opposition. It is not so to-day. Many of the ablest medical men in Europe and America now declare phrenology a true science. In its infancy its strongest opposition came from medical men. For the credit of the profession I regret that this was so. But the contest is over; truth prevailed. Now educated people generally admit the truths taught by phrenology, and its opponents generally are illiterate. Such opposition had astronomy; and some of them yet say the earth is as flat as a pan-cake.

In conclusion, I must say that my fond desires have long been to see empiricism perish, and the study and practice of medicine conducted in the light of science,—pathology being the guiding star; to see learned men everywhere study and embrace the truths of phrenology; to see the fact recognized that the lower animals possess the faculties of intellection and the powers of reason. These desires are being realized. Opponents can get off the track or be run over.

PRESSURE ON THE CAROTIDS TO CONTROL INTERCRANIAL CIRCULATION.

By ROBERT B. MCNARY, M. D., Holden, Mo.

It is exceedingly strange to my mind, that the very simple and efficient means by which the intercranial circulation may be controlled, by means of digital pressure upon the carotid arteries, has been so universally overlooked. The pulsation of these arteries may be plainly and easily felt on either side of the trachea, and the circulation through them may be almost as certainly controlled by properly applied pressure, as if they were held between the thumb and forefinger.

The applicability of the principle to the great variety of diseases in which it is indicated, will of course suggest itself to the mind of any physician, and I will therefore not occupy your space by any expatiation upon the subject, but will remark, by way of illustrating its practical applicability, that I have succeeded in relieving a great many cases of violent headache, a convulsion or fit in a young man. But the stronger proof of its value as a remedial means was afforded in the case of a boy, eleven or twelve years old, who had been very dangerously ill for several days, with what was supposed to be congestion of the brain. He had had several convulsions, and had been perfectly blind since his illness began. I was requested to see him at night, and remain the next morning, till the physician in whose care he was, could meet me in consultation.

When I examined him, the symptoms were of such a peculiar nature, that I was utterly at a loss as to what I should do, in which unpleasant condition of my own mind, the above idea occurred to me, and I had hardly got my fingers well and firmly fixed, when he told me that his headache, (which I neglected to mention with the other symptoms), was better, and within less than five minutes I think his sight had perfectly returned, he was free from all pain or uneasiness, and continued to recover rapidly, without *any medicine*.

A good many cases in previous practice, have since occurred to me in which the same principle *might* have been applied with similar results, had I known it. I have never heard it from a medical man, or seen it in a medical journal, but it does seem to me to be of sufficient importance to be suggested, and at the command of every medical man, when the necessities of a case require it.

DIFFICULT OBSTETRICAL CASE—CEPHALO-
TMOY, ETC.

In the Practice of F. A. BAILEY, M. D.; reported by JOHN VITE, M. D.,
Hillsboro, Oregon.

May 2.—First saw Mrs. T. *æt* 35. Primipara of good health. Learned from the midwife in attendance that she had been in labor three days; that the membranes were ruptured on the first day of the labor. The os uteri was found well dilated, the presentation being the first in Bandaloque's classification.

The touch revealed a preternaturally narrow pelvis to be the cause of delay of the labor; the exact dimensions were not ascertained, but that the malformation was too great to be overcome unaided, was evident; hence the patient was chloroformed and the forceps applied with difficulty, and to no purpose, ossification of the cranial bones being too far advanced to allow them to yield to the pressure of the blades. It being evident that the mother or child must be sacrificed, cephalotomy was determined upon, and performed in the usual way, but with more than ordinary difficulty, in consequence of the preternatural consolidation of the cranial bones, the fontinelles being closed as in a child two years old.

The lady made a good recovery, leaving her bed in fifteen days. This case is reported to show that poor humanity is put to the same straits in these ends of the earth as elsewhere.

Hospital Reports.

ST. LOUIS (SISTER'S) HOSPITAL.

Clinic of Prof. E. H. GREGORY, reported by Dr. CHARLES GARCIA.

CASE I. A child 2 years old is presented, having a sore mouth. It seems not to be the result of hot water, or of a caustic of any kind. Its teeth are black, and the gums are red, but not tumified; the tongue is covered with white pellicles, but does not seem to be swollen. The fluid escaping from the mouth is a little bloody, caused by congestion and effusion from the capillary vessels. The child has not been taking calomel. I examine the cheeks to ascertain if there is any thickening of the walls of the mouth, or changes of the connective tissue. The mother has been using borax and honey.

Remarks. Borax and chlorate of potash are the popular remedies for sore mouth. Carbolic acid is now coming into use somewhat for the same cases. The child's bowels are regular and its appetite good. I can feel the crown of a tooth that is cutting. I will cut down freely on that tooth, as all swelling on that side may be connected with it. It will bleed and relieve the congested vessels and do good so far. Quinine is sometimes good for sore mouth. I have not disparaged the use of borax and chlorate of potash. A weak solution of muriatic acid ℨi, to ℥i of water, makes a very good local application. Also, sulphate of copper gr. i, to an ounce of fluid; or sulphate of copper grs. x; cinchona powder ℨi—mix and sprinkle a pinch on an ulcer. Tannic acid ℨss, in ℥iij tar water, makes a good wash; or even salt and water. A mercurial purge would be of benefit, notwithstanding the sore mouth. I would give calomel grs. iij, pulverized rhubarb grs. vii, and if it does not operate in six hours give a dose of castor oil; and after the operation give calisaya cordial and quinine for two or three days.

Case II.   A boy 5 years old, with glandular swellings about
the neck which first appeared in July last.   There are also in-
crustations about the eyelids and on the face.   This little chap
is restive, and has a discharge from the borders of the eyelids
and slight pains about the neck; has clear skin, blue eyes, and
light hair; we might say he has a strumous constitution.   If
the scabs on the face be rudely broken off and a wash applied
at night it would heal them rapidly; or we might poultice for
a few days, and then dress with Goulard's cerate.   Give the
child a teaspoonful of cod liver oil three times a day; give it
fat meat, cream, and let him live well generally.   Bathe the
eyes with warm water, or foment them, and then apply simple
cerate and citrine ointment, equal parts, to the edges of the
lids.

Case III.   A swelling on the left leg in a girl 13 years old.
She says it has been there for eight years, and has been more or
less sore.   She recollects when it first came.   It has been constantly increasing in size; but since last August it has been
growing more rapidly; previously it had been a hard lump, and
sometimes painful.

This tumor is attached to the surrounding soft parts, but not
to the bone; it does not seem to fluctuate, is deeply seated, and
not very well circumscribed.   It became painful four months
ago, and still remains hard.   The foot feels natural, and the
limb is not reduced in size.   This is a case for observation, and
not one to be operated on hastily; it is a serious case.   It may
be in the substance of the muscle.   There are no swellings in
the groin.   It may be simple in character, it may be a lym-
phoma, or it may be of a worse character.

Case IV.   A tumor on the neck.   From the characters presented we diagnosticate this as an abscess.   There are none of
the peculiar symptoms of aneurism present.   The knife is
introduced into the abscess, cutting from me; I usually cut
towards me.   Always carry the knife "home."   In lancing an
abscess on the finger, if the patient pulls away, he only assists
the operation.   Some years ago, I commenced opening an
abscess, cutting from me, and the surgeon in charge told me that
was not the way, and I have never forgotten the lesson.

CASE V. Traumatic cataract. This patient received a blow about the eye, sufficient to knock him senseless. Sometimes violence displaces the lens with the anterior chamber by rupturing the capsule of the lens; and disturbs the nutrition of the cornea, and leads to rapid changes in the transparency of the eye. This looks like a traumatic cataract. He says he could see immediately after the accident happened, but that he sees better now than he did some time ago. If he sees better now it would be the height of folly to interfere. The sight will probably be restored by the solution of the lens in the aqueous humor and its absorption, for the lens matter is soluble in the aqueous humor. Surgeons sometimes take a couching needle and admit the aqueous humor to the lens by rupturing the capsule. In this case there has been a rupture of the capsule, as frequently occurs from injury.

The first operation for cataract was performed by a goat which ran against the sharp end of a corn-stalk, rupturing the cornea and the capsule of the lens, thus admitting the aqueous humor to the lens. In such cases do not forget the use of atropine, as the recovery of vision often depends upon its use, and negligence in this matter is criminal. As you keep shingles in your office for surgical splints, so also keep atropine, as it may meet inflammatory action half way. Atropina is just as necessary in ophthalmia as a knife is to remove a cataract. We sometimes admit the aqueous humor to the lens through its covering, and if the lens swells and produces inflammation, we open the cornea and let it out; otherwise the compression on the iris and ciliary processes might produce sympathetic inflammation of the other eye, and both might be lost. Quiet and atropine may restore sight in this case. We must not forget the importance of watching these cases, so as to operate should it become necessary. The eye does not pain him, and is getting better every day. He feels perfectly well. Use the atropine three times a day.

CASE VI. Traumatic inflammation in the right leg of a boy 8 years old. There seems to be a contusion about the middle of the tibial shaft. The whole leg is hotter than normal. He seems to have been extensively injured; has been struck with some sharp body, probably a nail. The parts are inflamed.

He has been sitting up, with the leg hanging down, when it should have been elevated. Make hot applications. It may suppurate somewhere. It will probably soon be well.

CASE VII. A boy 3 years old. The child has been sick about two years. Here is a peculiar condition of the foot known as talipes valgus. Talipes in connection with knock-knee is nearly always valgus. The child is young, and you are aware that a great deal of growth is yet to take place. The child walks a little, and the condition might be ameliorated by a steel instrument extending up to the hip and having the limb bound to it; in this way the limb would sustain the body by being kept in a proper line with its axis. I have not seen in my practice, half a dozen cases of this kind. This child's general condition is not good, and one bad condition predisposes to another.

CASE VIII. Varicose veins. The patient is a cook, and has to be on her feet much of the time, standing near a hot range. She says these ulcers (varicose ulcers), opened last June, and have been increasing in size, notwithstanding the application of ointments, etc.

Patients sometimes object to coming before the class to show their infirmities, as they think it peculiarly uncongenial, and we should try to impress upon them that they are doing good for their day and generation. Always treat them with the utmost decorum, without noise or sign of pleasure on your part, for they are often in pain, and any indication of indifference or jest is disagreeable to them. One of your qualities should be a feeling for the suffering of your patient. There is no doctor so popular as he who sympathizes with his patients; it enables him to perform his *whole duty*, and we should always endeavor to do that.

There is no teaching comparable to clinical teaching, for a student may be made a perfect physician in this way and in no other. Patients are accomplishing some good in coming to the clinics, for they are doing something towards the advancement of physicians. There are in these enlightened days, laws enacted against dissecting, when everything should be done to assist it. There are a great many physicians perfectly indifferent to anatomy; but no man is great in medicine unless he has a good knowledge of anatomy; it is the basis, the foundation stone of medicine.

The veins of this leg have been swollen for nine years. This patient knows no cause for these ulcers. In all cases varicose ulcers are perpetuated by the incomplete circulation in the veins. Sometimes the circulation is so tardy, and the vitality so low, that at some spot a coagulum is formed, called a thrombus, which latter is the immediate antecedent of ulceration.

These ulcers would close in a short time if the patient would rest the limb, as it would improve the circulation which returns the blood. In applying adhesive strips over ulcers we support vessels and diminish their calibre, and the bandage acts in the same manner, and maintains the strips in position. In a large community like this, a physician might make a specialty of diseases of this kind, as the treatment which we have indicated might be successfully conducted without loss of time to the patient.

CASE IX. Chorea. Observe this young girl! She is in constant motion. Her limbs jerk, and she sometimes makes grimaces unconsciously. I suppose at first flush it is a case of chorea. In this case the general health seems to be good. I generally give such patients a purge in the beginning, and follow it with quinine. If that fails I give cimicifuga, which is the scientific name for black cohosh. Some say it is a specific for this disease. Tonics are indicated: muriated tincture of iron or arsenic. Hydrate of chloral and bromide of potash are favorably mentioned. In prescribing cimicifuga, you are giving a medicine famous for chorea. ‾

CITY HOSPITAL.

Clinical report by CLAYTON KEITH, M. D., Assistant Physician.

Gun-shot wound of right chest. Pneumonia (Traumatic), supervening. Randolph McCormick, aged 20 years, steamboatman, was admitted November 23d, 1872, and died November 26th, 1872.

Previous History. COULD GET NONE. Was accidentally (?) shot to-day in the right chest with a small, smooth bore, single barrel pocket pistol, in the hands of an associate.

Treatment. R Morphiæ sulph. ½ gr. every 2 or 3 hours. Rest—perfect quiet. Warm fomentations and wide bandage about the chest. Spirits frumentic occasionally.

Post-mortem examination 18 hours after death revealed the following facts:

1. On inspection of the body no external injuries were observable, save a small wound in the right chest, between the fourth and fifth costal cartilages, and about one inch to the right of the median line.

2. On opening the thoracic cavity, it was discovered that a small pistol ball had passed between the fourth and fifth costal cartilages, and penetrated the thoracic cavity.

3. That it had passed through the right pleura, middle mediastinum, along the edge of the middle lobe of the right lung, through the pericardium and superior vena cava, and had lodged beside the fifth dorsal vertebræ, where it was picked out with the hand.

4. The right pleural cavity was found filled with blood, containing 3 or 4 quarts of partly coagulated and partly fluid blood. The right lung was compressed into about half its normal space.

2. Pneumonia of the right lung existed, the evidence of which, minute crepitation and dullness on percussion, were heard prior to death.

6. The pericardium was found filled and distended with half coagulated blood, causing acute pericarditis.

7. The ball had perforated the superior vena cava within the pericardium, and about three-fourths of an inch from the entrance into the right auricle.

8. The remaining thoracic and all the abdominal viscera, were found in normal condition. The ball had passed directly backward.

9. No examination of the brain was made.

10. The case presents no points of special interest, other than the length of time intervening between perforation of the vena cava and death,—72 hours, or 3 days and nights.

Report of Cases from the Erysipelas Ward,

CASE II. Erysipelas of the face, head and neck; idiopathis: Charles M., *æt.* 43 years; admitted December 11th.

1. *Previous History.*—Health generally good prior to present attack. Was never sick before. While laboring in the wind, on wharf-boat, five days ago, was suddenly seized with rigors— alternate chills and flushes, headache and nausea soon followed accompanied by diarrhœa. In 48 hours afterward the rash or "erysipelatous blush" appeared on his forehead and in his temples. Says it was of a bright rosy red color and accompan- ied by an intensely burning sensation. The redness and œdema extended rapidly until it involved the entire face, scalp and part of the neck. Both eyes were entirely closed.

2. *Present Condition.*—Is a man of full, plethoric habit, accus- tomed to active life, having been surrounded by favorable hygienic conditions—a juggler by vocation. Pulse 112 and full. Temperature 102¼° F. Has no cough. Bowels are costive. Both eyes are closed. On account of the loose cellular tissue in the eyelids the œdema is most marked in that locality. Patient looks like a hideous monster. Has been delirious for two days and nights—is still delirious at intervals. The most prominent symptom complained of at this stage is the acute burning sensa- tion in his face and scalp. Has had no sleep or rest for three nights. Complains of headache and pains in the fauces; also of pain in his ears, and is somewhat deaf. Says his fever has been much higher than now. Urine contains neither sugar nor albumen. Urine is highly colored.

3. *Physical Examination.*—Heart and lungs present nothing abnormal. Spleen normal. Liver is somewhat enlarged. Has been a moderate drinker, but had used no alcoholic stimuli, he says, for months previous to present attack.

4. *Other Details.*—Has received no wound or injury what- ever about his head. This seems to be a typical case of idio- pathic cutaneous erysipelas, involving only the skin and sub- cutaneous cellular tissue. No abscess has yet formed.

December 12, a. m.—Pulse 88; temperature 100°. One eye partly open. Is more rational. Resting easier. Has less pain in head. Disease shows no disposition to extend farther.

P. M.—Pulse 100 and full. Temperature 102½°. Bowels costive. Throat is sore. Thirst is intense.

5. *Treatment.*—Quiniæ sulph. gr. ij every 3 hrs. Tr. ferri chloridi gtt. xxx every 8 hrs. Sol. Magnes. sulph. ℥ iv at once. Ammon. carb. gr. x in mucilago every 3 hrs, during the delirium. Beef tea twice daily. Syr. chloral ℥ ss (gr. xv) at bed time.

Cut the hair off, and applied Sol. Sodæ Silicate over face, scalp and neck twice daily. This treatment was continued for five or six days following.

December 13, a. m.—Pulse 88. Temperature 99½°. Has less pain in the head and face. Bowels moved three times last night. Right eye still closed. Disease shows no disposition to extend farther down the neck. Its limit is now circumscribed.

P. M.—Pulse 96 and strong. Temperature 101¼°. Delirium is subsiding. Face is greatly swollen. Tongue is dry.

December 14, a. m.—Pulse 80. Temperature 98¼°· Complains of constant thirst, but no pain in head or any part of the body. Fluctuation beneath right orbit. An abscess has formed in the subcutaneous cellular tissue of the cheek. The right eye is endangered by the abscess. Opened the abscess and evacuated the pus.

P. M.—Inflammation is subsiding. Desquamation has begun.

December 15.—Desquamation advancing finely. Rested well, only after taking chloral last night. Complains only of sleeplessness.

December 16.—Rested well, feels well, eats well. Pulse 64 and full. Temperature 98°. Tongue moist. Bowels regular. Complains of no severe pain. Is convalescing.

December 17.—Improving. Another abscess, over right eye and one behind right ear, and one over left parietal bone Opened all the abscesses and discharged pus.

December 19.—Doing well. No fever. Appetite good. Bowels regular. Another large abscess formed in the scalp; opened it and discharged pus. Applied poultices and continued quinia and iron.

December 21.—Convalescent. Is able to be up, dressed and walking about the ward. Abscesses about the head and neck are still open and pus is being evacuated. Complains of no other pain.

December 25.—Is well. Disease has run its course in two weeks.

December 30.—Discharged.

Reviews and Bibliographical Notices.

PRINCIPLES AND PRACTICE OF SURGERY. By Frank Hastings Hamilton, A. M. M. D., LL. D., Professor of the Practice of Surgery with operations, and of Clinical Surgery in Bellevue Hospital Medical College, etc. Illustrated with 467 engravings on wood. New York: Wm. Wood & Co., 27 Great Jones street. 1872. pp. xxvi—943.

In the volume before us, we have a work "intended as a text-book for students, and, at the same time as a direct and complete guide to the surgeon," and to supply a demand suggested by experience in teaching and in practice. Of the author, it is not necessary that we speak to the profession; his name is too well known from works already in the hands of nearly every practitioner in this country, to require of us any words of commendation. By his works he is known.

The task, however, of writing a work on general surgery, at this time, to comprise all that "belongs properly and exclusively to surgery" is indeed a difficult one; and at this time the competition is sharp and able. The nomenclature is that of the Royal College of Physicians and Surgeons of London, and marked (R. C.).

The work is divided into two parts: General Surgery and Regional Surgery. It is further judiciously divided into chapters and sections.

The first subject treated of—as it is first in importance—is inflammation. This part of the work, we think, is entirely too brief, comprising only about fifteen pages, while Gross has more than seventy on the same subject. The discoveries of Cohnheim and Stricker are passed over in a manner much too brief, and the names of these great workers are not mentioned.

Teaching for students should always be clear as well as correct. On page 21, we find, in speaking of the elevation of temperature in inflammation, the following language: "While the temperature of the blood at the heart in man, is never much above 98° Fahrenheit, the temperature of the parts suffering under acute inflammatory action may arise to 112°." The student would be very likely to draw an incorrect inference from this language.

On page 38, we find the following : "The source of pus corpuscles is not yet definitely ascertained. Among the earlier opinions entertained, we may enumerate the doctrines which ascribed its production to a disintegration or dissolution of the solids, to decomposition of the serum, and to changes in the coagulating lymph, and still later to secretion, the vessels of the part inflamed being supposed to assume an action analagous to that of the glandular system, causing thus a morbid secretion. This latter theory, suggested first by Simpson in 1722, received an apparent confirmation in the observations of Gendrin, who discovered within the capillaries of an inflamed tissue white corpuscles resembling pus globules.

"Subsequently, it having been ascertained that these white corpuscles constituted an invariable element of normal blood, a new theory arose, which to the present moment counts a large number of adherents, namely, that pus corpuscles are merely extravasated, colorless blood-cells, which have escaped by a species of endosmosis." This statement of the question *seems* to imply that the observations of Cohnheim and others on the escape of white blood corpuscles from the vessels, in suppuration, is a theory. We protest against calling facts theories.

The above indefinite language is in remarkable contrast to the positive and emphatic teaching of Prof. Gross as given on page 74, Vol. I, System of Surgery, last edition : "Coincident with the exudation of blood-liquor, the other vascular changes above described, the white blood corpuscles, leucocytes, lymph corpuscles, nomadic or wandering cells, as these protoplasms are variously termed, apparently increase in number, and adhere to the inner surface of the vessels, forming upon it an almost motionless layer, while the red corpuscles circulate slowly along the centre in their accustomed channel. Thus situated the white corpuscles begin to wander out or immigrate into the inflamed tissues through the stomata and invisible pores of the softened veins and capillaries, by virtue of the remarkable faculty which they possess of changing spontaneously their form and position, peculiarities, which, from their similarity to those of amœbæ, are designated as amœboid movements. This faculty, as well as the diffusion of the white corpuscles in the tissues, was first demonstrated by Prof. von Recklinghausen, without, however, his being aware of their vascular origin. Dr. Addison, in 1842, enunciated the fact that in inflammation the white corpuscles first pass into and then out of the walls of the vessels; and Dr. Waller, four years later, by experiments performed upon the tongue of the frog, confirmed the statements of his contryman. Although, subsequently, Prof. Stricker, of Vienna, discovered that the walls of the vessels, are permeable both to the white and red corpuscles, it remained for Dr. Cohnheim, in 1867, to establish the correctness of these observations, by demonstrating conclusively that white blood corpuscles wander from the vessels into the irritated and inflamed tissues, and that, in incipient inflammation, all such morphological elements as can not be distinguished from the pus corpuscles, are derived from the blood and not from the tissues. To Cohnheim, therefore, is due the credit of having correctly interpreted his own observations, and of developing the researches of his predecessors. * * *

" Thus, for example, the recent investigations already alluded to, of Professor Stricker and of Dr. W. F. Norris, of this city, have demonstrated the proliferation of the germinal matter of the cornea corpuscles ; Dr. Güterback has shown the division of the nucleus of the cells of tendons ; and Dr. Redfern, as is well known, first observed that the germinal matter of the normal cartilage cell is replaced by a mass of mobile cells, which are identical with white blood corpuscles." Again, page 124 : " It has been demonstrated by Virchow that, under the influence of assimilation of an excess of blood, liquor which has escaped from the dilated vessels at the focus of the inflammation, the connective tissue corpuscles proliferate and assume the characters of pus globules. This theory of the formations of pus, however, is too exclusive, and has been placed in doubt by the discovery of Cohnheim, who has shown by a series of well-contrived experiments that pus is in a great degree the product of the colorless blood corpuscles, which have wandered out of the vessels into the tissues. The results of these experiments have been confirmed by the researches of Koster, Vulpian, and other observers, and they carry the mind back to the days of Gendrin, who, in 1824, in his great work on the Anatomical History of Inflammation, enunciated almost precisely similar views, based upon his own investigations. It has, moreover,

been demonstrated that other cell elements enter into the formation of pus, as, for example, those of the cornea, muscles, glands,
mucous and serous membranes, which by their germination aid
in the process." This is plain, precise language, such as is necessary for students, or indeed for practitioners. Ashurst, in his
recent work on Surgery, has spoken very explicitly on the
subject.

In practice, the advice is generally very judicious, and at once
indicates the practitioner and careful observer.

In point, on page 40 : "Acute abscess should be opened freely
so that the matter may escape at once and without obstruction,
and, if possible, at such a point as will permit it to continue to
flow without the aid of bandages or pressure. We cannot too
*severely reprobate the practice of thrusting out the matter from
abscesses by violence ;* in consequence of which inflammation is
reawakened and suppuration is increased, or the interior becomes
filled with blood which, by decomposition, becomes in its turn a
source of inflammation, and often of hyæmic poisoning." [The
italics are our own.]

In hospital gangrene he recommends highly, as statistics justify, the use of bromine. On page 69, we find a table of 33
cases treated, with the following results :

> "Number treated with nitric acid,   -   -   18
> Average duration of disease,   -   -   16 days.
> Number treated with sol. bromine,   -   -   14
> Average duration,   -   -   -   -   6 days.
> Number treated with iodine,   -   -   -   1
> Average duration,   -   -   -   -   - 7 days.

"The cases were under the care of Drs. Caldwell, Peck,
Graves, and myself, respectively, and the sanitary surroundings
were as nearly similar as could be possible." He ascribes the introduction of this remedy, in this disease, to Dr. M. Goldsmith,
justly so we think, and we can most confidently recommend its
use in the worst cases.

Again, with his remarks on the treatment of tetanus (traumatic) we fully agree, taking the conditions as set forth fully
into account: page 74. "Nor do we hesitate to say that, in
case the disease has made but little progress, especially if only
the muscles of the jaw are involved in the spasms, amputation

will often afford a reasonable ground for hope; *particularly when* the *amputation does not* involve *parts near* the *body* as where the wounds are situated in the fingers or toes, or even in cases of injuries of the fore arm or lower portions of the leg." Further; of remedies, "by far the largest mass of testimony having accumulated in favor of nutritious food, tonics, stimulants, and opiates; the latter of which, if employed at all, must be given in the most liberal and persevering manner;" we would say to complete narcotism.

On *fractures* and *dislocations* our author is at home. We perceive a steady advance, by plaster-of-Paris as a dressing in fractures generally, upon the ground once occupied by apparatus more or less complicated. In speaking of the treatment of fractures of the femur we find the following, page 298: "During the last few years I have employed in my wards at Bellevue Hospital, in a large proportion of the cases of fractured thighs, plaster-of-Paris dressing. Most of my collegues have done the same, some of them having used this to the exclusion of all other forms of apparatus. For myself I must say that the practice has been adopted with some degree of hesitation and solely for the purpose of determining whether it possesses any qualities of superiority over other methods. The results thus far have been, as a rule satisfactory, since most of the persons thus treated have recovered in the usual time, and the limbs have generally been straight or nearly so. The average shortening has not been determined in a large number of cases, but from the report made by Dr. Bryant, late house surgeon, and from my own observation of a considerable number of additional cases, I would conclude that that the shortening was less than in an equal number of cases treated by any other method which I have yet seen adopted."

The use of the aspirator and needle for puncturing the bladder in cases requiring operation, has been omitted. Dieulafoy has, together with others, done much to introduce the use of this instrument into practice, and we think mention should have been made of its use. Other omissions might be mentioned; but all cannot be said on surgery in one volume.

Our author is cautious; an excellent quality in a surgeon; in no haste to adopt either new theories or new practice. We hope he will live long enough to enlarge the work from his own observations and experience, and add everything new that may be really valuable. The work is valuable, safe in its counsel, eminently practical, and a credit to our professional literature. The plates are excellent, and the typography clear; a credit to author and publisher.   H. Z. G.

THE PHYSICIAN'S VISITING LIST, FOR 1873. By Lindsay & Blakiston, Philadelphia.

Is an acknowledged necessity to all practitioners of medicine, in city or country. Really the only account book for *medical services* needed, if the doctor makes up his bills frequently, as he should if he expects to live by his profession. It has passed through so many revisions that its present size and arrangement meets the views of the great body of the profession. Physicians using it for the first time wonder how they did without it, and would not dispense with it again for ten times its cost.

CAMPBELL'S NEW ATLAS OF MISSOURI; with descriptions—historical, scientific and statistical. Maps constructed and drawn on the polyconic projection. By R. A. Campbell, Civil Engineer.

Letter press articles by G. Engelmann, M. D.; Hon. G. C. Swallow, A. M., M. D., late State Geologist; Capt. J. P. Cadman, A. M.; Prof. C. V. Riley, State Entomologist; Hon. John Monteith, State Superintendent of Public Instruction; Prof. William T. Harris, Superintendent of Public Instruction for St. Louis; Hon. John F. Wielandy, Corresponding Secretary of the State Board of Agriculture; W. H. Parker, Esq., Editor of the *Industrial Age;* also from the leading clergymen of the city of St. Louis in relation to the founding and present condition of the various religious denominations in the State.

The State is then shown in all its minutiæ on a series of about thirty full-page maps, exhibiting on a uniform scale of six miles to an inch, the counties with boundaries shaded, the municipal townships, in colors and named, the Congressional townships, with the range and number of each, and their sub-divisions into sections and fractional sections are all shown, so that a complete and faithful copy of the original survey of the State is placed upon exhibition.

There is accurately and clearly located every city, town, village, post-office, business point, railroad station, side track and river landing in the State, showing upon which sections and parts of sections each one is situated.

Few States in the Union are favored with so complete an epitome of valuable information—historical, scientific, and political. A glance over the title page will convince any citizen of Missouri that the author secured the services of exactly the right men, to inspire confidence in the accuracy and certainty of the scientific facts promulgated. The author has been equally successful in obtaining his *statistical facts* from the most undoubted sources of information, both from the State authorities and General Government—the list of post-offices of the United States being revised and corrected at Washington, D. C.; also the population of the various towns and counties from advanced sheets of the recent census returns.

The work deserves a place in every public and private library, business house, and drawing-room. Everywhere it should be as accessible to the sojourner or citizen as Webster's Dictionary.

The mechanical execution of the work, by A. W. McLean, Lithographer, No. 118 North Third Street; Barnes & Benyon, Printers and Stereotypers, No. 215 Pine Street, and Van Beek, Barnard & Tinsley, Binders, No. 316 North Third Street; all of St. Louis, would do credit to any of the Publishing Houses in the country.

HALF HOUR RECREATIONS IN POPULAR SCIENCE. No. V.—Nebulæ, Comets, Meteoric Showers, and the Revelations of the Spectroscope, concerning them, by Prof. H. Schellen and others. Coral and Coral Islands, by Prof. J. D. Dana, of Yale College. Dana Estes, Editor. Price 25 cts.

[For Sale at the St. Louis Book & News Co.]

This periodical is highly esteemed as a popular exponent of the progress of science, in the departments of which it treats.

BOOKS AND PAMPHLETS RECEIVED.

SURGERY—Principles and Practice. By Frank Hastings Hamilton, A. M., M. D., LL. D., Professor of Surgery, etc. Illustrated with 467 engravings on wood. Wm. Wood & Co., New York. 8vo. pp. 943.

WOMEN—On the Diseases of. Pathology, Diagnosis and Treatment. Including the Diagnosis of Pregnancy. By Graily Hewitt, M. D., London, F. R. C. P. Second American, from the third London edition, revised and enlarged. Philadelphia: Lindsay & Blakiston. 8vo. pp. 751.

WOMAN—Diseases Peculiar to. Clinical Lectures. By Lombe Atthill, M. D., University of Dublin. Philadelphia: Lindsay & Blakiston. 12mo. pp. 241.

FŒTICIDE OR CRIMINAL ABORTION—Lecture on. By Hugh L. Hodge, M. D. Philadelphia: Lindsay & Blakiston.

OVARIAN TUMORS. Their Pathology, Diagnosis and Treatment, Especially by *Ovariotomy*. By E. Randolph Peaslee, M. D., LL. D., Professor of Gynaicology, etc. With Illustrations. New York: D. Appleton & Co. 8vo. pp. 551. For sale by the St. Louis Book and News Company.

WILLIAMS' EXAMINATION of Prof. Ruse's Review of the Trial of Mrs. Wharton. By Philip C. Williams, M. D. Baltimore: Turnbull Brothers.

Extracts from Current Medical Literature.

Prophylaxis of Hydrophobia.

The *British Medical Journal* calls attention to the measures recommended by the Council of Hygiene of Bordeaux, for the better protection of people against the danger of hydrophobia. It is well known that the madness of dogs has a period which is premonitory and harmless. If these periods were generally known, the dogs could be put out of the way before they become dangerous. On this subject the Council of Hygiene has issued the following instructions:

"A short time, sometimes two days, after the madness has

seized the dog, it creates symptoms in the animal which it is indispensable to recognize:

"1.—There is agitation and restlessness and the dog turns himself continually in his kennel. If he be at liberty, he goes and comes and seems to be seeking something, then he remains motionless as if waiting, then he starts, bites the air, as if he would catch a fly, and dashes himself howling and barking against the wall. The voice of his master dissipates these hallucinations, the dog obeys, but slowly, with hesitation, as if with regret.

"2.—He does not try to bite, he is gentle, even affectionate, and he eats and drinks, but gnaws his litter, the ends of curtains, the padding of cushions, the coverlids of beds, carpets, etc.

"3.—By the movement of his paws about the sides of his open mouth, one might think he was trying to free his throat of a bone.

"4.—His voice undergoes such a change that it is impossible not to be struck by it.

"5.—The dog begins to fight with other dogs; this is a decidedly characteristic sign, if the dog be generally peaceful.

"The three symptoms last mentioned indicate an advanced period of the disease and that the dog may become dangerous at any moment, if immediate measures are not taken. It is best to chain him up at once, or, better still, to kill him."

It is desirable that this advice be inserted at least once a year in the public papers. It would also seem particularly desirable and practicable that these rules should be printed on the back of the notices and receipts for dog taxes. These excellent measures ought to become generally adopted.—*Boston Medical and Surical Journal.*

LYNN, October 18, 1872.

Messrs. Editors:

In the number of the *Journal* for July 4th, you quote from Dr. Williams's work on Consumption, "the medicine we have found to act as a specific on night-sweats is the oxide of zinc, in doses of two or three grains, in the form of a pill at night;" and you ask, "how closely will the experience of the American physician coincide with this statement?" While the surgeon of

the National Military Asylum, Eastern Branch, 1868-70, there were under my care many cases of consumption, mostly from two to five years' standing. Night-sweat was a very common symptom, and for its relief I learned to rely entirely on the oxide of zinc, three grains in a pill at night, combined with a little hyoscyamus. It seemed as nearly entitled to the name of specific as any medicine in the Pharmacopœia.   J. O. WEBSTER.
—*Ibid*.

Morbid Anatomy of the Epizoötic. Communicated by FRANK WOODBURY.

Prof. Gross, at the Jefferson College clinic, recently exhibited the post-mortem specimens obtained from a horse which died during the late epidemic, upon which he made the following remarks: "The horse was of medium size, and fourteen years old; he had been previously healthy during seven years in the service of Dr. Maxwell, his last owner. During the prevalence of the horse disease he suffered in common with his solipede brethren, and, although treated with the greatest care, he relapsed, when apparently convalescent, and died. This may be taken as a typical case of death from the disease, complications having been avoided by the treatment.

"The examination, carefully made by Mr. West, disclosed a large quantity of serous fluid in the thoracic cavity; the lungs were partially adherent, and a section sank in the water, showing a condition of infiltration or hepatization. In the trachea and larger bronchial tubes spots of lymph and numerous ecchymoses indicated the severity of the inflammation, and the mucous membrane, as far as the anterior nares, was discolored and covered with a muco-purulent secretion. Many of the bronchial lymphatic glands were enlarged. There was no evidence of disease discovered in the œsophagus or remaining viscera, and death evidently resulted from pleuro-pneumonia. The sweeping character of this disease and its rapid spread over the continent lead me to consider it of the nature of dengue. It is not communicable by ordinary contact; the morbific germs float in the atmosphere, making it epidemic rather than contagious."—*Medical Times*.

A Sure Test as to whether Life is Extinct or not.

A few years since a price was offered by the Paris Academy of Science for a sure and easily-applied test of the presence of death. In answer to this, Dr. Hugo Magnus, of Breslau, contributes a paper on this subject to Virchow's *Archives.* Dr. Magnus directs his attention to the vegetative phenomena, since among these may be found those peculiar to functions which will bear being reduced to a minimum, but upon the stoppage of which death follows at once. Now there are two systems, the functions of which are never completely suspended during life, *viz.:* the circulatory and respiratory. Choosing the former of these, Dr. Magnus resorts to a very simple method, which is thus described:

"If a limb of the body—a finger is best for the purpose—be constricted by a strong ligature quite tightly, there will be seen if the subject be yet alive, a reddening of the constricted member. First, the part in question becomes red, and the red color becomes darker and darker, and deeper in hue, till it is finally converted into a bluish-red, the whole limb being, from its tip to the ligature which encircles it, of a uniform color, except that at the region immediately around the ligature itself there is to be seen a narrow ring, which is not bluish-red, but white." On those whose skins are thickened and hard from work it may be necessary to choose some other part than a finger, as, for example, a toe or the tips of the ear. This evidence is as sure, to be brought about in the living body as it is certain to be absent in the corpse. The bluish coloration of the finger-tips, so often observed in the dead body, need not be regarded as a source of fallacy, for after ligation of a finger, as long as life is present, the whole limb, from the point of ligation to the extremity, will be uniformly blue-red. Large limbs, on account of offering facilities for the flow of the venous blood through the deeper veins, do not serve as well as the small extremities, in which the tissues are more easily compressed against bone."—*Medical Record.*

Diet of Literary Men.

The London correspondent of the Birmingham *Morning News* alludes to a new book that has recently appeared, containing remarks about the diet of certain literary men; and he states that he is acquainted with a well-known writer who cleaves to oatmeal porridge when he is in working trim. In this respect the said writer imitates Gerald Massey, who swears by oatmeal porridge, as a brain-inspiring compound. "There is a deal of phosphorus in oatmeal," Mr. Massey says, "and phosphorus is brain. There is also a large amount of phosphorus in fish. Consequently I never miss having a fish dinner at least once a week, and take a plate of good, thick, coarse, well-boiled Scotch oatmeal every morning in my life."—*Medical and Surgical Reporter.*

On Longevity.

Dr. Grey, some years since, published some statistics showing the average age at which the following classes died, after they had attained the age of fifty-one:—

Clergy....................................74 years.
Lawyers...............................72¾ "
Medical men............................78 "
Learned professions collectively. 76½ "

He afterward added the following observations, which embrace only the most eminent of these professions, with the following results:—

Clergy (bishops and archbishops)...70¼ years.
Lawyers, judges, etc ....67 "
Medical men (baronets, etc.)..........74½ "

From his observations he makes the following deductions:— 1. That members of the three learned professions occupy, in respect of the duration of their lives, a favorable position among the educated classes. 2. The difference in the duration of life among the three learned professions is not considerable. 3. That the three learned professions occupy the following relative position in respect to the duration of their lives, the longest being placed first: medical men, clergymen, lawyers. The vital statistics of Boston, show that "gentlemen," or those living on their incomes, are still longer lived than either professional men or farmers.—*Ibid.*

Population of the Globe.

There are on the globe 1,288,000,000 souls, of which 360,000,000 are Caucasians; 522,000,000 are Mongolians; 190,000,000 are

Ethiopians; 176,000,000 are Malayans; 1,000,000 are Indo-Americans. There are 8,642 languages spoken, and 1,000 religions. The yearly mortality of the globe is 42,043,000 persons. This is at the rate of 145,200 per day, 4,800 per hour, 80 per minute. Among 10,000 persons, one arrives at the age of 100; one in 500 attains the age of 80; one in a 100 to the age of 70. In 100 persons, 95 marry.—*Cincinnati Clinic.*

Treatment of Asthma.

George Goskoin, surgeon to British hospital for Diseases of the Skin, has had success in treating this disease by rubbing briskly into the chest, for the space of an hour, a chloroform liniment. The counter-irritation produced by the liniment was of benefit, but this benefit was increased by the jolting resulting from the rubbing. Anything that leads to the displacement of the air stagnant in the vesicles has proved able to relieve in many instances. It is advised that the friction be made with as much roughness as the case admits. Slight blows with the palm of the hand or the end of a towel on the ribs are quite allowable; and the friction should be extended to the front of the neck at the lower part, where the vagi enter the chest. The composition of the liniment need not trouble us, provided it be warm and work well.—*British Med. Jour.*—*Chicago Med. Journal.*

Carbolic Acid in Scarlatina.

Dr. Chapin (*Mich. Univ. Med. Jour.*) is very partial to the internal use of carbolic acid, and has come to consider it almost a specific in this disease. He is accustomed to use something like the following formula: R. Acid carbolici, tr. opii, ætheris chlor., aa dr. j.; glycerinæ, aquæ cinn., aa oz. ij. M. Sig. A teaspoonful every four hours. He also uses the acid as an application to the throat.—*Chicago Journal.*

Epidemiological Society.

The first meeting of the Epidemiological Society this season was held on the 13th ult., when the President, Inspector-General LAWSON, after some preliminary remarks, gave an outline of the epidemics in various parts of the world during the past twelve months.

The great diffusion of small-pox in 1871-72 was noticed, there having being epidemics at various parts—in Africa and Europe, from South of the Equator to the Arctic Ocean, in and from Southern India to Siberia, in America from Chili to Canada.

The hæmorrhagic form had been met with extensively through Europe, in Siberia, and in the Western Hemisphere from Trinidad to Canada. It was suggested as a subject for inquiry whether this might be connected with the influences which, of late years, have led to cerebro-spinal fever. It was shown that the epidemic, which recently passed over this country and North of Europe and Canada, was met with in Southern India in 1868, in Northern India in 1869 and in the South of France in 1870, and in London at the end of that year.

The course of measles and scarlatina in this country was traced, and the remarkable frequency of diphtheria in Scotland noticed, where in Edinburgh the ratio of mortality from this disease alone for 1871 amounted to $\frac{7}{8}$ in 10,000 living. Its presence in other countries was also referred to. The epidemic of whooping-cough at the end of 1871 and in the early part of 1872 in this country was next considered; and it was mentioned that it had been experienced at Shanghæ and Formosa in 1871, at the Cape Mauritius, and in the West Indies and Nova Scotia early this year.

Fever, with a few local exceptions, had been low since the middle of 1871, in Great Britain and Ireland. The typhus became less frequent, the enteric more common, and within the last five months relapsing had nearly disappeared. Cerebrospinal fever had attracted considerable attention in New York and Canada since January. Yellow fever had appeared, though nowhere in very great activity, from Monte Video along the Brazilian Coast, in the West India Islands, and Spanish Main. A febrile disorder described as typhus or plague had been very extensively diffused in Persia since 1871, and dengue had shown itself at Mecca, in many parts of India, in Burmah, and even in China. Cholera resumed its activity at the end of last and early this year, and there have been outbreaks on the East Coast in Western Hindostan, and in the country south of the Himalayas, from the delta of the Ganges, to near Peshawur, and in the districts of Nepaul and

Cashmere. In the middle of April (1872), it broke out in
Turkestan, and by July was in Samarcand and Bokhara, on the
one hand and on the other passed along the Amoor Duria to
the sea of Aral and the North East of the Caspian. In Russia,
cholera prevailed from the Black Sea to Finland with varying
intensity in different localities, it crossed the frontier into the
neighboring districts at various points in the course of the summer, and still remains in Poland, though decreasing greatly in
Russia. It has lately appeared at Buda, and single cases or
small groups have shown themselves at various points, more to
the West, indicating a disposition to occupy fresh ground, but it
is not likely to display much activity until the return of warm
weather.—_The Doctor._

Worms in Urine and Blood.

It will be remembered that, during his investigations on cholera in India, Dr. T. Lewis discovered the embryo of a round
worm in chylous urine, which is figured in his Report on
Cholera. Dr. Lewis has since continued this inquiry in Calcutta, and has not only detected these embryo in large numbers
in chylous urine in many cases, but has found them in very large
numbers in the blood of patients suffering from chyluria. A
single drop of blood from the finger has contained as many as
nine live worms. And the identity of these blood-worms with
those of the urine is, we understand, beyond doubt. Dr. Lewis's
observations will be published in the next Report of the Sanitary Officer with the Government of India, and will be looked
forward to with great interest.

A specimen of the embryo of the chylous-urine worm has
been submitted to Mr. Busk, who considers it some kind of
Filaria; and it may not be inappropriate to christen the new
entozoon "Filaria sanguinis hominis." It is remarkably like
some of the common tank-worms; and the mode of entrance
into the body (probably with the water), its growth and increase
there, and the effects it produces, are matters of the highest
interest, which we hope Dr. Lewis may soon clear up.—_London
Lancet._

Physiology of the Bile.

Some years ago Nasse demonstrated that the bile of the pig
was capable of converting starch into sugar. He was unable to

obtain evidence of the presence of any similar ferment in other
kinds of bile. Von Wittich showed how the ferment could be
isolated.   Jaconson observed the saccharifying power of the
fresh bile of the frog, pike, carp, sheep, ox, pig, rabbit, cat,
horse, goose, duck, and fowl, but was unable to exhibit it in the
bile of man; and this he attributed to the decomposition of the
ferment after death (Pflüger's *Archiv*, Heft 3, 1872). Owing to
the kindness of Dr. Hertz, von Wittich has recently had the
opportunity of examining some fresh bile of the human subject
escaping from a fistula; and his experiments prove conclusively
that it possesses a ferment capable of converting boiled starch
into sugar.—*Ibid.*

Quantity of Nitrogen in Muscular Tissue.

Nowak (*Wien. Akad. Ber.*, lxiv., [2] 359) finds that the
method usually employed for the determination of nitrogen in
muscular tissue (conversion into ammonia by combustion with
soda-lime) does not give accurate results. The percentage of
nitrogen is always too low, and varies by as much 0.8 per cent. in
the same sample.   The method of Dumas (combustion with
copper oxide, and measurement of the nitrogen as gas) is thoroughly trustworthy, and by employing it Nowak obtained the
following percentages of nitrogen in dry flesh: Horse, 13.48—
15.01; dog, 12.40—16.43; ox, 15.00—15.92; man, 14.61—16.02.
If this observation is correct it will necessitate the revision of a
great many important analyses. The flesh-formers of food are
often estimated by determining the percentage of nitrogen and
multiplying it by 6.3. It is clear that this calculation can no
longer be employed if the above figures are correct, for one
sample of dog's flesh would appear to contain 103.51 per cent.
of flesh formers. Of course a part of the nitrogen in flesh is
not present in the form of albuminoids.—*Ibid.*

*Aspirating Puncture of the Bladder in Cases of Irreducible
    Hernia.*

Aspirating puncture of the bladder in cases of irreducible
hernia is one of the important medical novelties now being investigated in France. Several strikingly successful cases have
already been published, and the *Lancet* in one of its late numbers contained the original relation of a case operated on by Dr.

Léon Labbé, of Paris. Dr. Demarquay has just presented a paper on the subject to the Academy of Medicine, wherein he states his intention to carry out the application of the proceeding to the following cases: (1) To all congenital herniæ, and to recent herniæ which become strangulated at the time of their formation; (2) to old cases of herniæ perfectly reducible a few days before the strangulation, and in umbilical herniæ recently strangulated. Dr. Demarquay adds that this aspiration of liquids and gas, with the object of rendering taxis more easy, must be practiced at an early time, when we are almost certain to put back into the abdominal cavity an intestinal fold which is not yet altered and is still capable of resuming its functions. —*Ibid.*

Origin of Pus Corpuscles.

Dr. R. H. Fitz (*Boston Med. and Surg. Journal*, Oct. 17) says that F. A. Hoffmann, (*Virch. Arch.*, vol. liv., 4 Heft), with P. Langerhans, has already shown that some time after the injection of cinnabar into the blood vessels, grains of the same could be found in the fixed cells of the connective tissue, and that whenever an irritation had occurred, the accumulation of pigment in these cells became so great that one could recognize the place with the naked eye, by the red color.

Hoffmann (in the present article) states that wounds were produced and afterwards cauterized, or dilute acetic acid was injected; twenty-two to twenty-four hours after inflammation was thus excited, injections of cinnabar were made.

The pus from the wounded surface contained no cinnabar, yet the tissues from which the pus came contained cells in which were numerous particles of cinnabar; these cells corresponded completely with the so-called fixed connective-tissue cells. The pigment was also found in clumps, imbedded in a dense fibrous stratum; tearing apart these clumps, there were found grains of cinnabar, free or sticking to the tissue-fibres, cells containing pigment and débris of cells. These were, doubtless, the remains of encapsuled abscesses. Apart from them, free cinnabar granules were not found in the connective tissue. Hoffmann infers that the fixed cells take no part in the production of pus, but remain wholly passive. Were they destroyed, the cinnabar must be set free after seven to nine days' suppuration, and be found as such or taken up by the wandering cells. Were they active, it would be probable that cinnabar would appear in the pus, especially as the pigment was found in large amounts in the vicinity of the suppurating surface. Hoffmann had previously shown that cell-proliferation in the extirpated cornea occurs, and, from negative testimony, he inferred that the increase proceeded from the fixed corneal corpuscles.

Stricker has found that the wandering cells are capable of division after leaving the vessels, so that the previous inference cannot be regarded as doubtful.

In conclusion, he states, "Up to the present time, any other source for pus corpuscles than the blood-vessels has not been proven nor placed upon a scientific basis."

Prof. Schiff, in a lecture before the Academy of Sciences at Florence (*Berl. Klin. Woch.*, 1872, No. 14), asserts that in extensive suppuration the white blood corpuscles might be replaced in a manner suggested by the experiment of enucleation of the spleen. When this operation is performed on dogs, these corpuscles increase if the animal remains healthy; much more so if peritonitis follows the operation. He asserts that the increase of these depends upon an irritation of the inner coat of the blood vessels; the more extensive this is, the greater the increase. One can, therefore, regard these as the product or transformation of the epithelial cells clothing the intima. This condition might be called a catarrh of the same.—*Medical Times.*

Cider in Rheumatism.

It has come to light, that in certain parts of England, working people, and even little boys employed to frighten birds away, are compelled to take a considerable part of their wages in cider. Common laborers are required to take three pints per day, carters and shepherds four pints, and boys one pint. Women who work out are required to take one quart daily. Aside from the moral evils of the practice, it is found that the health of the laborers is seriously affected, and that rheumatism is a frequent result; as might be expected on the prevalent theory that that disease is caused by, or associated with, lactic or uric acid in the blood. The subject has elicited the attention of the House of Commons, and proceedings have been instituted for the purpose of correcting the evil.—*Ibid.*

Disease of Ear Attributed to Quinia.

In the *Transactions American Otological Society,* recently published, is described the case of a physician who was cinchonized for malarious disease, and who afterward suffered from violent disease of the ear. His trouble began with laryngeal inflammation and chronic naso-pharyngeal catarrh. When the malarious affection supervened, he took 25 grains quinia every other day, until ringing in the ears and dizziness came on, followed by severe otitis. The otitis was subdued by antiphlogistic treatment, and facial neuralgia followed, for which he took 15 grains quinia, with the effect of producing pain in the ears. Every repetition of the dose was followed by pain. The nasopharyngeal disease increased, with returning neuralgia and otitis. The last was brought on within twenty-four hours by a dose of quinia. He suffered for several years, spending a portion of the time in Europe. He became deaf, and his ears filled with inspissated wax. At length, after long and varied torment, he was restored to tolerable health by judicious treatment. Dr. St. John Roosa, of New York, who describes the case, attributes much of the ear disease to quinia.—*Pacific Medical and Surgical Journal.*

Atropia in Night Sweats.

Dr. J. C. Wilson, in the Philadelphia *Medical Times,* calls attention to the efficacy of atropia in arresting the night sweats of phthisis, in doses of one-sixtieth of a grain once or twice a day. It was promptly successful after the failure of sulphuric acid, tannic acid, oxyd of zinc, and other remedies. Dr. Sidney Ringer also furnishes similar testimony in the *Practitioner,* he having injected it in the skin in doses of the hundredth part of a grain. Dryness of the fauces and dilatation of the pupils result from a continuance of the treatment.—*Ibid.*

Editorial.

WE invite attention to *Hayden's Cold Concentrated Saturates.* That heat is objectionable in the preparation of many vegetable extracts, is well known to Pharmaceutists, but the extent of the objection is not well defined, hence it is safe to discard *heat* where there is a possibility of its impairing the quality of the medicinal principlels to be extracted. Again the presence of inert matters obtained by boiling, necessitates a larger proportion of alcohol to prevent fermentation than would be otherwise needed, which is often a serious objection to say nothing of the retention of offensive extractive matters, at the expense of the more active medicinal principles disengaged by heat.

We believe cold saturates both more grateful to the stomach and uniform in strength. Also that they are more convenient to druggists in putting up prescriptions, as they unite more readily with the ordinary tinctures.

If the New York Pharmaceutical Company exercise the care in the *selection* of their medicines as well as in their *preparation* promised; their articles only require a trial to insure their use in future. See Advertisement.

PHYSICIANS engaged in the practice of medicine who decline to take *any* medical journal on the score of *economy,* are simply attempting to "save at the spigot while they lose at the bung." Such economy will bankrupt any physician in time. We sometimes meet with the objection that "they have not time to read a journal." We are sorry for the *patients* of any physician who can not spend half an hour a day, or even a week, to keep advised in some slight degree of the improvements and discoveries in his profession; as surely as the farmer or mechanic who neglects the means of improvement in their departments fall behind the age, and lose caste with their more intelligent and enterprising neighbors, will the doctor fall behind and ultimately lose caste by such neglect, as all know who give a moment's thought to the subject.

CORRECTION.—We regret the omission, in the December number, to credit the *London Practitioner* with an extract on the use of *Cannabis Indica* in the treatment of Migraine; also the *Medical and Surgical Reporter* with an article on the nature of the epidemic among horses.

Meteorological Observations.

METEOROLOGICAL OBSERVATIONS AT ST. LOUIS, MO.

BY A. WISLIZENUS, M. D.

The following observations of daily temperature in St. Louis are made with a MAXIMUM and MINIMUM thermometer (of Green, N. Y.). The daily minimum occurs generally in the night, the maximum about 3 P. M. The monthly mean of the daily minimum and maxima, added and divided by 2, gives a quite reliable mean of the monthly temperature.

THERMOMETER FAHRENHEIT.

NOVEMBER, 1872.

Day of Month.	Minimum.	Maximum.	Day of Month.	Minimum.	Maximum.
1	46.5	63.0	18	13.5	28.0
2	40.0	59.5	19	32.0	40.5
3	31.0	53.0	20	12.0	27.0
4	44.0	51.0	21	25.0	38 0
5	42.5	46.0	22	31.0	42.0
6	38.0	45.0	23	37.0	58.0
7	35.0	60.5	24	43.0	57.5
8	39.0	54.0	25	29.0	36.0
9	37.0	60.0	26	27.0	40.5
10	44.0	68.0	27	15.5	23.5
11	39.0	51.0	28	18.0	29.0
12	34.5	54.0	29	3.0	19.5
13	39.0	46.0	30	14.0	29.5
14	22.0	30.5			
15	24.0	31.0	Means	29.9	43.7
16	21.5	30.5	Monthly Mean		
17	20.0	38.0	36.8		

Quantity of rain and melted snow:

Rain 1.62
Snow 0.06
—————
1.68 inches.

E. BREY, Linguist and Instructor in the Classical, Biblical and modern languages, especially the German. Teaching rooms, 118 North Third street; 1319 Franklin avenue; 12 South Fifteenth street; (Haydn Conservatory of Music.) He is the originator of a NEW SYSTEM of teaching languages thoroughly and rapidly, which, consisting of translating not only verbatim, but also by ROOTS and AFFIXES greatly assists the memory, and is perfecting in ENGLISH.

Etymological queries on MEDICAL or general terms, as well as geographical or personal NAMES will be answered, more or less satisfactorily, by the above.

Mortality Report.

DEATHS FROM DEC. 1st TO DEC. 28th, INCLUSIVE.

DEC.		White.		Col'd.						AGES.								
	Date.	Males.	Females.	Males.	Females.	Under 5 yrs.	5 to 10	10 to 20	20 to 30	30 to 40	40 to 50	50 to 60	60 to 70	70 to 80	80 to 90	90 to 100	Total.
Saturday	7	141	102	10	6	124	24	14	33	25	18	10	7	2	2	...	259
"	14	148	104	15	7	116	18	18	34	39	20	15	6	8	1	...	274
"	21	123	103	17	3	108	14	19	34	29	29	9	9	5	1	1	254
"	28	145	97	12	1	109	17	21	20	30	25	20	8	5	4	...	269
Total,		557	406	54	17	457	73	72	121	123	92	54	30	20	8	1	1066

Atresia, Intestinal . 1
Abscess of Liver... 3
Accidents, Burns .. 1
Albumenuria 1
Anemia 3
Angina. 3
Apoplexy. 3
Atelectasis.......... 1
Acute Mania.. 1
Alcoholism 1
Asthma 1
Atrophia 2
Burns 2
Bronchitis 12
Cancer........... 7
Catarrh of Lungs. . 1
Cerebritis. 1
Chill, Congestive. 1
Cirrhosis 1
Congestion...... . 1
Conges. of Brain ...14

Conges. of Lungs ... 5
Consumption.......69
Convulsion..........47
Croup 11
Debility 10
Delirium Tremens. 1
Diarrhœa 2
Disease of the Heart 7
Diptheria 8
Dropsy 7
Drowned. 1
Dipsomania 1
Dysentery 7
Eclampsia 1
Empyema 2
Enteritis.... 2
Epilepsy.... /...... 4
Erysipelas 9
Fever, congestive.. 4
" puerperalis.. 2
" remittent... 2

Fever, typhoid.... 17
" irritative.... 1
Gastritis gastro en-
teritis. 8
Hemiplegia......... 3
Hemorrhage........ 7
Hepatitis 5
Hydrocephalus...... 3
Hypertrophy 1
Inflammat'n of brain 3
" stomach 1
Insanity 2
Injuries 5
Laryngitis.......... 5
Lockjaw............ 5
Marasmus 24
Meningitis 18
Metritis 3
Measles 6
Nephritis 1
Œdema 4

Old Age....... . ..13
Puerperal peritonitis 1
Perecarditis 2
Paralysis. 10
Peritonitis........ 9
Pyæmia 1
Pleuritis 5
Pneumonia. 49
Premature birth· . 2
Rheumatism 3
Scarlatina 3
Septicæmia. 1
Scrofula............ 3
Small pox ... .518
Softening of brain.. 2
Typhus 1
Ulcerat'n of stomach 1

Total........1066

Stillborn........ .. 23

TO ADVERTISERS.

This is one of the oldest and most widely circulated Journals in the United States. Those who wish to communicate with the Medical Profession, particularly *West* and *South*, will find it to their interest to use our columns.

Cards will be inserted on reasonable terms.

THE SAINT LOUIS

Medical and Surgical Journal.

FEBRUARY, 1873.

Original Communications.

EXTRACTION OF CATARACT BY THE LINEAR METHOD.

By H. Z. GILL, M. D., of St. Louis, Mo.

The method of *cataract extraction* by *linear incision*, in some of its *forms*, is now largely practiced, though the *flap* method is by no means abandoned ; but of the latter we shall speak only incidentally.

As early as 1707, Charles de Saint Yves extracted a chalky cataract from the anterior chamber, into which it had fallen spontaneously, by making an incision in the cornea below the centre of the pupil, and then extending it transversely to within half a line ($\frac{1}{2}'''$) of the margins of the cornea. He operated in this manner on several cases.

Pourfour du Petit, in 1708, performed a somewhat similar operation on a priest, by puncturing the cornea and extracting a cataract which had fallen into the anterior chamber. In 1716, he made a similar operation by piercing the cornea with a grooved needle, below the pupil, then following the groove with a lance, incising

from the point of entrance to the point of exit. Both
cases were operated on by the same method, as it appears, and both recovered.

Saint Yves and Petit were certainly among the first,
if not the first, to extract by linear incision. They, it
seems, applied the method only to cataracts, or rudiments of cataracts which had fallen into the anterior
chamber.

About the middle of the last century, George Friedrich Siegwart, Professor of Surgery at Tübingen, practiced a method by which an angular flap was made, first
incising the cornea below, then from each end of this
incision, extending it towards the periphery, and, at the
same time, towards the horizontal diameter of the cornea. The result was a flap composed of a short, horizontal incision below, and two lateral oblique ones.
But none, so far as we can learn, and as Graefe has well
stated, seemed to have the idea of sacrificing the advantages of a gaping wound or flap, to those of more rapid
healing in a small incision.

Palucci, at Paris, in 1750, had an instrument made
after his idea, and practiced a method somewhat similar
to St. Yves and Petit, and applied it to capsular cataract also. He made a curved incision in the cornea,
below the level of the pupil, the chord of which was four
lines (4‴), and the height of the curve, or arc, about
one and a fourth lines (1¼‴). He was not pleased with
the results of his method, and still favored the operation by the needle.

At the beginning of the present century, 1809, James
Wardrop, reported in the *Edinburgh Medical Journal,* a
method of incision of the cornea which, very like

Seigwart's, was really a flap with three nearly straight incisions.

In 1811, Gibson, of Manchester, England, proposed also a method of extraction, not only for the rudiments of cataracts, but for the soft variety after the couching needle had been used without success. The incision was made about one line (1‴) from the margin of the cornea, and three lines in length (3‴).

Travers wrote his observations on cataract in 1814. He first detached the lens by means of the needle—preparatory operation,—then made the incision in the cornea to the extent of one-fourth its periphery, through which the detached and divided lens was extracted.

Friedrich and Edward Von Jaeger seem to be the first who gave the name *linear extraction*, and adopted it instead of the term *partial extraction*, which the former had applied to extractions of the capsule through small incisions.

These various incisions had fallen almost entirely into disuse at the principal ophthalmic clinics, both on the continent and in England, by 1850, except for capsular cataracts. About this date several operators began modifications of linear section for lenticular cataract — Bowman, Von Graefe, and Critchett. And Mooren, Jacobson, and Waldau added modifications of the flap extraction. Mr. Critchett says (1): "Thus there suddenly appeared three new methods of operating for cataract, bearing the name of their several champions—the method of Mooren (2), Jacobson (3), and that of Schuft (Waldau) (4); but justice compels me to state

(1) Royal London Ophth. Hosp. Reports. iv, 319.
(2) Preliminary Iridectomy.
(3) Simultaneous Iridectomy.
(4) Scoop Extraction.

that these gentlemen lighted their tapers at the torch of
their great master, Prof. Von Graefe. Each of these
methods had been previously suggested and practiced
by him, but only in exceptional cases, instead of as a
general rule."

The linear incision and extraction with the scoop was
first extensively and successfully employed in London,
by Messrs. Bowman and Critchett, and on the Continent by Von Graefe. The last operator said he chose
the *English method*, almost exclusively, for his cases during the months of January, February, March, April,
and half of May, 1865, and became quite familiar with
it, for it coincided in many respects, with what he called
his *primitive method*. At the close of the above date,
namely, May 19, 1865, Von Graefe operated on his
first case by the *modified linear extraction*, a brief description of which we will here give : (1)

With the narrow, straight knife, known by the name
of the distinguished author, he enters at *a point* in the
sclerotic, *two-thirds of a line* from the margin of the cor·
nea, and *two-thirds of a line* below the level of the summit of the cornea,—below a tangent to the summit of
the cornea. This is the situation of the puncture, and
the counter-puncture corresponds to it, on the opposite side. An incision joining these two points is to be
completed in such a manner that in the anterior chamber it will be in the periphery of the corneal structure,
and in the external wound slightly in the sclerotic coat
beneath the conjunctiva. The external wound of such
an incision is from four and a half to five lines long;
and the little flap of conjunctiva at the top, will be

(1) *Clinique Ophthalmologique.* Edition Francaise. 1866.

about two lines broad. Such an incision deviates so slightly from a strictly linear cut, that it gives the height of a flap about the quarter of a line only. In cases of small nucleus the external wound may be reduced, and brought within the cornea at the summit, thus avoiding altogether the flap of conjunctiva.

This operative method became very popular, and its results undeniably favorable. However, some operators, of large experience, never adopted this method, of whom we may mention Prof. Von Hasner, of Prague, and Desmarres, of Paris, and others in our own country.

The *modification* of Graefe was the iridectomy; and the operation is now generally termed *peripheric linear* extraction.

There has been in the minds of ophthalmic surgeons, a desire to avoid iridectomy, and preserve the iris intact; in other words, to mutilate the eye as little as possible. Wecker expressed the opinion some years ago, that the operation for cataract would probably end in the preservation of the iris entire.

In 1867, Dr. R. Liebreich, then of Paris, now of London, began a new method of operating. We had the pleasure of witnessing some of the operations, and observed that he was not following Graefe. He has now completed, as he thinks, his method, and has given it to the profession in the *St. Thomas's Hospital Reports,* *Vol. II.,* from which we have *a reprint* sent us by Claxton, Remsen & Haffelfinger, of Philadelphia. These enterprising publishers were good enough to furnish, at our request, electrotypes of the original engravings, by which the operation can be made quite clear. We will now let the author speak for himself:

On page 8, he says: "No wonder that, in consequence

of these advantages of Graefe's method, the flap extraction became soon more and more abandoned. To me, however, it appeared that the mechanism of Graefe's method was still too complicated, and too violent, that prolapse of the vitreous body, and hemorrhage into the anterior chamber, were too frequent during the operation, iritis, and strangulation of the iris in the corners of the wound too frequent after it, and that the most favorable results, compared with the most favorable results in flap extraction, were not perfect enough. If these inconveniences are carefully inquired into, it is found that they can all be brought back to one and the same principal cause; namely, the peripheric position of the incision. The peripheric position explains why—

" 1. It is impossible to remove the lens without iridectomy.

" 2. The excision of the iris must be very extensive, else the iris tends to prolapse.

"3. It is necessary to perform the operation above, in order that the enlarged part of the pupil may be covered by the upper eyelid; the removal of the lens upwards is far more difficult on account of the tendency of the eye to roll upwards; and consequently,

"4. During the whole operation, the eye has to be kept open by the speculum, and to be drawn downwards by the forceps. This is not only painful and injurious to the eye itself, but causes

"5. Not unfrequently, prolapse of the vitreous body, to which a peripheral incision itself already tends. Prolapse of the vitreous body, and hemorrhage into the anterior chamber, are the chief impediments to a careful removal of all the *débris* of the cortex and cause

"6. Those grave forms of iritis which are kept up by

the permanent irritation caused by the tumefied remains of the lens behind the iris.

"Of these disadvantages I was perfectly aware, after I had followed for a short time Graefe's original plan, and I proposed some modifications, therefore, in 1867, in an article on cataract which I wrote for the 'Nouveau Dictionnaire de Médecine et de Chirurgie,' Paris, Baillière. They, however, were but a first step, and during the last four years I have by a large series of systematic experiments arrived at a method, which now, after more than 300 operations performed by it, I consider definitely settled.

"Gradually I removed my incision more and more from beyond the margin towards the centre of the cornea, so that it is now entirely situated within the cornea, with the exception of the points of puncture and contra-puncture, which are placed about one millimetre beyond it in the sclerotic(1)—the whole remaining incision passing with a very slight curve through the cornea, so that the centre of it is about 1½-2 millimetres within the margin of the cornea, and, consequently, nearly in that place towards which the equator of the lens is turned, when by a slight pressure on the margin of the wound the lens is brought into that rotation of which I have spoken above in flap extraction. In this form and position of the wound a broad excision of the iris could be avoided, and consequently I cut off smaller and smaller pieces of the iris, until at last I entirely gave up iridectomy. I now saw that without actual formation

(1) Of course only as regards the outside of the wound. As regards the inside, all the wound, even the puncture, is situated in the cornea, the peripheral part of which cannot be reached by a knife introduced in the indicated position without previously passing through a small portion of the sclerotic.

of a flap that mechanism can be brought about, by
means of which the advancing equator of the lens overcomes the obstacles of the iris and of the sphincter pupil-
læ in order to enter the wound.   Avoiding iridectomy,

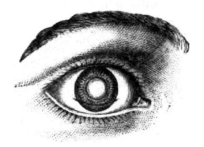

I could do without elevators and forceps, and thus
change the whole operation into a less violent and
almost painless one. Made with Graefe's knife, the most
perfect regularity can be very easily obtained without
fixation.   My operation is now made in the following
way :—

"The patient lies on his back ; chloroform is administered only on his express desire ; the pupil having been
dilated with atropine the day previously, if possible.
For the right eye the operator stands behind the head
of the patient ; for the left, at his left side.   An assistant is not necessary.   All the instruments required are
two, namely, the smallest Graefe's knife possible, and a
cystotome which has a common Daviel's spoon at the
other end. The whole may even be united in one instrument, which has at one end Graefe's knife, at the other end
Daviel's spoon, and within the handle a cystotome which
admits of being pushed in and out. Supposing the right
eye is to be operated upon. In that case the operator takes
hold of the upper eyelid with the index finger of his
left hand, whilst he slightly presses the middle finger

against the inner canthus of the eye. The knife, held
in the right hand with its back horizontal and backwards, the plane of the blade making with the horizontal
meridian of the eye an angle of about 45°, enters the

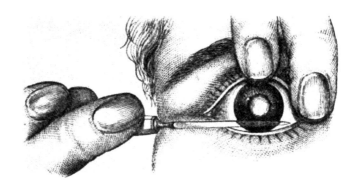

sclerotic with its point about one millimetre externally
to the margin of the cornea, at the place shown in the
accompanying woodcut. *Without altering the direction*,
the knife passes through the anterior chamber in order
to make the contra-puncture on the opposite side, so
that the point of the knife becomes visible in the scler-
rotic about one millimetre (or less) distant from the
cornea. The knife is now pushed forwards, so that its
retraction finishes the incision. As soon as the incision
is made, the eyelid is to be dropped.

"The second part of the operation consists in the
careful opening of the capsule.

"In the third part Daviel's spoon is slightly pressed
against the inferior margin of the cornea, and the index
finger of the left hand, which holds the upper eyelid,
through it exerts a very slight pressure on the highest
point of the cornea. Thus the lens is made to rotate

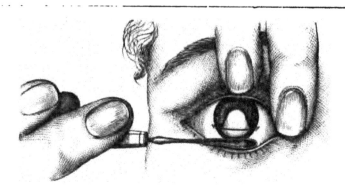

a little, its lower margin presses in the manner already described against the posterior surface of the iris, pushes the iris forward, passes along it to the margin of the pupil, overcomes the obstacle and places itself freely in the wound, which is made to gape by Daviel's spoon pressing against it. A slight pressing movement of the index finger of the left hand, by means of which the upper eyelid is shifted from above downwards over the cornea, serves to expel the lens. Similar movements of the lids are employed for the purpose of forcing out any remaining *débris* of the cortical substance, after pushing them from behind the iris towards the pupil, by gently rubbing the shut eyelids. Should the pupil then not appear round, but its margin drawn towards the wound, it regains its normal position by an outward shifting of the lower lid ; or, if that be not sufficient, by the introduction of Daviel's spoon. Immediately afterwards I put some atropine into the eye, and close it by my compressive bandage.

"What are the advantages of my method of operating ?

"1. It is undoubtedly of all methods the simplest and the least painful.

"2. It is unconditionally the easiest to perform, and

requires the least practice; it may, therefore, be performed by those who have only occasional opportunities of operating; and those patients will profit by it who are unable to reach a central point in order to place themselves in more practiced hands. On account of the greater facility of operation, the last pretext for reclination of cataract is removed, which, though almost universally and justly condemned, is still here and there performed.

"3. It is preferable to the flap extraction, on account of the safer and constantly regular incision. The flap incision scarcely ever acquires the regularity which may theoretically be demanded, even if made by the most practiced operator, with the best assistance, the most enduring patient, or under chloroform by the use of the elevator and fixation instruments. At one time, its height or breadth is not what it is intended to be; at another time, its position is incorrect or the wound irregular. Indeed, part of the irregularity is due to the difficult form of the incision, but by far the greater part, according to my conviction, is due to the mechanism by which the cuneiform cataract knife makes the incision. A small Graefe's knife would make a flap safer and more regularly than any wedge-shaped cataract knife. The incision I designed can easily be made, in every case, exactly in the desired form and position, even if the patient is very restless, without assistance, without elevator or fixation. This mainly depends on the facility with which the place of the contra-puncture can be chosen, the knife drawn back and made to pierce at another point, if a mistake is made in the selection of the place for contra-puncture, and in the freedom with which in terminating the incision the inclination of the knife can be changed, if necessary.

"A little practice will enable every operator to avoid those corrections, and to make the contra-puncture, as well as the whole incision, correctly, according to his original plan.

"4. Compared with Graefe's method, it has the advantage of a more favorable position of the field for the operation, and avoids through it all the inconveniences to which I have referred as arising out of the peripheral position of the wound.

"5. In regard to the mode of healing, it favorably contrasts, like Graefe's method, with the flap extraction, on account of the diminished influences which age, constitution, general state of health, season, and other causes exert: also on account of the less demand made upon the patient to remain quiet after the operation, and, above all, on account of the lesser tendency to suppuration of the cornea.

"6. The advantages of my method over that of Graefe are shown by the ultimate results obtained—by not furnishing a greater percentage of total suppuration than Graefe's method my best results are in regard to optical and (if I may use the term) anatomical perfection, identical with the best results obtained in flap extraction.

"The method is well-adapted for the different cataracts, with the exception of—

"1. Those laminellar cataracts, which need only be treated by iridectomy.

"2. Cataracts which in earliest childhood have to be operated upon by repeated division.

"3. Perfectly liquid cataracts (division with a broad needle).

"4. Partial cataracts, without a nucleus, already absorbed to a great extent, and therefore chiefly traumatic cataracts, for which also division suffices.

" In all other cases of cataract my proceeding can be adopted, only the breadth of the incision and its obliquity may vary very slightly, according to the size of the nucleus, the consistency of the cortex, and especially to the proportion which the size of the cataract bears to that of the cornea. In cases of equally softened cortex, with a smaller nucleus and sufficiently large cornea, puncture and contra-puncture may be made low down and closer to the margin of the cornea, and thus by slighter inclination of the blade, the incision obtains a strictly linear form. With a large and hard nucleus and tough immature cortex it will be necessary, especially if the cornea is exceptionally small, to make the wound somewhat larger and a little more curved. For that purpose puncture and contra-puncture must be made a little closer to the horizontal meridian of the eye, and the blade somewhat more inclined (a little more than 45° from the horizontal meridian).

" In this way it is in every case possible to make the wound sufficiently large for the easy passage of the most voluminous cataract, without incurring the tendency to gape. Even for the removal of the lens with the capsule (without opening the latter), the wound is sufficient.

" If Pagenstecher's procedure is followed, my incision must then be combined with iridectomy. Delgado's procedure can be followed out, even without iridectomy. Delgado introduces a small instrument into the anterior chamber, before he makes his incision, and presses with it on the lens, in order to free it from its natural connections and to remove it, together with the capsule, after the incision has been made.

" I intend to propose another method of extracting the

lens together with its capsule; but a more extended series of experiments is required before I can definitely decide the question, whether and in what cases this procedure can be usefully combined with my incision.

"The question, if and in what cases my procedure is to be combined with iridectomy of more or less extent, can be solved only after a larger experience of my operation without iridectomy than I yet possess. I have performed several hundred operations with iridectomy, but as yet scarcely 100 without.

"I hope that I shall not be left alone to work out this question, but that other surgeons will accept my proposal, which, to recapitulate shortly, is as follows:—

"To avoid the disadvantages in Graefe's operation, arising out of the peripheral position of the wound, and the disadvantages in flap extraction, arising out of the height of the flap, I propose a new method of extraction, which is to be made in the following manner:—

"Puncture and contra-puncture are made in the sclerotic about 1 mm. beyond the cornea; the whole remaining incision is to pass, with a very slight curve, through the cornea, so that the center of it is about 2 mm. distant from its margin. This incision may be made upwards or downwards, with or without iridectomy, and the lens may be removed through it, with or without its capsule.

"If, as I now operate, the extraction is made downwards without iridectomy, the whole proceeding is reduced to the greatest simplicity, and does not require assistance, elevator, fixation or narcotism, and only two instruments.

"In this latter form my procedure has the advantage of being, on the one hand, the least dangerous mode of extraction; and on the other, of being able to obtain the most perfect results, viz., that condition in which the eye operated upon differs from the normal eye only by the absence of the lens, and the cicatrix of the cornea difficult to be seen."

This *new* method has, indeed, certain features which recommend it theoretically; and the question of superiority in practice, is one which is now being worked out by a number of operators.

The results of Graefe's method, when compared with that of the flap, or the scoop method, may be judged of by examining the results. Loring has brought the facts together in the form of comparison as given in the *Transactions of the American Ophthalmological Society*, 1871, p. 108 : " Making, now, a comparison between the final results of Dr. Knapp's series of cases by peripheric linear, and Graefe's by the flap, we have, arranged in tabular form, something like the following:

	Knapp's Linear.		Graefe's Flap
1st series	46	against	80
2nd "	46	"	84
3rd "	59	"	91

This average gives 35 per cent. in favor of the flap, with vision $\frac{1}{4}$ taken as a standard in each case."

Unless a uniform standard of vision after the operation were adopted, it is difficult to estimate the comparative degree of perfection obtained by only one of the methods now adopted. If one takes vision $\frac{1}{4}$, and another $\frac{1}{10}$, we shall never arrive at the exact condition, or the superior merits of one method over others. It seems to me quite clear that some forms of linear incision expose the eye less to the dangers of inflammation of the various tissues most frequently involved; and as a consequence, fewer cases of entire loss of vision will be found to result from this method than from the flap. Whether, however, a higher degree of vision is attained in case the eye is not lost is quite another question, and is not yet settled. If Leibreich's method, which has been called the *median flap* extraction, shall be found to combine at once the fewer dangers and the more perfect eye; that will be the one to be adopted. It certainly recommends itself theoretically, and time alone can prove its real value. My own experience with the new method, though not numerous in cases, has been entirely satisfactory. The operator should select any *form* (1) of the *new method*, which the circumstances or conditions seem to indicate. If the iris does not dilate freely under atropine, or if there has been previous inflammation of the deeper structures of the eye, I should, as I have done, make the iridectomy. We have been the first here, so far as we know, to perform this method, and can confidently *recommend it for trial.* Since commencing the preparation of this article, I have written to Dr. H. W. Williams, of Boston, for his views and experience with linear extraction, knowing that he had been very successful with the flap operation; and he has given his opinion so fully and freely, that we deem it but proper to insert the letter in full:

(1) Liebreich, l. c. page 19

" THE NEW METHOD OF EXTRACTING CATARACT.

" By HENRY W. WILLIAMS, A. M., M D., of Boston, President of the American Ophthalmological Society, First Vice President of the International Ophthalmological Congress, at London.

" The favorable results reported to have been gained by the " linear extraction " of Graefe, as compared with those of other methods of operation for cataract, have made every ophthalmic surgeon feel bound to give this method a fair and ample trial. · But here, as in the trial of the "out-scooping", also formerly advocated by Graefe, my own experience has been only one of disappointment. Nor can I impute the less fortunate results obtained merely to personal *maladresse* for I have had opportunities for observing a considerable number of cases treated by others, among which direct failures as well as subsequent accidents have been by no means exceptional. I have heard the same dissatisfaction expressed by skillful operators in other American cities,—and during and after my attendance at the recent Ophthalmological Congress, I witnessed the growing disfavor with which linear extraction is coming to be regarded by European oculists. It was, therefore, with great pleasure that I saw, especially at the Clinique of M. Liebreich, a large number of operations by a new method, termed by MM. Lebrun and Warlomont, "median flap extraction", and advocated by these authorities as well as by Mr. Critchett. The claim to good results seemed to be fully confirmed by these cases, and by a large number operated on some months previously, where the eyes were in excellent conditions as to vision.

"The narrow knife, introduced by Graefe for his linear extraction, and which is an unquestionable improvement upon any of the modifications of Beer's triangular

6

knife, is employed in this method.   Lebrun and Warlomont favor the upward section of the cornea, Liebreich
practices the downward section.   I am inclined to prefer
the upward section in eyes which are full and prominent,
and the downward where the globe is sunken in the
orbit.   Liebreich operates without anæsthetics, and without fixation of the globe, or separation of the lids by a
speculum, raising the lid and preventing rotation of the
eye by slight pressure with the fingers of his left hand.
The knife is entered at the outer margin of the cornea
(or by Liebreich in the sclera just beyond this margin),
carried across the anterior chamber to the opposite point
in the horizontal diameter of the eye, and it is held
obliquely, instead of parallel to the plane of the iris, as
in the old method.   The incision is completed in such
a direction that the apex of the flap is opposite the
margin of the pupil when in a state of moderate dilatation.   The cystotome is readily introduced, and the
capsule of the lens extensively incised.   Slight pressure
upon the globe, opposite to the wound of the cornea,
whilst at the same time the outer edge of the wound is
slightly pressed backwards with the curette, allows of
an easy exit of the lens, without iridectomy, and without the contusion of the iris or risk of loss of the vitreous, sometimes accompanying the former methods of
flap extraction.

"It will be seen that the position of the wound is
anatomically most favorable for the ready passage of the
lens, while at the same time its small size, as compared
with the former semi-circular flap, allows of immediate
union in nearly every case, thus abolishing the dangers
arising from prolapsus of the iris or ulceration of the
edges of the wound.   The slight scar is so placed as not

to interfere with vision, and in a short time scarcely a trace of it can be perceived.

·" The advantages claimed for linear, as contrasted with extraction through a large peripheral incision, were, that the small size of the wound was favorable to immediate union, and the excision of a part of the iris facilitated the removal of the lens and lessened the dangers of subsequent prolapse. Its evident defects were, the mutilation of the iris, the necessity for long continued manipulation of the eye to effect the expulsion of portions of the cortical substance of the lens, which did not readily escape through the small incision, the frequent and not always harmless evacuation of considerable quantities of vitreous, and, above all, the situation of the wound, so near the ciliary region. We all know · the serious consequences often resulting from accidental injuries in this situation, and, though these are not to be expected after a simple incision, like that for linear extraction, if immediate union is obtained, yet, where from any cause healing is delayed, the ciliary region is liable to be involved in the cicatrix. This, as I have already seen happen, may lead to separation of the retina, or to an affection of the other eye, with sympathetic inflammation.

"Since my return home, and within the past eight weeks, I have performed the median flap extraction at the Boston City Hospital in thirteen cases. In the last, operated on two days since, the corneal wound is already well united, and the patient counts fingers readily. Four other cases, operated on a week ago, might even now be safely discharged, scarcely any reaction having attended the healing process. All the other cases followed a similarly favorable course, and obtained excellent vision, remaining in the Hospital an unusually short time. For most of them reading glasses have already been selected.

"A series of thirteen cases is not a large one,—and, though everything connected with the operations and the after-treatment has been so remarkably favorable, I should perhaps have formed a less decided opinion as to the merits of linear extraction, had not my former exceptional performances of a similar method in some peculiar instances, afforded me similar experience as to good results.

"This method is free from most of the objections attaching to both the other principal modes of operating. The wound is smaller than in the peripheral flap operation, and of a form better adapted to secure complete apposition of its edges and a prompt reunion, while it allows of an easy removal of the lens without much pressure and without contusion of the iris. It almost wholly obviates the chances of loss of vitreous, and of hernia of the iris with its attendant dangers. As compared with linear extraction, it seems to offer the same facility in healing of the incision which is claimed as the great merit of the linear method, it leaves the iris intact to perform its normal functions, and there is no cicatrix so placed as to be a source of future mischief."

ON TETANUS AND TETANOID AFFECTIONS, WITH CASES.

By B. Roemer, M. D., St. Louis, Mo.

The following cases are taken from my diary as they occurred in my practice during the years from 1862 to 1868. The remarks which I have added, form rather an expansion of short notes taken at the bedside of my patients, than an elaborate comment,—the result of after thought. References are freely given, and if the reader notices familiar faces in these pages, he should remember that experience and study are valuable only in comparison with the labor of others, who, as common property, are our guides and commentaries, and whose opinions should be subject to the maxim, "*creta an carbone notandum.*"

Case I.—Robert B. entered hospital with vuln. sclopet. of left arm: entrance of ball on ulnar side of wrist, ranging upwards near interosseous space, and passing through elbow joint, with exit at middle third of humerus July 1, 1862. Omitting treatment of wound, I state that on August 25th, his bowels having been constipated to require active medication, the pain in his arm and epigastrium, and his general listlessness, with uneasiness at the præcordia induced me to pay him strict attention. In the night of August 25th, I was called to see him; he complained of violent cramps in his bowels and stiffness in his jaw, and on the following morning he lay immoveable, stretched out and having contraction of the muscles of the larynx and neck. Distressing pains darted over the whole body, and during the vio-

lent paroxysm of the spasm, of from two to six minutes interval, the contents of the bladder were forcibly
ejected.   Perspiration, difficult and labored respiration,
and increased pain at the lower sternum and from the
ensiform cartilage towards the spinal column were
added.   At 5 P.M. his voice was sensibly altered, face
sardonic and pulse accelerated.   There was neither re-
nor pro-curvation.   The wound had become hot and dry.
The intermissions between the exacerbation became
shorter, and spasms were provoked by touch and muscular volition.   His mind remained unimpaired, and
the successful issue was in no small degree due to his
prompt and anxious obedience to my directions.   The
temperature was for the first fourteen hours 105° F.,
and afterwards 100°.   The treatment up to the evening
of August 26th, consisted in the repeated exhibition of
cathartics: castor oil, ol. tiglii, elaterium with calomel,
aided by enemata of progressive strength.   Meanwhile
he was ordered,

        ℞ Ext. Cannab. Indic. gr. ss.
          Quinine,   grs. ij. M

every hour, increasing the extract after the third dose,
to one and one and a half grains every hour.   His
bowels responded Aug. 27th, 12:30 A. M.   Has taken
twenty-three grains of ex. cannab. ind.   On Aug. 27th,
at 5 A. M., the treatment having been continued and
the symptoms materially abated, I reduced the extract
to its primary dose.   The condition of his arm necessi-
tating an operation, I amputated at 3 P. M. on the
same day.   Trismus remained for five days, with an "in-
explicable" stiffness of the whole body.   Cannabis ind.
was reduced to one-fourth and one-eighth grain doses at
longer intervals.   Total amount taken 146½ grains.

The arm on dissection disclosed a spiculum of bone pressing on the median nerve, without, however, affecting its calibre or condition. The patient was about the ward on Sept. 6th, and the stump had healed on Sept. 18th. Tetanus followed the injury in 56 days, and amputation had no share in the recovery.

Case II.—Wm. B. A.; vuln. scl. Ball entered left inferior maxilla, midway between its angle and coronoid process, ranging horizontally forward along maxilla to the last right incisor, destroying bone and teeth in its course, and fracturing by concussion the inferior right maxilla at the second molar; exit on right half of lower lip, which was much torn. Ligaments implicated: left buccinator, pterygo-maxillary, left superior constrictor and right buccinator. After removal of all spicula of bone, I resected the angle of the left inferior maxilla; a fistulous opening forming on the right inferior maxilla, point of fracture, it was sufficiently enlarged to clear it of pieces of bone and two teeth, after which Barton's fracture bandage with fixed chin and maxillary band of leather was adjusted. In the second week symptoms of opisthotonos appeared under obstinate constipation and pain at the præcordia. The spasmodic contractions were intermitting and every ten or fifteen minutes. The treatment consisted of ex. cannab. ind. one-half to one and one-half grains, every one or two hours, combined with quinine and active cathartics. His bowels acted upon repeated enemeta in thirty-six hours. Made a perfect recovery, tetanus being relieved on the fourth day.

Case III.—F. C. A.; accidental vuln. sclop. of left wrist. Amputation below elbow necessary on first day. Trismus appeared on the third day after admission in the hospital, and on the fourth day after injury. Tonic spasm marked in subacute form. *Treatment :*

R Ext. Cannab. ind. grs. 1 to 3
Quinine, grs. 2 M

every half to one hour. Made a good recovery in six days, after taking 63 grs. of the extract. Dissection of wrist disclosed no alteration in the nerves implicated.

Case IV.—W. H. D.; v. s. through right wrist. Had been furloughed from another hospital (Richmond, Va.), fainted on his way to the railroad depot, and was brought by citizens to my hospital. The primary injury was undoubtedly much aggravated by his fall. Tetanus in a subacute form set in on the eleventh day after reception of gunshot wound. Amputation became necessary five days after the appearance of tetanus. The treatment was the same as in the preceding case. Spasm disappeared on the fifth, and he fully recovered on the ninth day.

Case V.—T. P.; v. s. Ball entered radial side of left forearm, a little below elbow, traversing the joint. Tetanic spasm commenced on the fifteenth day; amputated arm above elbow on the second day after admission. The treatment consisted of opium in 1-2-3 grs. doses every one and two hours. Spasm with recurvation recurred at longer intervals, but with increased violence. Substituted ex. cannab. ind. gr. 1 to 3, with quinine grs. 2, every hour. Recovered in eleven days Took thirty-five grs. opium and afterwards fifty-one grs. of the extract. Temperature, for two days 103.5°, then 101°, and 99.5° F.

Case VI.—Thos. B.; ball entered ulnar aspect of right arm, middle third, ranging towards and traversing elbow joint, with exit one inch below external condyle, and fracturing external condyloid ridge. After removing many spicula of bone, it was found necessary to resect the partially detached portion of the fractured condyle. The patient improved rapidly, although amputation was daily held before him. An abcess of the triceps m. was freely opened. On June 9th (the gunshot wound was received May 12th—entered hospital May 20th), prolonged constipation supervened, and during the succeeding night trismus. . Active cathartics and enemata were at once ordered, with a desired effect on June 11th, or 46 hours after trismus. Having divided *my* supply of Indian hemp some time previously with other surgeons, and having no confidence in the article at command, prescribed

> R Quin. sulph, ℈ i.
> Chloroform, gtt. L.
> Mucil. acaciæ, f. ℥ ss.
> M. S., a teaspoonful every two hours,

and applied chloroform to the arm and spine. Warm poultices were actively resumed. Tetanus in a subacute form developed itself on June 10th. 9 P. M., and a persistent anæsthesia by chloroform failing to control the spasm, I applied morphia in grain doses to the openings in the triceps m. The third dose, in the course of as many hours, had a decided effect. On June 14th he was much relieved; the before scanty discharge of pus became profuse. Trismus continued for one week, until June 20th. Morphia was continued in reduced doses, and tonics added with stimulants. The wound healed well, leaving the arm anchylosed at an angle of 110 degrees, but with full use of hand and fingers. Temperature, 101.5°, 103° and on June 13th, 99° F.

Case VII.—N. B.; Tetanus in consequence of a minute punctured wound in the heel from stepping upon a
nail.   Had his shoes on at the time, and the hole in the
leather was scarcely perceptible.   Two days after the
accident he felt stiffness of the jaw and an unusual cos-
tiveness of the bowels, to which, however, he paid no
attention.   A botanic physician advised a liniment, etc.,
without indicating the nature of the case.   Had the first
tetanic spasm on the 5th day at 7 P. M.   Living twenty-
three miles from the patient's house, I saw him about
seven o'clock next morning.   Found the botanic practitioner engaged in preparing poultices of peach tree bark
(he declared that with the leaves the case would be quite
a simple one), and giving Mr. B. repeated hot plunge-
baths.   Acute tetanus fully developed.   Temperature,
104.5°, and an hour afterwards, or half-hour before death,
106° F.   A previous attempt to forcibly separate the
clinched jaw resulted in the loss of two teeth, which
were shown me.   Spasm extremely violent (with hydro-
phobic spittle around teeth), and mixed with tonicity of
muscle and convulsive tremor; shoulders raised upwards
and slightly backwards at each paroxysm; muscles of
larynx and pharynx violently and persistently contracted
so as to produce a quick succession of gurgling sounds;
the eye drawn backwards and injected; face red and a white
foam around lips.   The case being hopeless for medication per os I confined myself to endermic applications of morphia, cannabis indic., and inhalations of
chloroform combined with enemata.   The inhalation of
chloroform seemed to call forth violent spasm of the
glottis, and a labored or spasmodic inspiration.   The
tobacco enema and the $\frac{1}{20}$–$\frac{1}{15}$ drop of nicotine, showed
no effect whatever.   The patient died a little more than

an hour after I arrived, having been comatose for the last twenty minutes. Mode of death: apoplectic spasm. Autopsy refused.

Case VIII. J. B. H.; admitted to hospital February 14, 1864. Presented 3 cystic tumors upon left thigh, internal aspect, extending from lower edge of middle third of thigh to the groin near pubic portion of fascia lata and saphena opening; overspreading sartorius, pectinæus, abductor magnus and gracilis muscles; with a base of oval form; longest diameter (along axis of femur) 10 inches, shortest diameter at right angles with former 5.5 inches, and with a vertical radius of 5¾ inches. Had been operated upon twice within five years, but the tumor returning he was ordered to hospital for treatment. 'The great press of surgical business (just after a battle) compelled me to postpone the case in favor of more urgent ones, and I placed him upon the general list for future attention. On March 2d, at 8 A. M., and probably also during the night, he gave symptoms of trismus and in a few hours afterwards of tetanus, increasing rapidly in violence. Believing tetanus to be due to pressure upon a nerve, he was at once placed under the influence of chloroform, and the whole tumor excised, which amounted now to four cysts. Tetanic spasm set in while under anæsthesia, trismus only having been noticed before chloroform was exhibited. Temperature before operation 101°, immediately after removal to his bed 102.5° F. Respiration became greatly embarrassed, and I resorted once during the operation to artificial inspiration, finishing the enucleation of the tumor without anæsthesia. Tetanus assumed its full vigor after the patient's removal to his ward, opisthotonos interchanging with tetanus erectus. In the treatment I had prescribed early in the morning ol. ricini in full doses with croton oil, followed by injections, and a volatile liniment was freely applied over the maxillary articulation, region of the mastoid process, nuchæ and spinal column, aided by the local use of morphia in 2 grain doses. Internally I ordered,

> ℞ Chloroformi, Ether. Sulphur. āā f. ʒ i
> 　Tr. Opii.　　　　　　　　　　f. ʒ ss.
> M. S. a teaspoonful with mucilage every hour.

At 10 A. M. (operated at 9 A. M.) deglutition became impossible, every attempt inducing an instant and violent spasm. Temperature 103°. The above mixture was repeatedly applied to the lips with a sponge and the following enema given:

> ℞ Sodæ Chlor.　ʒ ss.
> 　Tr. Opii.　　f. ʒ vj.
> 　Chloroformi, gtt. xxx.
> 　Mucilag.　　f. ʒ j.　M.

Chloroform was also brought in contact with the spinal column upon raw cotton. Bowels acted at 12 M. Hemorrhage from a superficial artery of the wound required the removal of the dressing, and the bleeding vessel being secured by torsion, a solution of morphia was injected along the edges of the wound, while in apposition. The spasm, however, continued unabated. Temperature at 2 P. M. 104.5° F. Respiration became more and more irregular and stertorous, and the patient died at 6 P. M, under spasm of the glottis. Temperature at 5:30 P. M. was 106° F. The continuance of tetanus was about 10 hours. The whole of the tubercular mass weighed 4 pounds and 7 ounces.

Careful dissection gave no alteration of the nerves implicated or adjacent. The post mortem examination of the brain and spinal column was made 12 hours after death; body well nourished; rigor mortis fully developed; veins superficial to the brain distended; substance of the brain healthy; about one drachm of a serous fluid was collected from the lateral ventricles, of a specific gravity of 1007—cerebro spinal fluid; lining membranes of the ventricles normal, under the microscope showing no traces of inflammation; similar condition of choroid plexus, septa and fornix. The spinal cord was free from inflammatory evidences; the arachnoid close to the opening irregular and distended; blood-vessels healthy; pons varol. normal; slight vascularity of dura mater. The microscopic examination of the spinal cord was made especially in the cervical region, the condition there being more strongly marked. The instrument used was one of fine powers, giving 400 diameters. I feel obliged here to return my warm thanks to Assistant Surgeons Goodwin and Goldsmith for their continued and valuable assistance, also to Mr. J. M. Tomlinson, whose late return from his studies of the paintings in Italy enabled me to secure his services in copying the microscopic results, which I shall give on a future page.

Case IX.—I. N., a laborer, was visited by me on the night of Aug. 29th, 1868. Found him lying upon the floor, able to answer my questions, but, as he says, obliged to be quiet on account of "sudden pain over his body." On examination diagnosed trismus and opisthotonos. Had a fixed jaw for two or three days and remembered, on my directing his attention properly, that he had received a slight injury to one of his feet about a week ago, of which, however, no trace remained. Bowels constipated for several days. Ordered a full dose of castor oil with two drops of croton oil at once, to be followed by enemata, if required, and the folowing local and internal remedies:

> R Tr. Aconit. Rad.   f. 3 ss.
> Glycerin., Chloroformi, āā. f. 3 vi.
> M. F. Lin. S.

Use freely over muscles of jaw and neck, and,

> R Tr. Aconit. Rad.   f. 3 ij.
> Quin. Sulph.   Ə iss
> Syr. Limon,   f. 3 i M. S.

a teaspoonful every 3 hours.   Six hours afterwards, two doses of the mixture being taken, and the liniment applied three times, I found the symptoms unchanged; spasm more prolonged and epigastric pain intense. Temperature 104.5° F. Gave two teaspoonsful of the liquid, to be repeated in one hour.   No relief being obtained, I substituted the ex. cannab. ind. in ½ grain doses every hour, and injected hypodermically a solution of hemp (10 grs. to 2 drachms water), 10 minims as a dose.   In six hours, 9 grains having been used internally, and 5 grains hypodermically, the patient slept 20 minutes, and woke up under a severe spasm.   Continued the hemp in 2 gr. doses every hour, and repeated its hypodermic exhibition every two hours as indicated by the violence of the spasm.   Twenty-four hours after the first exhibition of cannabis ind., the patient took 4 grains at a dose every hour for four hours, with two injections of one gr. each.   Spasm of shorter duration; masseter muscles sensibly relaxed and the patient in better condition. Temperature 101°.   The extract was now diminished to

2 and 1 grain doses, which he continued for five days. Took internally 174, and by the syringe 21 grains of the extract. Recovered fully in two weeks.

Although Wunderlich's observation on a high temperature in fatal cases of tetanus and at their termination is fully verified in the foregoing cases, yet it should be borne in mind, that many persons give a temperature during health much above or below the accepted average, and that, consequently, without anterior data no implicit reliance can be based upon the thermometer.

Tetanus was not of common occurrence in the Crimean war. Macleod saw there 6 cases in camp, and 7 in Scutari; he estimates the percentage to gunshot wounds below that given by Alcock, 1 in 79. Its fatality was universal; nor could a predisposing cause be detected in the locality of the wound. Prof. Busch of Bonn (in Verhandlung des Naturh. Vereins für Rheinland u. Westphalen, 1867, s. 15) gives the following reports on tetanus during the late wars :

From the fights in Paris (1848) among 1000 wounded, no case.
Stromeyer in the Schleswig-Holstein war (1849), - 1 "
Demme (Austrian army), Italian war (1859), - - 86 cases.
Demme (Italian army) Italian war (1859), - - - 140 "
Busch, Crimean war, among 12094 wounded. - 19 "
Busch American war* (1861–5) - - - - 363 ··
Busch Bohemian war (1866) - · - - 21 ··

In Guy's Hospital during 7 years tetanus occurred as follows :

After 856 case of contusions - - - 1 case.
" 1364 cases of operations - - - 1 "
" 456 cases of burns - - - 3 cases.
" 594 cases of wounds - - - 9 "
" 398 compound fractures - - . 9 "

---

* See below.

Busch considers the percentage of recoveries greater in tropical climates, although there the liability to tetanus is greater. Thus is the negro race more predisposed than the white race; and Mr. Peat gives in his Essay on Tetanus in the East Indies (Poland in System of Surgery, vol. 1., p. 321), these estimates among castes: Hindoos 1.63, Mussulmans, 1.09, Parsees, 1.005, and Christians, 0.75 per cent.

In the Indian campaign unextracted balls seemed to favor the advent of tetanus, especially if underlying strong fasciæ. Mention is made of sudden changes in temperature, as after the battle of Ferozepore and Chillianwallah, and a like cause was adduced by Baron Larrey in the Egyptian and German campaigns (1809), 100 cases following the battle of Bautzen, and a still greater number after Dresden. Baudens reports that in Africa, during a north-east wind in December, 40 slightly wounded soldiers gave fifteen cases of tetanus, of which twelve died, and the recovery of the remainder was ascribed to their removal to a warm place. Yet, after the battle at Alma, although the opposite extremes in temperature prevailed, no such results were noticed; and Hennen, to reconcile these differences in meteorological causes, taught that cold air in motion predisposed to tetanus, and cited the battle of Muskau as an example, after which few of the French soldiers had tetanus, although the heat was great; whilst after Dresden, the weather being cold and wet, a great number died with it, even after primary operations. In both Indies heat predisposes the native and foreigner alike, and according to Dr. Kane the same obtains in the Arctic regions.

Dr. F. Sorrel sums up from his special reports that in the late war there occurred in the Confederate armies

66 cases of tetanus, with 6 recoveries, out of 56,775 wounded—a mortality of 91 per cent., giving 1 case for every 860 wounded. This statement, however, is incorrect, since a number of cases are omitted. (In December, 1864, to which period the report is here quoted, Dr. Baer, an assistant to Dr. Sorrel, informed me, that the cases of tetanus under my charge were not included, because my report had not been received; and a similar fate befell, undoubtedly, that of others.) The Guy Hospital Reports by Poland, give from 1825 to 1858 exclusive 72 cases of tetanus, an average of .063 per cent. of all cases treated, of which terminated fatally 62 or 86.1 per cent. Of these 72 cases were 69 of traumatic and 3 of idiopathic origin. Peat and Morehead report from the Iepeeboy Hospital, at Bombay, 0.8 per cent. tetanus of all patients in charge with a mortality of 93.95 per cent.. and from the City Authorities (Dr. Leith), we have in six years 1716 deaths from tetanus, a mortality of 92.3 per cent. According to Busch (loc. cit.), Blanc saved 43; Demme, 7, and he himself, 33.33 per cent., whilst in the American war only 7.4 per cent. recovered. In London, out of 345,132 deaths in six years, 110 were from tetanus, the whole number treated being 117, a mortality of 94 per cent., and in England, for the same years, 759 died from this disease out of 811 cases, in a total of 2,431,602 deaths, a mortality of 93.53 per cent. Additional tabular results show (Am. Journ. Med. Sc. Oct., '58, page 477,) that tetanus is more common in the United States, even in the more northern latitudes, than in England. Of the 16 cases by Turner, 12 were of traumatic origin with 4 recoveries, 66.6 per cent. (perhaps inclusive of trismus and subacute tetanus), 2 cases were idiopathic, with 1 recovery, 50 per cent., and 2 cases were trismus

nascentium with 100 per cent. mortality, or an average
of 68.74 per cent., much below the ratio of other Reporters, showing how uncertain statistics appear if derived from a limited number of cases. The discrepancy will
be more distinct from the per centage of my cases now
reported, 5 cases of a subacute and 2 of acute tetanus
recovering, with 2 deaths, giving an average mortality of
only 22 per cent.

Macleod's opinion on the absence of predisposing
causes in certain gunshot wounds over others to tetanus, is verified by most observers. Watson reports a
case of tetanus fatal in fifteen minutes after an injury
of the thumb from the breaking of a china dish. T.
Spencer Wells, after it had been recorded that in 300
cases of Ovariotomy only one resulted in tetanus, had
in one month two cases to follow that operation. D.
Gordon relates a successful case of uterine tetanus,
witnessed by Prof. Simpson. The Bombay Reports
state that no ratio exists between the violence of tetanus
and the severity of the injury, and that 86.56 per cent.
occurred after wounds of the extremities. John Hunter
believes that all cases seen by him resulted from wounds
of tendons, for "these parts heal less readily." Prof.
Fonssagrives, of Montpellier, had two fatal cases, a
child and an adult, following the hypodermic injection of
quinine dissolved by the aid of sulphuric acid. A
third case occurred in New Orleans, resulting fatally
two months after a similar operation, the injection having been made in the deltoid muscle. Travers relates
cases dependent on the ligation of the umbilical, spermatic cord and of the anterior crural nerve, and he considers tetanus after tying the umbilical cord common
in hot climates—yet in the Dublin Lying-in Hospital,

the infants died, at one period, within two weeks at the rate of 17 p. c.,* and the *Berlin Monatschrift für Geburts-kunde,* 1864-5, gives 95 fatal cases of trismus nasc. among 380 births in the practice of one midwife. In the belief of Travers a clean cut never results in teta-nus. S. Cooper, per contra, gives an instance where it followed the amputation of the mamma, and the Earl of Darnley died with tetanus from the amputation of two of his toes. A slight wound of the ear, a cut from a whip below the eye without abrasion, the paring of a corn, a bite on the finger from a tame sparrow, the ex-traction of a tooth, the injection for hydrode, cupping without scarification, and similar trivial causes have led to fatal tetanus, so that the enumeration of exciting causations seems to amount to a *gratis dictum.*

Sir James McGregor, (Med. Chir. Transact. vol. VII. and vol. VI. p. 453), fixes the latest term of tetanus supervening upon an injury on the 22d day. The *Bombay Hosp. Reports* sum up as follows:

10 days' interval in 148 out of 306 cases, or 48.366 p. c.,
10-22 "   "   " 134 "   " 306 "   " 43.790 " "
+ 22 "   "   " 24 "   " 306 "   " 7.843 " "

and deaths occurred after 5 days in 62 cases; in Guy Hosp , the 3 fatal cases died—2 after the 28th and 1 after the 32d day. Poland (loc. cit. page 319), gives

130 cases up to the 10th day, mortality 101 or 77.69 p. c.
126 "   "   "   " 22d " . "   65 " 51.50 " "
 21 " beyond the 22d "   "   8 " 38.09 " "

and in 327 fatal cases died—

---

*2944 infants died out of 17550 in this Hospital. (Dr. Jos. Clarke.)

in 2 days - - - - -	79
" 2 to 5 " - - - -	104
" 5 " 10 " - - - -	90
" 10 " 20 " - - - -	43
" + " 22 " - - - - -	11
Total, - - - -	327

Hence, the second and tenth days embrace 59.33 p. c. of the whole mortality—still the favorable prognosis in tetanus is not, as some authors insist, commensurate with a long incubation.* Sir Brodie (Med. Gaz. Clin. Lect. vol. II. 344) holds the 17th day as the latest period, and Blanc (Chelius' Surg. I. 415) saw a case one month after the injury. The case of Robt. Byrd now reported (No. I.) had 56 days intervening between the reception of the gunshot wound and acute tetanus. Watson gives the range of incubation from the 4th to the 14th day, and also B. Travers (in Further Inquiry Concerning Constitut. Irritation, tetanus p. 292) limits the accession of tetanus to a fortnight. Curling refers to a case recorded by Ward (Copland's Med. Dict. vol. III. p. 1114), in which tetanus supervened 10 weeks after a burn in the axilla.

---

* Dr· O'Beirne saw in the Peninsula 200 cases, all of which proved fatal, and Hennen affirms, that he never witnessed a case of " acute symptomatic Tetanus " to recover. Of the same opinion are Dickson and Morgan.

[To be Continued.]

NOTES ON THE SURGICAL USE OF ELECTRICITY.

By David Prince, M D., Jacksonville, Illinois.

Supposing that any contribution upon this developing subject may be interesting, I submit the following notes:

The subject in its present aspects is new. Though it is nearly a hundred years since Galvane discovered the agent in the form which bears his name, the employment of galvanism to promote absorption of unhealthy growth, and to stimulate the growth of healthy tissue, is new. It may be well to premise a few distinctions adopted by those who now write upon the subject.

Electricity, electric, electrization, are terms employed to cover the whole subject, though sometimes confined to static or frictional electricity.

Galvanism, galvanic, galvanization, are terms employed to denote the form of electricity produced by chemical action, to denote the use of the agent, and the effects produced by its employment.

Faradism, faradic, faradization, are terms employed to denote the form of electricity produced by induction, the uses of this agent or the effects of its employment.

For illustration: if a galvanic current be passing along a wire and another wire be placed in close proximity without touching it, a current will flow in the latter wire in the opposite direction, at the closing and opening of the circuit, *i. e.*, at the starting and at the stopping of the primary current. While the primary current may flow constantly as long as the chemical decomposition continues, the secondary current can only exist momentarily and is repeated just as often as the

primary current starts and stops. It is always, therefore, an interrupted current. Faradization always sig-
nifies the employment of an interrupted current though
the interruptions may be so rapid as to destroy the
feeling of shocks. For the stimulation of nerves and
muscles, the high tension of this current and its shaking
character, render it most highly useful in arousing
organs from a sluggish condition.

The soothing or quieting effect of this current is
never direct, but indirect or secondary, as a lethargy
may follow such exercise as exhausts from its degree or
its duration. Faradization for paralyzed muscle should
therefore be of short duration, for the exhaustion of
an irritability already enfeebled, must do more harm
than good.

It is nearly or quite useless for surgical purposes, because it is impracticable to make the induced current
heat a metal for cauterization, or to make it effective in
electrolysis. By this term is meant the decomposition
of the tissues so as to set their elements free—hydrogen
and the alkalies going to the negative pole, and oxygen
and the acids going to the positive pole.

For the purpose of electrolysis the negative pole in
the form of a needle (or a number of them) is employed
to develop hydrogen in the tissues. If the action is
only continued for a very brief period, the vitality of
the tissue is not destroyed, but a new action is set up
which in many instances is sufficient to stop a morbid
growth. If the action is continued longer, the tissue
is torn apart by the development of hydrogen, and a
slough is the consequence of the disintegraton.

Ordinary steel sewing needles can be employed for
electrolysis for they are not corroded by the hydrogen

which is developed. When it is the object to produce coagulation and solidification, as in the treatment
of the contents of an aneurismal tumor, the needle
introduced is connected with the positive pole, and it
must be of platinum. The plating of needles for this
purpose is useless, because the galvanic current causes
the plating to peel off, and if not, the deposit of carbon
upon the needle holds with such closeness that the plating must become detached in the attempt to clean the
needle.

Needles connected with both poles may be inserted
into a tumor, and this may be advantageous when it is
wished not to subject the underlying parts to the
passage of the current. This may be the case when the
growth is upon the head or face. In other cases the
positive current (and *vice versa*), may be introduced
through a sponge in the hand, or applied to any convenient part of the body.

The momentary electrolysis of a morbid growth may
be borne without the previous induction of anæsthesia,
but the prolonged application is too painful for the
conscious condition. Electrolysis from its perfect manageability is to become the king of caustics, and is destined to rescue from the monopoly of quacks those morbid
growths which are not treated by the knife. Neither can
the induced current be made to produce that therapeutic
effect upon morbid material of low vitality, by which it
would seem that a higher vitality is imparted, and by
which, excessive growths are arrested, while those which
are too sluggish are stimulated. It is in this last direction that new interest has been excited in the employment
of galvanism.

The current is introduced so as to occasion the least

possible irritation upon the surface, large moist sponges
are employed in order to distribute the current over
large surfaces, and the part to be affected, whether external or internal, is within a stream of galvanism, which
would be electrolytic in its action if not so widely
diffused.

The following case may seem to illustrate the *therapeutic* advantage of the galvanic in distinction from the
electrolytic mode of application.

Case of infiltrated epithelial growth in sub-parotideal
region of two years' growth. Failure of dissection to
remove the whole of the tumor. Growth under the influence of electrolyzation. Partial removal again by the
knife. The current again employed with wide distribution, with rapid absorption of the infiltrated material.

May 28, 1873.—Elijah A. Reynolds, aged 40, in May,
1840, perceived a small tumor under the angle of the
right lower jaw, hard, but not sensitive to the touch.

In August it began to grow rapidly. In October it
diminished in size. In May, 1871, it began to grow
again. In January, 1872, it began to be painful, and
continues painful to the present time. It has grown
perceptibly during the last month. A small additional
tumor is perceptible under the jaw, near the median
line.

The accompanying cut, Figure 1, exhibits the appearance of the tumor previous to its dissection.

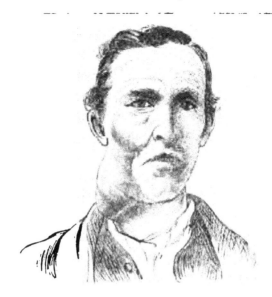

Operation under chloroform. The dissection was commenced from below, and the tumor was found to have no membranous enclosure, but to be incorporated with the tissues surrounding it. It broke up readily under the pressure of the finger, and its deep surface not only dipped into the muscles, but the muscles themselves were rendered hard and rigid by infiltration of the same material.

It was not thought prudent to attempt the complete removal of the morbid material, but to apply electrolysis after a few days. Under the glass no caudate cells were discovered, and such cells as could be distinguished, had very much the appearance of those found in epithelial growths. The history of the tumor, and the appearance of its contents to the naked eye, were those of encephaloid disease.

The patient had been prepared for the operation by a cathartic the night before, and five grains of quinine in place of breakfast. A few hours after the operation

¼ grain morphia and 30 grains hyd. chloral were given.
The wound was left open, and kept covered with pieces
of old muslin, saturated with a solution of carbolic acid
of four grains to the ounce.

June 1.—Wound cleaning out and granulating well;
the patient kept upon the use of 7 grains of citrate of
iron and quinine three times a day.

June 4.—The seventh day from the operation, galvanization was commenced with a 32-cell-platinum-2-inch
battery.

The application was varied on different days, and
averaged about 20 minutes, twice a day. The poles
were interchanged, to see which was most agreeable to
the patient. The flat, metallic plate, covered with wet
canton flannel, was soothing to the patient, producing
sleep. The indurated tissue apparently softened and
lessened in size.

June 29.—One month subsequent to the operation.
After employing the flat electrode for two weeks, the
platinum needle (negative), was employed to destroy a
tubercle in the centre of the open ulcer for several days,
and some increase of thickness being discovered upon
the upper and posterior margin, the needle was also
introduced here. A rapid increase of volume followed
the employment of the needle in the electrolytic way.
It became evident that this mode of application was
injurious. The patient became demoralized, and came
near leaving in order to try somebody's cancer salve.

SECOND OPERATION.

The new growth upon the upper and posterior margin (just under the ear), was removed. This time
again, no attempt was made to remove the whole of the

morbid material. Several vessels were tied or acupressed.

A minute portion of the mass showed under the microscope only compressed epithelial cells. No caudate cells were discovered. From this time on, the galvanization was kept up through the application of a sponge to the wound connected with the positive pole twice a day about half an hour. The tonic of quinine and iron was kept up. After about a month the

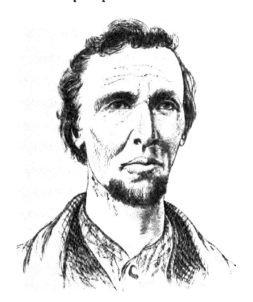

galvanic current was applied twice a week. A constant current 100-cell-battery was substituted for the 32-cell-battery previously employed. The full power of the battery was generally borne. Cicatrization went on rapidly, but a sinus remains open up to this time. Its surface has been occasionally stimulated by the application of carbolic acid. The painful condition soon disappeared after the second operation and has never returned.

The cut No. 2 illustrates the present appearance of the patient. He has, for a considerable time, performed his customary labor as a farmer and enjoys good health.

With regard to this case, it may be said that if the growth was not cancerous, but scrofulous, or cachectic, the power of the galvanic current to arrest this last kind of morbid degeneration is at least vindicated. As far as the reproduction of a tumor is evidence of cancer, so far any agent may be said to be a remedy for cancer, which has the power to arrest this secondary growth.

The history of this case shows that the power is not one of destruction, as the growth increased during the employment of the current for electrolysis, but an agent which directly promotes a more healthy nutrition.

The following are cases treated by electrolysis.

Miss Miller, aged about 20. *Electrolysis* of ganglion or weeping sinew on one of the tendons of the extensor longus digitorum, upon the left wrist, of 6 months' duration, originally caused by a sprain.

December 13, 1872.—A steel cambric needle was made to transfix the tumor, and was connected with the negative electrode. A sponge held in the hand was connected with the positive. The current of 100 cells was allowed to pass one minute and the needle was then withdrawn. Intense pain was experienced about the needle, which ceased with the cessation of the current. There was a manifest immediate softening of the little tumor.

Dec. 26.—The surface is entirely smooth, though there is still some pain at the place of the ganglion.

Jan. 7, 1873.—The swelling and lameness have entirely disappeared. In this case there was no sloughing only sufficient action to produce absorption of the exuded material, and a return of the tissues to a healthy condition.

John Ives, aged 21, living near Greenview. Lupus upon right cheek, first noticed 6 months ago. A dense scab grows upon the surface one-fourth of an inch in diameter, causing slight bleeding, as it is pulled from its rough base. Induration and thickening exist beneath the morbid surface, half an inch in diameter, situated half an inch behind the angle of the mouth.

December 14.—Four small cambric needles, threaded with small iron wire and connected with the negative electrode, were inserted into the indurated tissue just beneath the surface. The positive connection was made by a sponge held in the hand. The current of 100 cells was permitted to pass during one minute. The pain of this application was very severe, but ceased the moment the circuit was broken.

December 31.—Patient returned. The induration has nearly disappeared and the ulcer has healed, leaving no mark. The application repeated with two needles. The patient has not since reported.

More cases of rapid absorption after brief electrolysis might be detailed, but these are sufficient to serve as examples of this power of galvanism.

In the employment of galvanism for rheumatism, some degree of chronicity is favorable to the marked effect of the agent—indeed, it is doubtful whether in acute inflammation the galvanic current can be of any avail. In chronic rheumatism the relief of lameness by the passage of a strong current is often instantaneous. Frequent repetition is necessary, however, for permanent relief.   In neuralgic pains the strong current almost always alleviates and sometimes effects an entire abatement of the pain for the time.   The removal of the ultimate cause is, however, necessary to a permanent cure.   When this cause is mal-nutrition of the nerve itself, the galvanic stimulus may correct this mal-nutrition and thus effect a permanent cure.

In some neuralgic pains, and especially neuralgic headaches, the galvanic current interrupted (by clock work) affords more rapid relief than the continuous current.   In the case of headache, the best effects are produced by bringing the cervical portions of the sympathetic nerves and the 8th pair within the scope of the current.   For this purpose no stronger current is employed than can be borne without discomfort.

It has been the intention of this communication not to tell all that can be said, but only to make a few notes.

Hospital Reports.

CITY HOSPITAL.

(Notes as taken Oct. 10th., 1872.)

OVARIAN TUMOR.—MULTILOCULAR.

CASE I.—Amanda Edwards, (colored); aged twenty-three years; single; nativity, Commerce, Missouri; entered *City Hospital*, October 8th, 1872.

Patient, who is more than ordinarily intelligent for one of her race, gives an apparently candid, straightforward history, and says that she has never subjected herself to any practices, by which she could become pregnant.

General health good previous to three years ago. About that time, she noticed an enlargement, or, as described by her, " a lump as large as her fist, just below the ribs, on right side." Slight soreness at that time on manipulation, but no shooting pains either then or since. Growth was very rapid during the first year; since has been slower but continuous.

At present, abdomen is greatly distended, being about *double* the size of an ordinary pregnant woman at full term. On inspection, abdomen appears unevenly enlarged, with the distention most marked on right side above, but on left side below, and irregular in outline. Palpitation reveals different lobes of the tumor with dividing bands or constrictions between them; also a difference in its consistence, part seeming to be fluid, part semi-fluid, while another part presents an almost solid appearance. Breathing has been at times affected; and never during past two years could she lie for any great length of time on her left side. Has never been troubled with vomiting or derangement of digestive organs. Bowels frequently constipated; urine passed regularly and freely; menstruation at all times regular. She says that lower extremities have been swelled, but they are not so at present.

Pulse 74; temperature 98½° F.; heart and lungs normal; liver and spleen. Urine contains neither albumen nor sugar.

Vaginal examination, as made to-day, shows uterus to be from three to four inches in depth, but quite movable, and to present a virgin os and neck.

Patient's general health and habit of body continue good. Has never been confined to her bed a day by sickness since present trouble began. No cancerous diathesis or similar abdominal enlargement has ever existed in her family to her knowledge. She works about ward, and seems very cheerful. Eats and sleeps well.

After above was written, patient was examined at different times, by some of the principal physicians of the city: Drs. Hodgen, Maughs, Barrett, Lankford, Scott, Papin, and others, with varied results, and with as varied opinions as to the feasibility of an operation. For instance, the uterus was severally found to be three, four, or six inches deep, as the instruments were handled at different times and by different manipulators. To some the organ was movable; to others, immovable. Thus, as facts seemed to warrant, the tumor was variously located--but generally with an interrogation—in uterus, ovary, or broad ligament, or said to involve two or more of these organs in its growth. However, its multilocular character, and its varied consistence were agreed upon by all. Then, finally, after many examinations and discussions, it was decided that no operation for removal of growth was advisable.

Next the question arose as to the propriety of tapping the fluid portion and drawing off as much as possible. Here, too, diversity of opinion was rife; but while the doctors were disagreeing, and soon after several prolonged examinations, peritonitis set in on Jan., 12th '73, and closed the scene with the death of the patient, at 6 o'clock, A. M., Jan. 15 '73.

These details are thus noted, that the younger members of the profession and those who seldom meet with such cases, may see how the most skilled are puzzled to diagnose and to treat them in practice.

Post-mortem examination, made at noon of the 16th ult., in the presence of many of the above-named physicians, revealed an inflammation of the peritoneum, covering both tumor and viscera, with a sero-purulent effusion into abdominal cavity. Parieties of abdomen strongly adherent to tumor by old attachments, which on right side extended as high as ribs.

Latter considerably florid, with liver pressed well up under them. The tumor, after being in reality dissected out, was found to be multilocular and connected with left ovary by a thin pedicle, some ten inches long, and two to four wide. Lobes were greatly distended, with walls thick and firm, and on the left somewhat cartilaginous. Contents varied, such as greenish serum, brown, jelly-like liquid, large amount of sebaceous material, and a mass of irregular bones, closely agglutinated together, as large as the fœtal head at full term, with more or less scattered and smaller fragments. Whole weight of tumor supposed to be from 30 to 40 pounds. Right ovary somewhat enlarged. Uterus drawn upward and to the left. Length four inches; appearance otherwise healthy. Microscopical examination of contents of tumor, as made by Drs. Robinson and Michel, reveals sebaceous matter with dermoid epithelia, hair, bone of normal construction with fibro-cellular attachments, Haversian canals, concentric layers, lacuneal, and inosculating canaliculi. The pathological specimen when exhibited at a meeting of the St. Louis Medical Society, gave rise to a very interesting discussion as to whether it had its origin in a dermoid cyst, or from a blighted ovum.

Report of Case by CLAYTON KEITH, M. D., Assistant Physician.

FEVER INT. AND EPILEPSY. TREPHINE—DEATH.

I.—*Previous History.* Christian D., æt. 23; admitted Jan. 1st, 1873. Patient's general health has been excellent until within the last six years. No sickness prior to that time. Six years ago, while at work on the Delaware and Lehigh Canal, he was struck on the head with a loaded whip, which fractured his skull, driving in a portion of the left parietal bone, in front of the parietal eminence. In consequence of this injury he lay for five weeks in the Philadelphia Hospital, in an insensible condition. While there, he had several pieces of skull removed

About five months after leaving that hospital, he began to be troubled with " fits." These have continued at intervals since; at first being about two months apart, but gradually increasing in frequency until three months ago, when he had as many as thirteen in 24 hours.

At Keokuk he was again operated upon, the trephine being used a second time, and bones removed. Convulsions continued after the operation. Had several in the same hospital, and one since his arrival in this city, about one week ago. Has been suffering with fever, intermittent, for the past few days, and enters hospital to be treated.

II.—*Present Condition.*   Pulse 76; temperature $98\frac{1}{4}°$ F.; urine contains neither albumen nor sugar; has no cough or diarrhœa; bowels regular; habits temperate; condition of body good. Is troubled with shortness of breath and palpitation of heart on sudden exertion; complains of occasional pains in the precordial region. The scalp has entirely healed, leaving an extensive and thick cicatrix over the site of the trephine.

III.—*Physical Examination.*   Organs generally present no abnormity; heart's impulse is slightly increased; liver and spleen show no enlargement. Ordered Quinnæ Sulph. gr. iv. every 8 hours, and Kali. Bromid, ʒss, thrice daily.

IV.—*Other Details.   Jan. 5th.*—Convalescent from fever, intermittent. Patient continued in apparently good health, and free from any epileptic seizure until Jan. 9th, A. M. At 6 o'clock this A. M., was seized with an epileptic convulsion, which lasted several minutes. Remained in an insensible condition till 8 o'clock, when he had a second convulsion. Is at this time, 9 A. M., M., still insensible, ejaculating an occasional groan, and opening his eyes when sharply spoken to, but answering no questions. Pulse moderately full. Passes his urine in bed.

Jan. 9th, P. M.—Convulsions every 2 hours through the day. Is still insensible. Kali. Bromid. ʒ ss every three hours.

Jan 10th. A. M.—Patient continued to suffer with convulsions through the night and this A. M., rather more frequently. Convulsions recurring at intervals of an hour and a half. This morning the intervals are accompanied with more frequent and loud ejaculations. Calls for water occasionally, is otherwise apparently insensible. Involuntary evacuations from bladder. Bowels unmoved for two days.

Jan. 10th. P. M.—At 2 P. M., the convulsions continuing, an opening was made in the scalp (the usual crucial incision), over the skull where a portion had already been removed, to see if there yet remained any depressed bone, which might be removed with the hope of partial, if not entire relief. But no such portion could be discovered; only a considerable thickening of tissues over the site of the former trephining. No recurrence of convulsions during this P. M., after opening scalp. Is rational at times, asking for water, and answering direct interrogatories.

Jan. 11th, A. M.—Patient was much more quiet through the night. Continued Kali. Bromid. every three hours. Semi-rational this A. M., till he had a convulsion, at eleven o'clock. Stupor continuing it was deemed advisable on consultation with Dr. H., to remove another portion of skull adjoining the former operation.

P. M—Patient more rational this P. M., than for two days past.

Jan. 12th, A. M.—Spent a moderately quiet night. Still talks irrationally and occasionally cries out. Pulse 96. Took some milk this A. M., the first nourishment since convulsions began.

P. M.—Remained quiet through the day till five P. M., when he became very wild and delirious, his derangement manifesting great violence. Was put in a straight-jacket and ordered to the cells. Pulse 104 and full. Face flushed and hot. Bowels still unmoved. ℞ Hydr. chlor. mit., gr. x. followed by a laxative.

Jan. 13th, A. M.—Bowels moved freely this A. M. No convulsions to-day. Resting quietly. Taking food.

Jan. 14th, A. M.—Condition unchanged. Bowels still active.

P. M.—Pupils dilated. Still muttering. Tongue moist and white. Takes no nourishment. Coma, with occasional low, muttering delirium.

Jan. 15th.—Died this morning in a convulsion.

V.—Post-mortem examination; thirty hours after death. 1st. Body well formed, not emaciated. 2nd. *Head.* On removing the calvarium it was found that no portion of the skull was pressing upon the brain substance—no spiculæ of bone were found driven into the brain. That portion of the dura mater which had been exposed by trephining was indurated and thickened. It was adherent to the skull to the extent of an inch around the orifice. The dura mater and arachnoid membrane were intensely congested. The veins covering the hemispheres were everywhere turgid with blood. On removing the dura mater, the brain substance immediately beneath the site of the trephining was depressed one-fourth of an inch, presenting the

appearance of an ulcer. On cutting through the depressed surface, found the brain substance indurated to the depth of one-
fourth inch, while beneath the induration the brain was
slightly softened. No effusion was found beneath the arachnoid or in the ventricles. The remaining portions of the brain
were found in normal condition. No examination was made
of the thoracic or abdominal viscera.

ST. LOUIS (SISTERS') HOSPITAL.

Clinic of Professor F. H. Gregory.   Reported by Dr. Chas. Garcia.

CASE I.   A blind youth, with fracture of the right arm ; first
seen December 7th. This young man's arm was bent when he
presented himself. The callus was deformed, having been neglected four or five weeks. The Professor forcibly, and without
chloroform, rectified the deformity. In such cases as these we
do not refracture the limb, but we simply unbend the deformed
callus. This being done, it must be held in position by com-
presses and splints, properly applied and retained by bandages ;
or, if in summer, adhesive strips are more comfortable.

Dec. 14th.—Our patient again presents himself before the
class ; he is doing well ; we will now remove the dressing and
direct him to use the arm.

CASE II.   Patient aged twenty-three ; admitted December
7th. This is a fracture, compound comminuted, of the right leg,
and according to report, was produced by the passage of a car
wheel over it. We have here a serious case, everything seems
broken up except the vessels ; they are intact. The ankle joint
is not involved. The accident occurred last evening, and a large
splinter of bone was removed from the wound this morning.
Our patient is a young, healthy man, of temperate habits. We
have advised amputation which the patient has declined ; so
everything considered, we are justified in attempting to preserve the limb. We are here reduced to the question of a poor
limb or none at all. The dangers and uncertainties of the case
have all been fully explained to the patient. We have decided
to apply the immovable dressing in the form of plaster-of-Paris.
Carbolic oil is applied to the wound ; cotton batting is next applied on the limb to prevent too much pressure at certain

points—to equalize the pressure; and over this a strip of three or four thicknesses of cotton cloth on each side of the limb, thoroughly saturated with the plaster-of-Paris; wide enough to envelop it. Over all is passed several layers of roller bandage, the sides having been reinforced by pasteboard to ensure a sufficient degree of firmness, and then the thin liquid plaster rubbed over the surface. A shingle was placed against the sole to prevent the foot from dropping, which frequently causes much pain and deformity. We may be compelled to remove this entire dressing and substitute the bran-box; when the plaster is set we will cut a window in it opposite the wound, in order to apply dressings to it.

Dec. 31st.—The limb is still in plaster-of-Paris. He has erysipelas, commencing at the site of injury where the soft parts sloughed considerably, and the disease from that point extended up the thigh, involving the sub-cutaneous connective tissue quite extensively. It was necessary to incise the integument freely in several places to give exit to the pus and to facilitate the removal of the dead connective tissue which came away in large pieces. The foot is warm, the circulation in it good; and we are using carbolic acid dressings. The pulse is about 100 per minute; the tongue dry and coated; his thirst is urgent, and he sweats profusely

Jan. 7th.—Our patient slept well last night, and feels better to-day. The circulation is however feeble; he eats little; the general condition is bad; he sweats profusely, but has no diarrhœa. The pus is escaping from the incisions. The granulations are filling up the gap in the limb.

Jan. 11th.—To-day there are decided symptoms of pyæmia. He has diffuse inflamation, metastatic in the arms and shoulders. He has chills, occurring mostly in the day, sometimes irregularly. It may be distinguished from some other diseases with which it might be confounded, by the irregularity of the chills and fever. The thermometer placed in the axilla denotes unusual variations, thus differing from the essential fevers. There is no fever heat in any disease comparable to pyæmia, except in tetanus. He has no diarrhœa. The pleura and lungs are often involved in these cases. The leg has been retained in the plaster-of-Paris dressing, having a large window cut in it,

sufficient to give free access to the parts requiring applications.
The limb is dressed with powdered clay. It slips off readily
and is easily renewed and it does away with rag dressing. The
clay at once disinfects and prevents offensive exhalations, by
absorbing them, which, otherwise, might infect the ward. We
give him quinine and sustain him with nutritious diet.

Jan. 14th.—The physiological processes of the body are at a
very low ebb. The wound is inactive in consequence of the
depressed condition of the entire body. The surface of the
wound looks like a torpid ulcer. We have been feeding him,
and giving him tonics, also beer, porter and eggs. Always hope
so long as the appetite is sustained and no diarrhœa. The case
continued about the same till the 16th, when he had a decided
chill; and on the 17th he died.

MEDICAL SOCIETY PROCEEDINGS.

The St. Louis Medical Society held their annual election January 4th. The officers elected for the ensuing year are:

President—Frank G. Porter, M. D.
Vice-President—G. Hurt, M. D.
Treasurer—J. C. Gamble, M. D.
Rec. Secretary—John Bryson, M. D.
Cor. Secretary—John Green, M. D.

The St. Louis Microscopical Society held their annual election January 9th. The following officers were elected for the ensuing year:

President—D. V. Dean, M. D.
Vice-President—Homer Judd, M. D.
Treasurer—A. J. Steele, M. D.
Rec. Secretary—H. Z. Gill, M. D.
Cor. Secretary—Chas. E. Michel, M. D.

Meteorological Observations.

METEOROLOGICAL OBSERVATIONS AT ST. LOUIS, MO.

BY A. WISLIZENUS, M. D.

The following observations of daily temperature in St. Louis are made with a MAXIMUM and MINIMUM thermometer (of Green, N. Y.). The daily minimum occurs generally in the night, the maximum about 3 P M. The monthly mean of the daily minimum and maxima, added and divided by 2, gives a quite reliable mean of the monthly temperature

THERMOMETER FAHRENHEIT.

DECEMBER, 1872.

Day of Month.	Minimum.	Maximum.	Day of Month.	Minimum.	Maximum.
1	28 0	41.0	18	22.5	31.5
2	36.0	51.5	19	17.0	23.5
3	31.0	44.5	20	7.0	23.0
4	27.5	41 0	21	3 0	7.0
5	35.0	44.0	22	—10.0	22 5
6	26.0	44.0	23	—8.0	5.5
7	29.0	53.0	24	—14.5	—0.5
8	35.0	42.5	25	—7.0	11.0
9	10.0	22.0	26	7.5	18.0
10	14.5	23.5	27	—1.0	15.5
11	18.0	29.0	28	9.0	27.0
12	25.5	31.0	29	15.0	34.5
13	23.5	45.0	30	31.0	37.5
14	26.5	47.5	31	32.0	35.0
15	13.0	24.5			
16	21.5	31.5	Means	16.5	30.3
17	15.0	33.0	Monthly Mean 23.4		

Quantity of rain and melted snow:

Rain 1 02
Snow 0 79

1.81 inches.

E. BREY, Linguist and Instructor in the Classical, Biblical and modern languages, especially the German. Teaching rooms, 118 North Third street; 1319 Franklin avenue; 12 South Fifteenth street; (Haydn Conservatory of Music.) He is the originator of a NEW SYSTEM of teaching languages thoroughly and rapidly, which, consisting of translating not only verbatim, but also by ROOTS and AFFIXES greatly assists the memory, and is perfecting in ENGLISH.

Etymological queries on MEDICAL or general terms, as well as geographical or personal NAMES will be answered, more or less satisfactorily, by the above.

Mortality Report.

FROM DEC. 29th, 1872, TO JAN. 25th, 1873, INCLUSIVE.

Date	White Males	White Females	Col'd Males	Col'd Females	Under 5 yr.	5 to 10	10 to 20	20 to 30	30 to 40	40 to 50	50 to 60	60 to 70	70 to 80	80 to 90	90 to 100	Total
Saturday 4	137	95	10	5	93	23	15	39	28	18	14	10	4	3	...	247
" 11	119	71	8	4	78	16	15	29	24	12	11	7	6	2	...	202
" 18	126	91	16	10	98	10	15	41	34	14	11	12	5	3	...	243
" 25	101	84	9	4	89	10	6	31	19	18	10	9	3	3	...	198
Total.	483	341	43	23	358	59	51	140	105	62	46	38	18	11		890

Abscess of Liver.. 9	Delirium Tremens . 1	Hypertrophy 1	Pertussis 2
Accidents. . . . 2	Diarrhœa 4	Inanition 5	Pleuritis . . . 1
Anemia 1	Disease of the Heart 2	Intussusception .. 2	Pneumonia 64
Apoplexy. . . . 5	Diptheria.......... 2	Inflammat'n of brain 2	Premature birth.. ... 3
Aneurism of Aorta . 1	Dropsy 8	" bowels 3	Pemphigus 1
Asphyxia. . . . 11	Dysentery. 3	" liver. 5	Pyemia. 1
Asthma 2	Eclampsia 4	Injuries 4	Rheumatism 4
Bright's Disease .. 4	Empyema of Lung 1	Intemperance .. 1	Scarlatina 6
Bronchitis.. ... 13	Encephalitis 1	Laryngitis 6	Scurvy 1
Cancer 8	Enteritis. 3	Lockjaw. 10	Scrofula 3
Catarrh . . 1	Epilepsy 1	Marasmus ... 18	Scald 1
Cellulitis . . 1,	Erysipelas. . . 9	Measles 4	Shot wound . . 1
Chill, Congestive. . 2	Fever, congestive 4	Meningitis.. . 25	Strangulation 1
Cirrhosis ... 1	" intermittent .. 1	Melitis . 7	Stenosis . 4
Conges. of Brain 16	" puerperalis.. 15	Metro Peritonitis.. 4	Suicide 3
Conges. of Lungs 17	Fever, typhoid..... 16	Melancholia 1	Sync pe 1
Consumption. . . 50	Fracture 1	Nervous prostration. 1	Variola. 338
Convulsion... 47	Gangrene.... 1	Œdema 1	
Croup. . . . 11	Gastritis ... 3	Old Age 7	Total 855
Collapse 1	Hemorrhage ... 4	Paralysis. 7	
Debility 18	Hydrocephalus.... 5	Peritonitis 15	Stillborn 35

BOOKS AND PAMPHLETS RECEIVED.

SURGICAL DISEASES OF INFANTS AND CHILDREN. By M. P Guersant, M. D., Paris. Translated from the French by R. J. Dunglison, M. D. Philadelphia: Henry C. Lea. pp 354. 8vo. 1873

ORGANIC CHEMISTRY—Wöhler's Outlines. By Rudolph Fittig, Prof. of Chemistry in the University of Tübingen. Translated from the eighth German edition, with additions, by Ira Remsen, M. D., Ph. D. Philadelphia: Henry C. Lea. 1873.

OBSTETRIC APHORISMS, For the use of students, concerning midwifery practice. By Joseph Griffith Swayne M. D. Second American, from the fifth revised English edition, with additions, by Edward R. Hutchins, M. D. Philadelphia: Henry C. Lea. 1873.

THE SAINT LOUIS

Medical and Surgical Journal.

MARCH, 1873.

Original Communications.

ON TETANUS AND TETANOID AFFECTIONS, WITH CASES.

By B. ROEMER, M. D., St. Louis, Mo.

[Continued from page 92.]

The *symptoms* of tetanus are in general well marked, enough so at least in its typical form to allow a prompt and distinctive diagnosis. If we, however, compare the various subdivisions of this class of diseases, as evidenced by tonic spasms, we find as much difficulty here as in every other aspect of this affection. The majority of diseases can be traced from their symptoms to uniform and controlling causes, and *vica versa*, but in tetanus we have no such deductions for its successful study. The following classification of transitory tetanus seems to me to be proper:

I.   Tetanoid affections.

  1.   Spasmodic muscular action from systemic sympathy.

  2.   Tonic spasm, following and concomitant with other diseases of the nerve centres.

(Rigor, Trousseau's intermittent tetanus, tetanillus and rheumatic spasm are embraced under (1); the intermittent tetanus is perhaps a tetanic epilepsy, (*Vide Journal des Connaiss. Medic.* June 10, 1860.) The case of hysterical tetanus reported by Dr. Belcher in *Med. News and Libr.* 1866, p. 199, examplifies the affection under (2) ; in this instance tonic spasm blended with hysteria followed upon a slight punctured wound made by a pair of scissors.)

II.   Trismus.
 1.   Simple trismus.
 2.   Trismus nascentium *seu* neonatorum.

(This last affection is usually regarded as a *tetanus* of infants, and my reason for classing it here is its *superficial* similarity to a pure tetanus. To me it seems much nearer allied to uræmic intoxication, and might be termed a uræmic eclampsia of infants.)*

III.   Partial tetanus.
 1.   Opisthotonos.
 2.   Emprosthotonos.
 3.   Pleurothotonos.

IV.   Tetanus proper.
 1.   Acute.
 2.   Subacute tetanus.

V.   Strychnia tetanus.

(Tetanus from strychnia, etc., is allied to II, III and IV only by symptoms. Its pathology does, however,

---

* The epidemic occurrence of trismus nascentium, as above alluded to, militates much against the assumption of its being a true tetanus, which cannot be said to recur under such conditions.

warrant a deduction of treatment of one to the other.)

All of these different classes, with exception of the last, may be traumatic or idiopathic. Tetanoid affections are usually the result of idiopathic causes, and the idiopathy of *true* tetanus may justly be doubted, of which more hereafter.

The muscles generally first implicated are those of the jaw, throat and neck, constituting trismus. The beginning of tetanus, after an interval of variable length in which trismus seems firmly to establish itself, is marked by an acute pain at the sternum and ensiform cartilage. The muscles of the jaw give now in their distortion to the face a sciurous expression, as I have termed it, from the resemblance to the full pouches of a squirrel's neck. Pain near and dryness of the wound are an uncertain accession. The incipient general spasm extends from the diaphragm to the spine, most usually from above in a downward course, until slowly all the muscles of the trunk, face and extremities are implicated, the hands and fingers only remaining under more or less limited control of volition. The sphincter muscles finally are overpowered and from the combined result of an exhaustive action of the facial muscles and the beginning of a succumbing of the mental faculties the risus sardonicus is developed, which constitutes the acme of tetanus. We have three stages:

1. Premonitory or incubative symptoms of uncertain length of time and character.

2. Implication of the spinal cord.

   (a.) Spasm of distinct or isolated muscles. Trismus.

(b.)　Intermission in the progress of symptoms sometimes well marked.

(c.)　Spasm of general or unilateral muscles. Partial or general tetanus.

(This is evidently the most decisive step in true tetanus. If opiates, etc., can procure rest or a cessation of spasm, and if catharsis can be effectually brought about, we may assume a subacute form with more favorable prognosis.)

3.　Sympathetic or continuous implication of pons varolii and brain with spinal polarity.

Clonic spasm indicates a participation of the brain and the prognosis is more doubtful. The risus sardonicus and the persistence of spasm of the glottis evidence the centralization of the nervous erethism. If the transit upon the brain has been sudden, we may expect also asthenic sequences. Pari passu with the progress of tetanus, a general hyperæsthesia is added, so that spasm follows through the senses of touch, etc. Medullary apoplexy, as in other convulsive affections, must be regarded as a subordinate accession in tetanus, and is manifested by the loss of consciousness, involuntary epileptiform motion and sudden death. In apoplexy of the spinal cord, the attack itself is sudden, usually preceded by prolonged pain in the cord and by congestion, and its first symptoms are paralysis. Like tetanus, it affects the sphincter muscles; is rapid in its course and unaccompanied by contraction of the limbs. Reflex excitability is consequently destroyed, the respiratory act embarrassed, and we notice aphonia with impairment of speech. To this follows paralysis of sensation and sometimes the opposite, hyperæsthesia; one or both sides may be equally affected with an increased temperature in the paralyzed parts. In epilepsy, on the contrary, we have in the contraction of the cerebral blood-vessels from similar causes a loss of consciousness, the direct result of an increased volume of blood, which, by its downward pressure upon the spinal cord, produces a tonic contraction of the laryngeal and respiratory muscles; the latter being first acted upon, (evidencing the paroxysm by the usual premonitory exclamation), and shortly afterwards of the muscles of the body generally, causing the fall of the body. The acme comprehends an exhaustion of the nervous powers, and stupor, after which the slowly recurring respiration, sleep, etc., indicate a return to the cerebral equilibrium.

Asphyxia is the usual and legitimate mode of death in tetanus. The insufficiency of blood-oxygenation and the continued presence of venous blood in the nerve-centres, especially if the attack is violent and rapid in transition, lead at times to pressure upon the encephalon and to death from asthenia, or an arrest of the cardiac action through the medulla oblongata. Asthenia may also be supposed a casual mode of death from the great waste of tissue by metamorphosis after violent (*especially* after long continued) muscular action, and after increased and irregular excitability of the trophic nerves or their representatives. This deficiency in con-
. structive material is not only steadily augmented, but the pabulum is at the same time withheld in the non-arterialization of the blood during thoracic and diaphragmatic spasm.

Sudden death in tetanus is the result either of spasm

of the glottis or of structural changes in the nerve-centres during violent general spasm, and the post mortem
appearances of a vascular or inflammatory character
should always be carefully referred to the mode of death,
not only because they may point alone to the last phenomena of life totally differing from tetanic causes, but
they may be due to certain cadaveric changes: equaliza-
tion of fluids by their reduction to a level or to their
mutual points of resistance; influx of liquids through
orifices before spasmodically closed, especially in tetanus,
because of the non-coagulable character of the blood;
and chemical changes precursory to decomposition.
Moreover, it should be remembered that any prolonged
and intense functional activity must and does lead to a
corresponding structural abnormality, the result of a
cause utterly incapable of explaining the causation of
the functional aberration.* The complete muscular
relaxation after death, and the subsequent rigor mortis
furnish great objections to microscopic examinations.
Every deviation in the course of the disease from true
tetanus should be carefully noted, so that the observer
may be prepared for corresponding necroscopic conditions, and in view of the most common morbid appearances of the brain and spinal cord the question is open,
how many of the cases with congestion of the spinal
cord showed at the same time the greatest degree of
cerebral congestion, and what were the symptoms before
death between them?

In cerebro-spinal meningitis we find uniformly opisthotonos either fully developed or indicated by slight

---

* Niemeyer gives an account of a *waxy* muscle, in a post mortem of tetanus,
which owes its peculiarity to the spasmodic functional exaltation.

contractions and spasmodic twitches of the muscles of the back; tremor similar to consecutive electric shocks, and in some instances severe trismus are induced upon the slightest touch. The morbid appearances of the nerve-centres point to the true locality and pathology of this disease in revealing the blood vessels of the pia mater engorged, the membranes thickened, fluid in the ventricles, base of brain, and in the membranes of the spinal cord; we find lymph deposited over the pons varolii and along the medulla oblongata and spinal cord; fibrine along the fissures of the brain, etc., from which we are warranted to conclude that the tetanic affection was a secondary or progressive phenomenon of a disease, which under other phases, gives occasion to paralysis, coma, or convulsive contractions of muscles. We have effusions of serum beneath the cerebral membranes with opacity in typhus; yet tetanic spasm has never been recorded as being symptomatic of it. Tetanus in its milder form is sometimes observed during disordered catamenia as a hysteric tetanus; in such cases the lesions, or absence of lesions of the spinal cord, are in analogy with true tetanus. The same is true of some forms of chorea, in which the grotesque movements have gone beyond control and assume the type of tetanic spasm. The French school locate this affection in an excitability of the cerebellum, which fails to co-ordinate the muscular activity, but it is really, perhaps, an irritation of the excito-motor nerves. In it, also, we have no anatomical lesions. *Trousseau* speaks of a grave form of intermittent rheumatic contractions, in which the patient is seized suddenly with tetanic rigidity; the muscles of his neck, chest, and abdomen act convulsively and curve the trunk forward, and the spasm can be produced by compression. He ranks this affection among the neuroses with epilepsy, hysteria and eclampsia, and regards it due to the brain and spinal cord, without lesions of either. *Pritchard* in his Treatise on Diseases of the Nervous System gives instances of a convulsive tremor without cerebral or spinal disturbance. One of the effects of uræmic poisoning is opisthotonos and general tetanic spasm, not only the result of purely experimental, but clinic production. Carbonate of ammonia, if injected into a vein, produces these results, and the exhalation of ammonia and its presence in the blood has been supposed the chief cause of uræmic intoxication. Tetanic spasm can also be obtained after ligating the renal arteries or excising the kidney; the spasm continuing as long as urea is retained in the circulation. Trismus nascentium is supposed by *Simpson* to be due to albuminuria; autopsies, however, have given no morbid changes beyond a doubtful collection of serum in the spinal canal containing urea, and a doubtful cerebral anæmia. It is possible that it is of traumatic origin, with idiopathic causes, as filth, damp, and hot or cold air, but the position of Simpson is more probable, as already mentioned. *Richardson*, perhaps from such facts as above enumerated, classes tetanus among the zymotic diseases, produced as a specific poison in the wound, and which he is capable, as he avers, of creating at will, by the introduction of carb. of ammonia into the system, losing sight of the grave question, why tetanus under such genetic circumstances, is of so comparatively rare occurrence, and why it is not decidedly epidemic and inoculable. But tetanus is a concomitant symptom, not only in uræmic diatheses, also structural diseases of the kidney may lead to it. *Fincham* relates before the Western Med. and Surg. Society (*London Lancet*, Feb. 1861, p. 175), a case of renal abscess, in which the patient labored under the most violent spasm of the muscles of the neck, jaw, trunk, and extremities, *consciousness* and *rationality* remaining unimpaired; autopsy showing no structural changes in the nerve-centres, but numerous small abscesses in both kidneys. Add to this that we have tetanic spasm at times in delirium tremens, depending on inflammatory excitement or nervous erethism; in central hyperæsthesia, and in arterial hyperæmia; in anæmia of sudden occurence in diseases involving the brain, spinal cord, with (catalepsy), or without paresis (chorea), or the mesocephalon alone (hysteria), in the strictly local hypercinetic affections of the jaw (trismus), of the face, in strabismus as a symptom of intestinal or cerebral disease, in writers' cramp, in the administration of chloroform for anæsthetic purposes; following the mechanical pressure of the cerebro-spinal fluid in spina bifida, etc., and tetanus as an abstract pathological fact, appears surrounded by contradictory symptoms and negative vital phenomena. As in the case of N. B. (No. 7.) tetanus sometimes approximates hydrophobia* in its guttural spasm on attempting to drink, or in an adventitious horror of water and its rejection; in the flow of saliva, thirst, laborious respiration, with well-marked clonic spasm, hallucinations, delirium even to mania,

---

* Case 5 (Ogle's Collect. of Cases of Tetanus in St. George's Hosp., *Brit.* and *For. Med. Rev.* 1868, Oct., p. 485) is a combination of tetanus and hydrophobia. In the perusal of this case the reader will, however, discover tetanic and epileptic spasm so blended as to resemble hydrophobia. It exemplifies, also, the complication of spinal and cerebral symptoms.

etc. *Macleod* alludes to a thick spittle adhering to the teeth, leading one to look upon hydrophobia as a hybrid between tetanus and epilepsy. The interchange of rigor with tetanus has been noticed by most writers; if the former is a precursory anæmia of the cord depending on the toxæmia, the last might be considered an anæmia of the brain depending upon the spinal cord.

According to *Valentin* (*Physiol. des Menschen*, II. 2. p. 366) tonic and clonic spasm is induced by a direct injury to certain portions of the spinal cord. The same results from the loss of blood, as after ligation of the cerebral carotis. Its explanation lies in the diminution of repelling and equalizing pressure upon the cerebrospinal fluid, which is impelled forward to fill the vacuum. An evacuation of this fluid above the first cervical vertebra results in irregular movements like intoxication and circular motion, and according to *Magendie* (*Physiol. u. Klinische Untersuch. über die Hirn v. Rückenmarkflüssigkeit*, s. 43) and *Longet* (*Anatomie et Physiol. du syst. nerv. de l'homme et des anim. vertébr.*, and in his *Annal. médic. psychol.* VI, p. 160), symptoms of hydrophobia are developed with backward movements, which subside after healing the wound and reproduction of the fluid. Tetanic spasm from strychnia results from a paralysis of the blood vessels of the cord (congestion) and affects the system rapidly because the exciting agent has a certain and self-containing influence proportionate to the overdose taken. The greatest resemblance between tetanus proper and tetanic spasm from strychnia is in opisthotonos. Traumatic tetanus may be said to end where strychnia tetanus commences; the last invading the brain in its beginning (the hands and fingers also are very early contracted), while the first reflects its energy in that direction only in an advanced stage. The risus sardonicus is the opening in strychnia poisoning and in tetanus it is ushered in as the finale.

The instructive experiments of *Dr. S. W. Mitchell* are entitled to be mentioned here, as they have, in my opinion, an important bearing upon this subject. Similar results were obtained by *Dr. B. W. Richardson*, of London. The first phenomena noticed by *Dr. M.* were in consequence of his research on the cerebro-spinal fluid and its agency in producing convulsions under pressure.* ·Injecting half an ounce of water (66° F.) into the spinal canal of a rabbit, convulsions ensued and shortly afterwards death. By this injection the blood was displaced in the spinal vessels and caused bleeding from the exposed veins of the cord and head. A larger amount of water under 100° F. was borne in the second experiment, and spasms followed instantly upon the introduction of water at 32° F. Every variety of convulsive action was thus effected. Subsequent experiments proved that the local and external application of extreme cold upon the spine brought about similar results. The agent usually employed was rhigolene. As the reader is familiar with the nature of these experiments, I will confine myself to a cursory notice of the results : (loc. cit. p. 108) "it results from these experiments that at or about the fourteenth vertebra from above downward we cease to notice backward spasm and stupor, and see only signs of weakness or of tetanic rigidity in the legs." A jet of rhigolone thrown upon the spine of a frog (p. 110) "occasions spasmodic

---

* Amer. Journ. Med. Sciences, 1867, January, p. 103.

movements of the legs, and at intervals violent tetanic contractions." The pigeon, under the application of cold to the spine "may be handled or laid on its back and side, while at any moment a loud sound or a sudden motion will break the spell and it will abruptly run backward several feet" (p. 111). The following symptoms of partial tetanus (emprosthotonos and opisthotonos) should be marked: (loc. cit. p. 112) "in the spasm from chilled spine or cerebellum the head is carried at ease during the interval between the fits, but at the moment of attack the bill strikes the floor quickly, first on one and then on the other side, the head being drawn violently forward. Even in the most terrible of the summersaults caused by cold, the head was drawn forward, and the backward turn was produced by the action of the muscles of the legs and wings, rather than by those of the back, neck and spine." It is of some importance to ask, what influence the point of gravitation may have upon the spasmodic position of a pigeon, and what the results would have been in man? *Dr. Mitchell's* view is undoubtedly correct, that the tendency of a pigeon during spasm from anæmia is toward violent backward motion (op. cit. 1868, January, p. 31), and I would only add, that the phenomena resemble opisthotonos rather than epilepsy. He adds (op. cit. 1869, April, p. 334), "very little, then, of the convulsive acts is due to the direct effect of cold, much more to the intense and overpowering congestion which in turn wears off. The added proof lies in the fact, that local irritants which congest more slowly occasion in the spine the same phenomena after the lapse of a longer interval." Intense cold to freezing, and the injection of water produced, consequently, similar effects, that is, any displacing agency upon the spinal fluid gives tonic spasm.

Direct injury to the cerebellum and spinal cord conditions similar results. *Fodéra, Magendie, Flourens, Purkinje* and *Krauss* have observed tonic spasm and opisthotonic movements in mammals and birds after the loss of the cerebellum. *Mitchell* also has verified these experiments. *Hertwig, Lafargue, Volkmann* and *Nicolucci*, on the contrary, have denied them. This discrepancy in so direct and conclusive experiments originates, perhaps, in the peculiarity of certain animals. *Ecker, Burdach, Magendie*, a. o., declare the ebbing and flowing of the cerebro-spinal fluid, while *Haller* and *Flourens* deny it, owing to their selecting animals for experiments which in reality do not possess this quality (domest. rabbits). *Flourens* saw a backward movement five, and *Bouillard* only four times in eighteen experiments.

In this connection we will now consider some of the post mortem appearances of tetanus.

From the *Guy Hospital* we have the anatomical dissection of 34 cases, in 20 of which the brain was examined and found in a normal and healthy condition in 11, or 55 p. c.; in the remaining 9 cases it was congested, pinkish, with ulcerations upon the under surface of the anterior lobes and decomposed. The spinal cord was examined in 19 cases; in a few it was redder that usual, congested and softened, but in the greater number nothing abnormal was discovered. The condition of the nerves at the wound was noticed in 14 cases, of which 5 showed them to be inflamed. In addition to these data the heart was violently contracted in 1 case (laryngotomy having been performed to relieve suffocation; death took place on the second day), in 7 cases the lungs were congested; pneumonic appearances were discovered in

3 and apoplectic in 4 cases. In one instance the larynx was closed by folds of the epiglottis being caught in the rima glottis. *R. Froriep* (*Neue Notizzen*, 1837, Jan., No. 1) has observed in 7 cases a direct injury of a nerve from pressure or wound, with a peculiar inflammation, knotty swelling and redness. *Erichsen* (in his Practical Clinical Remarks on Tetanus, *London Lancet*, 1859, vol. I, p. 355) is of opinion that "in traumatic tetanus a certain condition of the nervous system is always to be met with, namely, an unhealthy state of the nerve-branch or twig running from the wound, . . , . . . congested, inflamed, infiltrated, its neurolemma thickened, softened and discolored, often for a considerable distance from the wound." *Friedrich* (Dissert. de Tetano traumat., Nov. 1837, in Casper's *Wochenschrift*) has collected a number of cases with inflammation of the adjacent nerves. *I. F. South* saw two cases (the preparations of which are in St. Thomas' Museum), in one of which thin plates of bone, and in the other similar plates of cartilage existed on the arachnoid coat of the spinal marrow; but, he adds, that in many other cases examined by him no such appearances were observed, nor any other characteristic of disease. *Demme* and *Flechner* describe the presence of a new formation of connective tissue in the cord, and the added investigation of *Rokitansky* sums up as follows: that the product of proliferation is a viscous matter; filled with nuclei; not capable of progressive formation; usually found in the white medullary substance; is microscopic; uniformly discovered in the medulla oblong., crura cerebri, inferior peduncles (corpora restiformia) and over the spinal cord; and the result, in his opinion, of persistent congestion. *Rouse*, Surg. Registrar to St. George's Hosp., traced in

a fatal case of tetanus the radial nerve into the wound, which had divided in three branches above the injury, two of which were cut across without morbid appearance. The brain and spinal cord were healthy. The same condition is reported by *Peck*, of the same hospital, in regard to the ulnar nerve. *My first case* now reported (Robt. B.) gave on dissecting the elbow joint, a mechanical pressure upon the median nerve without further lesions, and my eighth (J. B. H.) nothing abnormal in the nerves of or surrounding the tumor. Case No. 3 (F. C. A.) was similar to No. 8.

Fergusson, of King's College Hospital, found slight vascularity of the cauda equina and all other portions of the cerebro-spinal axis natural. *Curling*, London Hospital, saw only a small quantity of fluid in the lateral ventricles, and *Rodgers*, Infirm. of the Strand Union in England, reports in an idiopathic case the superficial veins around the spine gorged with blood, the dura mater congested, a small quantity of bloody serosity upon the pia mater opposite the fourth cervical vertebra, the pia mater much injected as far as the cauda equina, the cord vascular especially in the cervical region, and the membranes of the brain and the brain itself congested. *L. Clarke* gives in six cases disintegration and softening of portions of the cord in its grey substance, in some parts almost soluble. *W. H. Dickinson* (*Med. Chir. Transact.* vol. II. p. 265), gives a minute description of the microscopic appearances of the spinal cord, of which I transcribe the following: The blood-vessels distended with blood, dilated to many times their calibre; crammed with blood-corpuscles so as to look like solid cylinders; in some places blood-corpuscles were extruded; oftener only the fluid por-

tions of the blood traversed the wall, appearing translucent, in contact with and surrounding the vessels, lying
in the grey matter of the nervous substance, in the
white, in the fissures and occasionally outside the cord;
a certain amount of the nervous element disintegrated,
as if the exudation had a solvent action upon the tissue; the central and anterior parts of the grey matter
most extensively affected on the side opposite to that of
the injury; the irritative cause of tetanus on reaching
any column or segment of the cord appeared to diffuse
itself throughout its whole length undiminished in intensity; cervical region no more affected than the lumbar, etc. The accompanying diagram shows the micro-

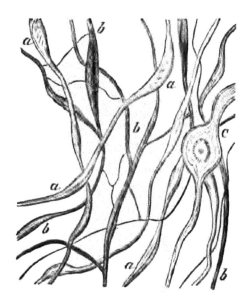

CASE No. VIII.—*J. B. Hartley.*—Longitud. section of posterior
spinal cord; cervical region. ($\frac{400}{1}$.) *a*—nerve tubes; *b*—
capillaries; *c*—nerve corpuscle and tubes.

scopic view of the spinal cord in the *case of Hartley* (No. VIII) above given; the portions subjected to the test were examined in their natural condition, and others, immediately adjacent, after being hardened with chromic acid; the blood-vessels presented uniformly an engorged condition, stagnation with coalescence of corpuscles and a predominance of the white bodies. The internal dynamis of the blood current must have been sufficiently powerful to enlarge the coats of the vessels at their weaker or less supported diameters, and to produce now and then a corresponding constriction. At these pouches or dilatations, the fluid portion of the blood was distinct from clusters of red and white corpuscles, which adhered together and to the walls of the vessels. The alternation of distention and constriction was in some degree only an increase of their relative size, and corresponded in this respect to the anatomy of the meningo-rachidian veins. The adjacent nerve tubes had a similar varicose appearance, at times flattened, and the interior of a changeable reflection of light—their periphery being invariably translucent, pearl-white and somewhat shaded, darker lines running longitudinally but without regularity to the neurilemma, which I took to be funiculi aggregating into the fasciculus. This gave rise to an imperfectly transmitted light. The accompanying blood-vessels adopted the shape of the nerve-fasciculus to their own diameters, giving a dilatation with a constriction and *vice versa*. The transparency of the neurilemma had a broader field, and its transmitted light was more distinct at a dilatation, but scarcely perceptible near the pouch of a blood-vessel. Minute hair-like fibres were visible in two localities, seemingly afloat and without terminus except in their origin, which lay in the centre of the tube.

The autopsy of a case by *Dr. Bodine* (Transactions of Pathologic. Society of Philadelphia, *American Medical Journal*, 1866, July, p. 130.) gave these results: the membranes of the brain without particularly abnormal appearances, though there was considerable pearliness of the arachnoid; the substance of the brain much softened with a punctuated redness; ventricles normal; some congestion at the base of the brain; spinal meninges somewhat congested; the cord throughout its whole extent softened, and in the cervical portions almost diffluent. (p. 132). I transcribe the second question suggested by the author: "Were the tetanoid symptoms, which were so prominent on the patient's admission, the indications of his real condition, and were the pathological appearances found after death owing to the continuance and persistence of tetanus, or was his real disease from the beginning an inflammatory affection of the cerebro-spinal substance and membranes, and was tetanus a mere epiphenomenon?" A somewhat analogous case (to which I shall refer hereafter) is that of *W. W. Keen*, (softening of the spinal cord, rigid and persistent contractions of flexors of lower extremities, *Amer. Jour. Med. Sc.* 1869, July, p. 128), and gives these cerebro-spinal lesions: "Dura mater not adhering; redness over entire pia mater, especially on outer and upper anterior half of left hemisphere; base of brain red without difference of consistence; puncta vasculosa abnormally marked, especially in posterior portion of each lobe; in lateral ventricles half a drachm of cerebro-spinal fluid; vessels from fornix forming the puncta vascul. large, numerous and distended; corpus striat. and thalam. opt. on both sides slightly vascular; dura mater of *spinal cord* vascular, adhering to the arachnoid from 1st to 6th dorsal nerve,. left side, and to 8th dorsal on the right side; entire cord vascular and softened; transverse sections almost diffluent, least so at the lumbar enlargement; below 5th cervical the outlines of grey matter indistinct from diffluency; *microscopically*, all the arteries of brain and cord with fatty degeneration; large number of compound granular corpuscles in the softened mass; no fibrous developments; nerve tubes of the softened parts narrower than usual, often deprived of their myeline, especially on the left side of the cord, but anterior and posterior portion alike; nerve roots wasted, and their arterial walls fatty; cylinder axes throughout, normal." The progress in this case was the reverse from that reported by Dr. Bodine.

[To be Continued.]

TRANSFUSION OF BLOOD.

By Dr. H. LEISRINK of Hamburg.

[Volkman's Clinical Lectures—translated from the German by Dr. Henry Kirchner, St. Louis, Mo.]

" Blood is a very peculiar juice."

There are few operations that deserve to be called life-preserving in such an eminent degree as transfusion, and among these few there is hardly one, that is technically so simple and so devoid of danger in its execution. Struck down by a sudden enormous loss of blood, a person lies breathing with difficulty, a face pale as wax, pulse hardly perceptible, amidst his relatives, who are frightened, expecting his end from second to second. Finally the long-looked-for physician comes and declares that an operation might save him.   Every one is willing to give his blood for the purpose.   A short operation follows and new life runs through the veins of one supposed lost.   The face reddens afrèsh, the pulse rises, the central organ receives fresh blood, as by a spell the scene is altered—the person's life is saved? How technically simple is the operation, how insignificant the instruments!   In case of need any syringe answers and a bistoury and forceps is all that is requisite. Indeed if any operation, this one deserves to become the common property of all physicians, for any one might be called upon at any moment to perform it.   To hesitate is out of the question, every moment bears danger, a precious human life hangs upon the point of the knife of the physician, he lifts the dying from the verge of the grave and brings him back to blooming pulsating life.

How seldom has a physician the opportunity to say: "I saved a human life!"   After making this operation, when necessary the consciousness of being the saver of a human life will proudly make your bosom heave.

The operation had many adversities before it could occupy its present position, secure for all times, in surgery.   We will not discuss the question, whether in the seventh book of the Transformations of Ovid, transfusion is spoken of, or whether the operation was performed on Pope Innocent VIII, suffice it to say that in 1666, *Lower* first made transfusion on the dog.   *Denis* in Paris made it on the human being, in 1667, with success.   After him, in the same year, *Lower* and *King* made it in England several times with success.   Phantastic, nonsensical ideas connected themselves with transfusion of blood from one being to another. In all earnestness the idea was gotten up that now a remedy was found to renovate the human species. In all these cases the blood of animals was used, mostly of the calf, and from this fact got the opponents of the operation or rather of the operator their weapon. The lowering of mankind was spoken of, the honor of the invention was accorded to the devil, and so the opponents of the 'operation succeeded to bring it into bad repute, especially as some mishaps discouraged the friends of the operation, and so it was excommunicated with the help of worldly and spiritual authorities.*

This operation, upon whose birth people entertained such high hopes, of which they had expected everlasting life upon earth,—when their unreasonable demands were not fulfilled, was cast into the darkness of oblivion, it was hardly known any more by name even to physiologists. But when a new era dawned upon physiology and a more finished technicality spread over our science, then the poor Cinderella was recalled to begin a new life at the hand of physiology and especially of the physiological experiment, to rise from step to step, to occupy a brilliant position in surgery, which, it may be said without wanting to be prophetic, will be more stable from year to year, never to be shaken permanently hereafter.

James Bleandell, it was who first in 1824 executed the operation with success upon the human subject, with human blood, and then made in quick succession three more successful transfusions.

---

* *Von Belina Swioutkowski, die transfusion des blutes,* 1869, p. 9.

In France and Germany the most illustrious names were connected with the regeneration of transfusion. *Dumas* and *Prevost* as well as *Dieffenbach*, and especially *Panum*, were very active. For the most important paper we are indebted to the last named author * who showed scientificially that for transfusion on man only human blood, and that defibrinated, should be used. Especially this last demand was in some measure an answer to *Martin's* paper (on transfusion in hemorrhage of parturients, Berlin, 1859), who only wanted to transfuse undefibrinated blood.

Kühne † gave a considerable extention to transfusion in his paper on poisoning by oxyde of carbon. Several practical physicians wrote on transfusion independent of *Martin*. *Neudörfer* employed it in chronic anæmia consequent upon purulent discharges; *Nussbaum* in chlorosis, etc. Of the most importance are the labors of *Hüter*, who first introduced arterial transfusion.‡ Of the method itself one may think as he pleases, but it cannot be denied, that the writings of this surgeon awakened a lively interest broadcast amongst physicians. In this consists its great merit. I myself am not enthusiastic upon arterial transfusion, but one must have read the paper of Hüter to know that there is nothing more full of genius existing in this branch.

So far a short sketch of the history of the operation, we have no room for more.

n looking at the practically important relations we have three questions to answer:

---

* Virchow's Archiv. XXVII. 1863.

† Central Blatt. 1864, No. 9.

‡ v. Langenbeck Archiv. Bd XII, Central Blatt, 1869, No. 25.

I.   What are the indications to-day for transfusion?

II.   Do we take defibrinated or undefibrinated blood?

III.   How do we execute the operation in the best and simplest manner?

As regards the first—indication for transfusion—we can formulate it thus: *Transfusion is indicated in all those pathological conditions, where all the blood in quantity and quality is so altered, that it is unfit to fulfil its physiological duties.*

A very wide range indeed, yet we hope to show it a perfectly justifiable one, for we have to accept *anæmia* acute and chronic, as also blood poisoning in its most varied forms, or the alterations of it when the corpuscular elements are diminished or increased in quantity (obstinate cases of chlorosis and leukæmia).

In the first instance anæmia ought to interest us, the alteration of the blood in quantity, and we have to distinguish here that anæmia occurring acute, by more or less considerable losses of blood, and the chronic produced by a long continued loss of material as in typhus, profuse purulent discharges, etc.

If we look at acute anæmia, we here have the most brilliant aspect of the operation and of that indication, that is the first, and was up to a recent date the only one.

Here transfusion will attain most, as in otherwise healthy people, the quantity of blood being only too little and a restitution of the necessary quantity will mostly be a *restitutio in integrum.* Above all we have to do here with hæmorrhages of parturient or lying-in women, further with anæmia after operations or injuries. Excepted are the losses of blood in consumption, intestinal hemorrhages in dysentery and similar diseases, here an increase of blood pressure would not be desirable.

Take a peculiar position in a practical point of view, the cases of loss of blood in lying-in or parturient women. It may have occurred to every practicing physician that in a precipitate birth, in abortion, in placenta prævia, relatively large quantities of blood are lost, for a time threatening symptoms ensue and yet pretty soon a complete recovery follows.

I believe that we do not go wrong to lay great weight upon the ability of the uterus to contract in the recently delivered or aborting woman. If the uterus is not able to contract, and the blood flows continually from its open vessels, do not hesitate a moment to make transfusion. For *the injection of blood is the best stimulus for the relaxed uterus.* Marked cases that bear on this subject can be found in the paper of *Martin ;* so is No. 6 of the dissertation of *Evers'* Rostock, 1870, very convincing. But when the bleeding of the uterus ceases, when it contracts with energy, then the transfusion may be given up for the moment, when no otherwise pressing indications demand it. It may perhaps become necessary secondarily, and just that possibility of delay is often not to be underrated in its moral effect. A few weeks ago I saw a case, in which through precipitate birth, a woman lost a comparatively large quantity of blood. The question here was, whether to transfuse or not ; everything was ready to make the operation. For a time the pulse was hardly perceptible ; she breathed with difficulty ; her face was as pale as death, but after two hours the scene was entirely altered ; pulse full and good, and her appearance considerably better. Full recovery followed in a relatively short time. But if the next day the pulse sinks again, and if, in weakly women, a continued illness is feared, then the operation may safely be made secondarily. In all cases where there exists any doubt, it is proper to make the primary transfusion; it is, when made with proper caution, absolutely void of danger and easily executed. We have to look differently upon large losses of blood in injuries. How slowly do patients recover in the usual way; often we see them suffer for years from the consequences; here is no time for hesitation, and we make the transfusion at once. The same holds good in hemorrhages during operations. In clinics we see transfusion performed as an every day occurrence.

Esmarch told me that he made transfusion on a person during the extirpation of a fibro-cavernous tumor from the base of the skull, where much blood was lost, by pumping back new blood into the arm. Also in a case of exarticulation of the femur, *Esmarch* caught up the flowing blood, and drove it back directly into the femoral vein.* So transfusion became an efficient help at other operations, and will become the more so after a time. A contribution to the utilizing of transformation I have given in the *Berlin Clinical Weekly*, No. 7, and in *Langenbeck Archiv.* vol. XIII; while for acute anæmia nothing more need be said. We meet for the chronic form, with opposition from different sides. Many who would not hesitate to make the operation in acute hemorrhage, bethink themselves a long time, whether to give the same benefit to a conva-

---

* This procedure was first recommended by Volkmann. See R. Volkmann, on three cases of exarticulation of the hip joint. German clinic, 1868, Nos. 42 and 43.

lescent from typhoid fever who cannot get well. And are not the relations in some measure the same?

I of course do not speak of patients who suffer from a disease that always diminishes the blood quantity anew. Even the most sanguine will not attempt to make a transfusion in carcinoma uteri or ventriculi. But there are cases where, from continued febrile disease, the vital powers are at so low an ebb that no convalescence can take place, or where the latter lasts so long that a small inter-current ailment is capable to extinguish the faintly-burning light of life. I admit that the several cases recently published in the dissertation of *Evers*, and later by *Jürgensen*,* are only partially encouraging, and yet, among them are such brilliant improvements and cures, that it is certainly remunerating to proceed in the same path. In this category belongs chronic catarrh of the stomach. In many of these cases exists a detrimental circulation. Because the quantity of blood is diminished, and at the same time impoverished, the secretion of digestive juices is badly performed, and because the materials for digestion are not secreted in sufficient as well as in good quality, of course good chyme is not sufficiently added to the blood. Transfusion takes a link out of the chain that encircles the patient, the blood is made capable of secreting good pepsin—hydro-chloric acid, digestion will be improved, and the patient begins to recover. We only have to modify the operation in these cases. Often we will have to make a derivatory venesection, and at the same time not inject a large amount of healthy blood at once, but we make *frequent transfusions in small quantities.* The heart, by degrees used to the poor quality and insufficient quantity, would be, as it were, surprised by a large mass of it, and by the poor quality it becomes of course, poorly nourished, like all the other organs. If we now impose too much work upon it *suddenly*, by injecting a larger quantity we might have bad consequences. We do not wonder when a badly-nourished biceps muscle cannot at once perform the labor of a Hercules. Therefore, in chronic anæmia *frequent smaller transfusions.*

As concerns the alteration of blood in quality, as indication for transfusion, the hospital physician has to contend above all with toxæmia from wounds, with pyæmia and septicæmia. It is not the smallest merit due to *Hüter* to have renewed the battle against these scourges of hospitals, and especially to have brought transfusion into action. The success is as yet not brilliant, but a temporary improvement is often enough obtained. One thing has to be understood—we shall only successfully overcome the septic and pyæmic alterations of the blood by transfusion, when we succeed in stopping the source of the poison. When from a wound the development of animal and vegetable organism is constantly renewed, if we leave a person suffering from pyæmia, to the poisons created by the same, we cannot save him by transfusion, if we would throw the blood by the bucket full into his veins. I always fear when I see such pains taken against the well-pronounced traumatic diseases, that the primary cause is lost sight of. In other words, the most effective warfare against this plague, consists in the most perfect hospital hygiene. So then, in the first instance, prevention of wound diseases; but if they yet appear in spite of all, then the inexorable foe must be fought upon his own ground, the blood, always presuming that a fresh poisoning of the already impoverished blood must be prevented. Here transfusion must be repeated, for we must replace, if possible, the old by entirely new and healthy blood.

Another qualitative alteration of the blood, that indicates transfusion is the poisoning of it by gaseous poisons, oxyde of carbon (charcoal gas), sulphureted hydrogen (coal gas). It is a known fact that it acts as a poison by entering into a closer chemical combination with the red blood corpuscles than oxygen. By it blood is robbed of its most important quality. By transfusion you attack the evil by its roots, in bringing new blood corpuscles into the circulation. In these cases we draw by venesection from the poisoned blood as much as possible and substitute for it an equal quantity of new, healthy blood. A second injection is needed when the first one proves insufficient. Of 3 cases of poisoning with oxyde of carbon that *Evers* reported, 2 were saved.

Transfusion further will have to be employed in the more rare cases of poisoning by opium, atropin and chloroform. It mostly depends upon feeding the central organs with new, not poisoned blood.

The composition of the blood in its corpuscular elements may be altered and this alteration may create a cause for transfusion. To this belong the obstinate cases of chlorosis and leukæmia. *Nussbaum* saw good success in chlorosis; *Mosler* in leukæmia although only partial in this latter disease, yet the experiments ought to be followed up, when other remedies fail.

II. Do we have to take defibrinated or undefibrinated blood for transfusion?

This question has thrown up much dust ten years

ago, especially after the appearance of the oft-mentioned paper of *Martin*, and caused many a battle, pro and con. Now it is settled, we believe, for good, and that in favor of defibrinated blood. Yet we will be impartial and weigh the advantages and disadvantages. *Martin* advances as an advantage of his method (l. c., p. 87) that by defibrinating, a good deal of costly time might be lost and that by using undefibrinated blood no disadvantage would arise. As to the first objection, we can hardly see the truth of it, for if the patient is gone so far that a few minutes will doom him to death, then we will be too late even with undefibrinated blood. The defibrination is so simple a manipulation, and one so quickly executed, that it certainly should be employed in opposition to the undeniable dangers of undefibrinated blood. And what are the dangers? Those of embolism and thrombosis. And if there never had occurred a case in whom embolism had hastened the end of the patient (the unfavorable cases being seldom published) the writings of physiologists such as *Prevost, Bischoff* and *Panum*, ought to deter us from using undefibrinated blood. Do we not wish to learn from science? *Panum* says in his eminent work, p. 249: "We never can be sure with undefibrinated blood, that we do not inject it partially clotted, if even this be in smaller quantities. The larger the quantity of undefibrinated blood to be transfused, the greater are the difficulties of execution and the greater are the dangers. The stirring of the blood has a special advantage, it makes the venous blood arterial, the blood corpuscles take up oxygen from the air and makes it so much the more fit for transfusion. All experiments to counteract coagulation, as supported by

Neudörfer, such as addition of alkalies, etc., are to-day looked on as child's play."

In what manner is blood best defibrinated? I have taken, in 5 transfusions made by me, a clean wooden stick for stirring the blood. After beating or stirring it for some minutes, I strained it through fine linen and then beat it anew. When I found no fibrin deposited on the stick I strained the second time, and now the blood was ready for injection. During the stirring, the vessel containing the blood is kept in another vessel with warm water of 38° C. temperature (100° F.). It is not necessary to be over anxious about one or two degrees, even if the blood cools down somewhat, it does not matter. This is in so far of importance to know, as in a country practice a thermometer is not always at hand to test the precise temperature.

So this question is answered; we take defibrinated blood for transfusion. Now the third question.

III. How is the operation in the best and most simple manner performed?

Of course the answer to this question must decide the fate of the operation, that is, the possibility of performing it easily, for if we have to do with a difficult and complicated operation it will never become the common property of all, and will only have a free sway in hospitals and clinics. Thank the Lord this is not so. This eminently life-preserving operation is at the same time the most simple and very easily executed.

First of all, what instruments do we need for the operation?

In case of need any syringe would answer, and a knife would do the rest. In case of need, said I; but the matter may be facilitated by instruments made especially for the purpose; we must only select the most simple.

Up to the appearance of *Belina's* paper inclusive, each writer on the subject held it to be his duty to invent a new instrument. Yet very few of them satisfy the demands of the surgeon.

What do we expect of a syringe for transfusion?

With the utmost simplicity it has to guard against access of air into the vessel. To satisfy this last, there were invented perfect monsters of syringes. One only needs to look at the paper of *Belina* to become frightened in this respect. The two most practical ones are those of *Eulenberg* and *Uterhart*, and perhaps the better of the two, the one of *Uterhart*.

Now for transfusion itself. In all cases in which the blood is altered in *quality* and not in quantity, then it is to be made a derivatory venesection at the time of transfusion, and the amount of blood drawn is to be a little larger than the quantity you wish to inject. But how much is to be injected? All quantities have been taken between ½ oz. to 12 oz. To establish a normal quantity for injection as *Hüter* desires, say 7 to 8 oz., is not objectionable. I believe that the indication has to decide this question also. In acute anæmia and in alterations of the blood in quality, as in poisoning, it will be an important point to inject as much as possible of healthy blood in order to dilute the poisoned blood. Here, of course, is not to be injected less than 250 grms. (about 7 oz.). In cases of chronic anæmia we have to make small infusions, say of 100 to 150 grms. (from 3 to 4 oz.) and repeat the same as often as may be necessary. I would here call attention to the fact that no one should hesitate to repeat the transfusion several times. You

must not fold your hands after the first effort to save
life, and leave the rest to God.

We should take example from *Hüter* in our perseverance. Suppose we are called upon to make transfusion.
A healthy, robust man, who is willing to lend his blood
for the purpose, is at hand. We draw blood from a
vein of his arm, and catch it in a clean vessel and defi-
brinate it in the above stated manner. Is it ready, you
must keep it warm while you turn to the patient, you
look for a favorably situated vein, say the median basi-
lic or cephalic, which is laid bare by an incision. With
a few more cuts you prepare it free in its circumference,
the distal end is now ligated, so as to keep the field of
operation free from blood. A little above you place a
second ligature, but without tightening it. You now
fill a Uterhart's syringe and also its canula, and carry
the latter through the incision into the vein. To the
canula you attach the syringe and drive with a slow ro-
tary movement of the piston, the blood into the vein.
Some person you will find to whom you can entrust the
pulse of the other side and who counts its beats aloud.
In doing this we are secure against accidents, and you
can see the breathing of the *not chloroformed* patient during the injection yourself. A slight deviation of the
pulse always occurs; it either becomes more full, or it
becomes for a moment smaller. This need not disturb
the operator, so a slight cough, or disquietude of the
patient. Strong oppression of the chest, irregularity
of the pulse demand caution, but syncope demands discontinuance of the operation. You will certainly guard
against some of these eventualities by quietly talking to
the patient, for the moral impression of the operation is
a great one. Accidents demanding a discontinuation of

the operation are very rare ; I only would not leave them unmentioned.

In the picture drawn I assumed that the surgeon operates by himself. If experienced assistants are at hand, of course this simplifies the whole procedure, so that while one prepares the vein, the other prepares the blood. This will shorten the time to one-half.

When the injection is completed you take out the canula, tie the vein above, and cut it through between the two ligatures, and sew up the wound ; one turn of roller bandage completes the whole simple manipulation.

A few practical hints may find a place here. It sometimes occurs that the canula stands against the walls of the vessel, and no blood is propelled into it. It suffices to draw the canula back a little, and to place it more into the longitudinal axis of the vein to overcome the impediment. A little pull at the untied ligature often suffices to facilitate the injection. But it may be said this is always venous transfusion ; is not the arterial transfusion better ? According to my views, the arterial transfusion is not at all suited to replace the venous, for manifold reasons. *Venous transfusion is a more simple operation and answers the same purpose as the arterial.*

Is this view a correct one, which I hope to show, then arterial transfusion never will gain ground. Transfusion unfolds its most brilliant side in the hands of the practical physician. The practical physician, who perhaps operates without sufficient assistance will not hesitate to open a vein, but he will probably be very careful how he cuts the brachial or radial artery in its upper part. Who guarantees that hemorrhage will not occur, when a physician after an operation has to leave his patient, and after the lapse of several hours may have

10

to go some miles into the country, when he has no experienced nurses; not to speak of the difficulty of the operation itself. Some weeks ago, an experienced surgeon in Hamburg tried arterial transfusion. The resistance was so great that the blood could not be forced in sufficient quantity, and he had to make a venous transfusion after all. These are unpleasant things that one would rather shun in private practice, even when the hospital surgeon cares very little about them. Similar obstacles *Hüter* describes himself. The access of air, whose danger of course in arterial transfusion is avoided, we do not fear when we operate with care and a good syringe, and phlebitis and its consequences are rare in private practice. Hence arterial transfusion will find no favor in private practice, if even it is practiced here and there in hospitals. A fundamental principle in surgery is, that of two methods leading to the same end, you must choose the one least complicated; and the most simple is venous transfusion. *Hüter* himself, does not emphasize his method, he says at the close of his paper: "Whether venous or arterial transfusion, remains with me a secondary question; but transfusion is a weapon against diseases, against which, we have heretofore fought in vain. This is the problem which we must try to solve. Success full of blessing will not be wanting."

And to work at the solution of this problem is the aim of these lines. May they be favorably received.

Hospital Reports.

ST. LOUIS (SISTERS') HOSPITAL.

Clinic of Prof. E. H. GREGORY, reported by Dr. CHARLES GARCIA.

CASE I. A little girl four or five years of age, with fracture of the arm. I saw this fracture yesterday, Dec. 11th. It was a "*green stick fracture*" and was very much bent. The mother discovered it by the deformity and brought it here. I straightened it and placed it on this splint. The operation of straightening is very painful, but it is quickly done, and seldom requires chloroform. The limb looks well. We use two splints, one above and one below the arm, and apply strips of adhesive plaster around them to keep them in position. It is important to see that the arm can be flexed without any undue pressure from the bandages; and the bandage should be narrower than is used for adults.

CASE II. In the same patient there is an erectile tumor, situated below the inner angle of the eye. It has been there twelve months, and is gradually increasing in size. It may be removed by applying nitric acid, or by picking it up on a small pin and strangulating it with a ligature. We here apply the former method. When tumors are to be removed, the sooner it is done the better. Every day they may be approaching some important situation, and if they are malignant, may implicate the system at large. However pathologists may differ in regard to the primary cachexia, there is no question about the secondary involvement of the constitution by malignant tumors.

Dec. 14th.—The case is doing well. The nitric acid seems to have destroyed the little erectile growth.

CASE III.—A man, aged fifty, from California, with necrosis of the radius. This patient fractured his radius about three years ago. I feel the enlarged lymphatic gland above the elbow joint. The patient says you seldom see a Californian without syphilis. Specific disease has modified this diseased bone. The

necrosed bone is not far from the radial artery, and it requires
caution in removing the sequestrum, otherwise its sharp edges
may injure the vessel. We should also choose an instrument
that can hold the bone firmly; even the granulations should be
respected. The sequestrum removed, I now oil my finger so as
to enter the cavity more easily, and search for more dead bone.
There is an immense case of new bone surrounding the sequestrum just removed. There may be some small pieces left, but
I think they are all out. Sometimes pieces of dead bone get
caught in the new case as in a vice. Lint saturated with carbolic acid is pushed into the wound.

CASE IV. *January 4, 1873.*—Tumor of the testicle complicated with hydrocele, in a middle-aged man.

Remarks.—I can count the constituents of the cord as they
slip under my finger, I feel for fluctuation but find little. Tumor
resembles the testicle in shape, and may be combined with hydrocele; rather a hydrosarcocele. He has had it for ten years.
Not malignant. Never had syphilis. Has been tapped and one
quarter of a glass of fluid escaped.

It is a tumor of the testicle, complicated with hydrocele. I
have never tapped it, but as he stops in the hospital, I will introduce an exploring needle. A yellow fluid escapes; the trocar
point is not free; little if any cavity. This is a case for observation.

CASE V. *December 5, 1872.*—Boy 2 years old.

This is a case of prolapse of the anus, distinct from prolapse
of the colon or rectum. I have seen prolapse of the colon six
inches. For this I sometimes blame mothers. The child is put
on the chair, and permitted to remain for hours amusing itself
with straining, till gradually a prolapse of the rectum occurs.
Mothers think they have no time to attend to their children,
and you see the results.

When prolapse once occurs, it easily re-occurs; but if the
little one is watched at the moment of defecation, and the anus
put upon the stretch by drawing it to one side, thus antagoniz-
ing the sphincter, the accident may be prevented. If this does
not do you must not allow the child to get up till after the
bowels have moved. Let the bowels move either in a standing

or lying position. It is well to use a gentle aperient. The following may be given to keep the bowels regular:

> R Mag. Sulph., Sacchar .Lactis., Sulph.
>   Pulv., Mag. Carb.,   āā ʒ ss
>   Anisseed pulv.   ʒ ss

M. S. ft. pulv. and give a teaspoonful for a dose.

(Child has not been seen since.)

CASE VI. *January 9, 1873.*—Spoiled eye; caused by a blow with a bottle, three months ago; eyeball was burst, but has no pain. Is it a proper case for an artificial eye?

I have said there is no pain; if there was pain I would recommend enucleation of the eyeball, because we know that sympathetic ophthalmia, is frequent, and by extirpation we save the other eye. As long as there is no trouble or degenerative process going on in it, let it alone; it makes a better stump for an artificial eye. After enucleation the conjunctiva and muscles remain as the stump for the artificial eye. In malignant disease it is right to remove the entire contents of the orbit, as a rule.

He has a scar here; and the flaccidity of this portion disposes the eyelid to drop, and I doubt if the lower lid would hold an artificial eye. A **V** shaped piece could be taken out of the lid, thus shortening it and causing it to sustain an artificial eye. He says he would not have one; therefore an operation is unnecessary. Observe the scar extends across the canaliculus. When the wound thus severs this canal, it is not possible to re-adjust the flaps so as to preserve the communication with the lachrymal sac; in such circumstances it is best to divide the canaliculus, making a direct opening into the lachrymal sac; thus anticipating the dribbling of tears.

Reviews and Bibliographical Notices.

A MANUAL OF QUALITATIVE ANALYSIS. By Robert Galloway, F. C. S. From the fifth London Edition. Philadelphia, H. C. Lea; 1872. 402 pp.

Some thirty years ago a method of instruction in modern languages, became very deservedly popular, which, leading the student from simple words and phrases, which at once enlisted his interest and attention, to more complicated tasks, by easy and imperceptible gradation, furnished him with a store of knowledge without once alluding to strict grammatical laws, reserving those for later periods, when they could be much better appreciated. This method has, with good success, been applied by the author to the acquirement of the principles of chemical analysis. The work is especially designed as a "guide to the beginner," to whom it endeavors to smooth the way and lighten the labor by giving tasks very easy at first, but made interesting by permitting the reason and utility of every operation to become at once evident. With such a design, it naturally excludes those elements or compounds which, from their rarity or want of useful application, are comparatively unimportant, thus sparing to the student the trouble of encumbering himself with the acquisition of tedious methods of research which he is never likely to need in a lifetime of practical analysis.

The first part begins with the analysis of the bases. The arrangement into groups is judicious, and the tables give a lucid exhibit in parallel columns of the deportment of the members of each group, with the re-agents. On pages 166 and 167, table VII gives a view of the general properties of all the six basic groups, followed by a number of practical hints how to avoid errors in the examination. Next follow the directions for the examination of the acids, to which upwards of fifty pages are given. Suitable questions and exercises are introduced from time to time as means of recapitulation, and for the purpose of inducing the student to think for himself rather than memorize only. Next in order come directions how to prepare substances for actual analysis by certain preliminary steps, which make them ready for the application of re-agents. Considerable space is deservedly given to flame and blow-pipe tests, and the various methods of the solution of solid bodies. We regret to miss here, and throughout the whole work, the valuable methods of research by the *spectroscope.* This instrument, which so much facilitates the preliminary examination, and which, in some cases, gives such definite indications where the best methods of wet analysis prove of doubtful value (as in the examination of blood and organic coloring matter) is not even mentioned. At the present time instruments of sufficient accuracy can be had at a very moderate expense, and should be in the hands of every analyst. We hope a future edition of the work will not omit the full description of the methods of spectral analysis.

The second part of the work is devoted to practical instructions for the analysis of the most important organic substances, and comprises seventy-seven pages of well-selected matter, treated in terse and lucid manner.

The third and last part treats of the manner of performing chemical operations, and the apparatus and re-agents required for their execution. This part is well written, and, as far as mere description can go, makes everything plain enough. A few extra wood-cuts might be advantageously added, but no amount of illustration will supersede the necessity of study with the apparatus in hand, and of personal instruction in mechanical manipulations by a competent teacher.

A list of the necessary apparatus, and a copious index close the work. Although we cannot endorse the author's unqualified condemnation of Fresenius' and Will's works, we cheerfully recommend his volume as being a most useful book for those who study analysis for use in the practical operations occurring in the laboratory of the pharmacist, the manufacturer of chemical and technological products, the amateur, the miner, or the physician. The latter, especially, will appreciate the simple and concise directions for the examination of such substances as are most interesting to him in his daily practice. Even he who studies science with a view to search its remotest recesses, will find this work a good introduction to his subsequent advances.

The typographical execution is good, and the proof-reader has done his duty much better than in the last edition of Fownes' Manual of Chemistry. The price is moderate, and within reach of every one who has an interest in the subject. We trust the work will meet with a ready sale, and that appreciation by the profession which it so amply deserves.   C.

Extracts from Current Medical Literature.

On the Value of Sulphate of Cinchona.

M. Briquet, the well-known author of an exhaustive treatise on cinchona, advocated the properties and uses of sulphate of cinchona at a recent meeting of the Paris Academy of Medicine. His conclusions were based upon 898 authenticated cases of cure by the sulphate, from Magendie and Chomel to our days. Its success was especially great in cases of intermittent fever of middling intensity. Furthermore, it arrests the paroxysms of typhoid, amends the symptoms of intermittent neuralgia, and is of great benefit in acute articular rheumatism. Dr. Briquet lays great stress on the mode of administering the drug. It should be given in a watery solution, in doses of from fifty centigrammes to one gramme (eight to fifteen grains), according to the intensity of the fever. The whole dose must not be given at once, but must be divided over five or six hours, and it is extremely important that the substance should be taken during the apyretic interval, and at least eight or ten hours before the return of the fit.—*London Lancet.*

On the use of stimulants in severe cases of febrile and inflammatory diseases. By Dr. LIONEL S. BEAL, F. R. S.

Summary.—The observations upon the action of alcohol on the "cells" or elementary units of the tissues justify us in concluding that its beneficial influence in very bad cases of disease is due in part to its action upon the pabulum and its tendency to render albuminous solutions less permeable, and partly to its direct action upon particles of naked and living bioplasm. Alcohol reduces the permeating tendency of the serum; it checks the disintegra tion of blood-corpuscles; it prevents the rapid growth of living matter; and it interferes with or modifies chemical changes taking place in organic fluids. When these changes are proceeding very rapidly, the capillary circulation beginning to fail, the heart's action becoming very weak and fluttering, and the strength ebbing fast, alcohol may save life.

In conclusion, the local and general action of alcohol may be shortly summed up as follows:

1. In internal wounds, and in internal diseases where alcohol acts beneficially, the good result is in part at least due to the alcohol checking the *increased action* already established.

2. Alcohol does not act as a food; it does not nourish tissues. It may diminish waste by altering the consistence and chemical properties of fluids and solids. It cuts short the life of rapidly growing bioplasm, or causes it to live more slowly; and thus tends to cause a diseased texture, in which vital changes are abnormally active, to return *to its normal and much less active condition.*

8. In "exhausting" diseases, alcohol seems to act partly by diminishing very rapidly the abnormally increased growth of bioplasm. The quantity required will depend upon the extent to which the changes alluded to have proceeded. In extreme cases half an ounce of brandy, or even more, may be given for a time (in some cases even for several days) every half-hour; and there is reason to believe that in desperate cases life is sometimes saved by this treatment.

Practical Conclusions.—Lastly, I shall venture to repeat here the conclusions I arrived at many years ago concerning the great value of the alcoholic treatment of low fevers and inflammations. Increased experience has afforded further confirmation of the correctness of the statements made in the paragraphs below. I do not, of course, refer to slight cases of fever, pneumonia, etc., in which no stimulant whatever may be required, but to *very severe cases of disease* only.

1. In what appeared hopeless cases, as much brandy as the patient could be made to swallow (an ounce and a half to two ounces in an hour) has been given for several hours in succession, and then as much as thirty ounces a day for several days, not only without producing the slightest intoxication, vomiting, or headache, but the treatment has been followed by recovery.

2. I would adduce the fact that a man not accustomed to drink, when suffering from acute rheumatism complicated with pericarditis with effusion, pneumonia at the base of one lung, and pleurisy on the opposite side, has taken twenty-four ounces of brandy a day for eleven days; the tongue being moist and the mind being calm during the whole time. While under this treatment, inflammatory products were absorbed, and the general state of the patient much improved.

3. I have been compelled to give a very weak child, weighing less than four stone, twelve ounces of brandy a day for ten days, while suffering from acute rheumatism with pericarditis and effusion. This quantity did not produce the slightest tendency to intoxication, or exert other than a favorable effect upon the disease. The patient did not begin to improve until the quantity of brandy, gradually increased, had reached the amount stated.

4. I would state that among the general conclusions I have arrived at, after carefully watching more than one hundred serious cases of acute disease treated with large quantities of stimulants, are the following: That intoxication is not produced; that delirium, if it has occurred, ceases, or is prevented from occurring at all in the course of the case; that headache is not occasioned; that the action of the skin, kidneys, and bowels goes on freely; that the tongue remains moist, or, if dry and brown, often becomes moist; that the pulse falls in frequency and increases in power; that respiration is not impeded, but that, where even one entire lung is hepatized, the distress of breathing is not increased, and it appears that the respiratory changes go on under the disadvantageous circumstances present as well as if no alcohol had been given.

The conclusion from all this is, most certainly, that alcohol does not do harm in fevers and acute inflammations; that it does not produce intoxication in persons suffering from exhaustive diseases; and that large quantities (from twelve to thirty ounces) may be given in cases which appear very unlikely to recover, and sometimes the patient will be saved. The conviction is forced upon the observer that, in desperate cases, these large quantities of alcohol are directly instrumental in saving life, not by *exciting or stimulating to increased action, but by moderating actions already excessive,* and at the same time by causing the heart to contract more vigorously, and so continue to drive the blood through the impeded capillaries.—*Medical Times and Gazette, May 25, July 13 and 27, 1872, pp.* 591, 29, 88.—*Braithwaite's Retrospect.*

On the Primary Dentition of Children. By Francis Minot, M. D., Harv.

* * * Authorities differ somewhat as to the order in which the first teeth appear, as well as to the time of their irruption. I have found the data given by Dr. Eichmann, founded upon the observation of 400 children, to correspond pretty exactly with my own experience; and it is sanctioned by the high authority of Dr. Schoepf Merei, of Pesth, by M. Trousseau, by Vogel, and others. Dr. Eichmann states that the twenty deciduous teeth make their appearance in *five groups,* at five distinct periods, and in the great majority of cases in the following order:—the first group consists of the two lower median incisors, which generally appear between the 28th and 33d week. In only three instances out of the 400 children did the first lower incisor appear as early as the 20th week, the next tooth, however, not appearing before the 31st week. Judging from my own observation, I should put six and a half months as the average date of the appearance of the first tooth. The second tooth frequently follows the first within a week, but it is not unusual for two or three weeks to elapse before the first group is completed.

The second group consists of the four upper incisors, of which the two central ones are the first to appear, the completion of the whole group requiring from three to six weeks. When a child has six teeth, therefore, there are four in the upper jaw and two in the lower. Trousseau observes that this fact, known to every woman who has had the care of young children, is strangely ignored by medical men, even by some who have written upon the very subject of dentition—and I am inclined to believe the observation is true of some practitioners of America, as well as France.

The third group includes the two lateral lower incisors and the four anterior molars. Generally, the upper molars are the first to come, next the lower incisors, and lastly the lower molars.

The fourth group consists of the four canine teeth, of which the two upper are called the eye teeth, and the two lower the stomach teeth.

The fifth group comprises the four posterior molars.

Although there are exceptions to the above order, yet they are rare in healthy children. There is more variation in the age at which each group begins to appear, as well as in the length of time required for its complete evolution; but within certain limits the period is tolerably exact. The average age at which the first tooth pierces the gum may be stated at six and a half months, and the group is usually completed at seven months. The second group usually begins to appear at the age of nine months, and requires six weeks for its completion. The third group appears at the age of twelve and a half months, and is completed at fourteen months. The fourth group usually begins at eighteen months, and often requires eight weeks, and sometimes longer for its completion. The fifth group does not commonly appear before the age of twenty-six months, and also takes at least eight weeks before it is finished.

An important fact in the history of the primary dentition, and which must never be lost sight of by the practitioner, is, that after the irruption of each group, there is a pause of longer or shorter duration, which is quite constant for each interval. Thus between the first and second group there is a pause of two or three months. Between the second and third group the interval is of about two months' duration. Between the third and fourth group the interval is from four to five months. Between the fourth and fifth group there is a pause of five months. I will arrange all these data in a tabular form, so that you may more easily comprehend them, and retain them in the memory.

1st group begins at 6½ months—completed at 7 months.
                    Pause of 2 or 3 months.

2d group begins at 9 months—completed at 10¼ months.

Pause of 2 months.

8d group begins at 12¼ months—completed at 14 months.

Pause of 4 to 5 months.

4th group begins at 18 months—completed at 21 months.

Pause of 5 months.

5th group begins at 26 months—completed at 80 months.

During the intervals between the successive groups the process of dentition is arrested, and the symptoms to which it often gives rise subside. The child is tranquil, sleeps well, is free from nervous and inflammatory troubles. Now is the time when any change which is to be made in the diet, mode of life, etc., should be begun. The important question of weaning should always be considered in reference to this period. If the mother be robust, and have plenty of milk, the child may be allowed to nurse, at least in part, with advantage until the fourth group is completed, when there will be an interval of five months in which he will be free from danger of convulsions or diarrhœa, and will have ample time to get accustomed to his new diet. Unfortunately, in a large number of cases, especially in cities, the supply of milk and the mother's strength require the child to be weaned earlier, and then, if possible, this should be done immediately after the completion of the third group, when the interval, though shorter than that which follows the canines, will yet be sufficient to permit the infant to get used to an artificial diet before the fourth begins to appear. Of course, you will not be governed by the state of the teeth alone in this important question; other considerations, especially the season of the year, the mother's health, and the supply of breast milk will have due weight; but I wish to urge upon you that in the case of delicate children, with a tendency to nervous or inflammatory symptoms, weaning can be much more safely accomplished during the intervals between the successive groups of teeth than at any other time. With perfectly healthy and robust children such precautions are not always necessary, but in delicate, town-bred infants, in those which show any disposition towards convulsions, diarrhœa, hydrocephalus, or that indefinite array of symptoms which are often styled "scrofulous," they cannot be neglected without risk. * *
—*Boston Med. and Surg. Jour.*

Chloride of Potassium in Epilepsy (Echo Med. et. Pharm. Belge).

Dr. Lander advocates this salt as better than bromide of potassium in epilepsy. He finds it is more active, costs five-sixths less, and has not the inconvenience of the secondary effects of bromide of potassium. He begins with small doses, and has continued the use of the drug for several months without any bad consequences, in daily doses of from 3 grammes 50, to 5 grammes 50 (1 to 2 drachms). Moreover, Dr. Lander thinks that the bromide is converted into a chloride in the stomach, so he suggests the immediate use of the chloride.—*Cin. Lancet and Observer.*

Renal Calculi in Children.

Dr. Jacobi, of New York, out of forty-six post-mortems of children under six months of age, has found renal calculi in six cases, and concludes that they are congenital, or date from the first weeks of life. He records two cases in which the passage of renal calculi through the ureters produced violent fits of pain and screaming. Generally these attacks of nephritic colic are overlooked.—*Gaz. Hebd.*, No. 29.—*London Lancet.*

Nocturnal Incontinence of Urine treated by Hydrate of Chloral.

Dr. Girolamo Leonardi has recorded, in the *Ippocratico*, of Naples, the results of the use of chloral in three cases of incontinence of urine. The administration of the drug very rapidly effected a complete and permanent cure. Together with the administration of chloral, Dr. Leonardi recommended very little drink to be taken in the evening. In the first case, a scrofulous woman, aged twenty-four, who had been constantly suffering from the complaint since the age of eighteen, chloral administered in doses of fifteen grains every night during five nights, and of fifteen grains every second night during ten nights, was remarkably successful. The incontinence was immediately stopped. A course of chloral was continued from time to time. The second case was that of a child, aged seven, who took only one-third of a grain of chloral for five nights. The third case was quite as successfully treated in the same way.—*Ibid.*

Prophylaxis of Scarlatina.

During a recent epidemic of scarlatina in my neighborhood, in which the prevailing type of disease was that of the simplex, yet a number being anginose, and two exhibiting symptoms of a malignant type, one of which proved fatal upon the fourth day, I was, as you may suppose, importuned to prevent by prophylactic measures the disease from spreading among the families as yet unvisited, several of whom resided in close proximity to that in which the fatal malignant case occurred. I accordingly began by sprinkling the floors with carbolic acid, placing large plates containing the acid upon the tables in the different apartments, and one family having a number of children, in addition to the above measures placed carbolic acid in the heater, so as to insure its thorough diffusion throughout all the apartments of the house. I also prescribed for all the children unaffected with the disease small doses of potassæ chloras, to be given three times a day. These measures were resorted to, as I frankly informed them all, with very little hope of their efficacy; but, judge of my surprise, when, as time passed on, not another case appeared in any of the families who had resorted to these means. One family, however, being in indigent circumstances, and living somewhat secluded from the others, by an oversight on my part, was overlooked in these precautionary measures; the disease prevailed in that family, all the children having it, and one in a malignant form. In regard to the measures instituted for the prevention of the disease I have no theory to offer, but the fact is certainly remarkable and worthy of note.

W. F. Dickinson, M. D., *Smithtown Branch, N. Y.*
—*Med. and Surg. Reporter.*

Tincture of Veratrum in Pneumonia in Children.

Dr. Jacobi, in a clinical lecture before the New York Medical Journal Association, says, "In acute pneumonia of a baby, I would give a drop of the tincture every hour; to a child four or five years old, perhaps two drops every hour. If the attendant is intelligent enough to count the pulse, I say bring down this pulse to 110, or 100, but not lower; because when the pulse falls lower, the drug is apt to cause vomiting and temporary collapse. To obviate local irritation of the pharyngeal or gastric mucous membranes, I give the tincture in barley-water. This drug has no cumulative effect like that of digitalis. It will bear combination with quinine, and I think this an important point. I often combine quinine with veratrum or digitalis where I want to get, not a speedy, but a continued effect upon the pulse, especially in the pneumonia of a debilitated child, where you are in doubt about stimulating to any great extent ; where you do not know whether you ought to commence with benzoic acid, camphor, etc., you will control the pulse better with quinine and veratrum than with the latter alone. I ought to add that, in most cases it is advisable to combine opium or hyosciamus with veratrum to obviate local gastric irritation."— *N. Y. Med. Record.—Rich. and Louisv. Med. Journal.*

The Treatment of Diptheritis with Carbolic Acid. (Dent. Klinik., 26, 1871.)—

Dr. Helfer employs carbolic acid in the proportions of 1 to 200 as a gargle and injection, in the proportion of 1 to 50 for inhalation, and in concentrated solution with the camel's-hair pencil. He had treated altogether sixteen cases of diptheria with carbolic acid; the majority of these cases were diptheritis scarlatinosa, a few, most probably, angina diptheritica sine exanthemata, and, as far as can be gathered from the reports of the cases, at the most, two or three were cases of idiopathic diptheritis. The results which Dr. Helfer reports, are of a nature to encourage experiments with the carbolic acid ; and he refers also to Prof. Henwig and Dr. Weikert, who had obtained excellent results from the same treatment. In two cases also, of pure croup, and in one of diphtheretic croup, the employment of carbolic acid resulted in a cure.—(See *Med. Chir. Records,* No. 161, 1871.)—*N. Y. Medical Journal.*

Pseudo-membranous Croup. By Ross C. Russ, M. D., Hillsboro, Ohio.

* * * In view of the true pathology of pseudo-membranous croup, we arrive at the following conclusion:

That any medicinal agent which has a tendency to depress the "vital powers" of the system, by deteriorating the blood, is highly contraindicated.

Emetics, clinical experience affirms, are generally of doubtful efficacy. It is to be remembered that it is rarely that the glottis is occluded by the copious infusion of the exudative lymph.

Indeed, experience affirms, that the greater part of the false membrane remains attached to the surface of the epithelium until death or convalescence is established.

If, however, there are detachments of false membrane within the air passages, cupri sulphas may be given in one or two large doses until emesis is produced; but it should not be forgotten that all emetic substances should be prescribed with great circumspection.

We have witnessed the most brilliant results from the alkaloid quinia in this exceedingly grave disease. We seldom give it as a tonic, but in one, two, or more large doses—from five to ten grains to children from five to ten years of age, given every one, two, three, or five hours, according to circumstances or indications to be met, combined with syr. aurantii and spts., lavandulæ comp., acidulated with aro. sulph. acid; these being suitable adjuvants for administration of quinia to children.

May not quinia act in curing this disease, by neutralizing the morbid principle in the blood or supplying one or more of the wanting elements to the blood, thereby preventing the blood changes? Indeed, it is a fact well established by chemical research (and one of the most remarkable of the age) that there is a principle in health analogous to quinia.

To illustrate more fully the beneficial action of quinia in this disease, I will subjoin the following case : Called in consultation with Dr. Holmes, of Lynchburg, of this county (Highland), to see a little daughter of Capt. H. C. Dawson, who had all the symptoms of pseudo-membranous croup; pulse 147 beats to the minute—quick, small, easily compressible; voice could not be raised above a whisper; efforts to cough, as it were, muffled—persistent, perilous; dyspnœa (which is always characteristic of this disease); pallid surface; agitation, with great anxiety, etc.

Quinia was given freely in the above case, together with beef essence, sweet milk, and coffee *ad libitum*.

Notwithstanding croupous pneumonia supervened, which called for alcoholic stimulants, with some auxiliary measures which are generally demanded in this complication of pseudo-membranous croup, our little patient made slow, but permanent recovery.

11

If the bowels should be constipated, a mild cathartic would be indicated; frequent sponging with tepid vinegar, immediately followed by friction with warmed flannel, is highly indicated in promoting healthy action of the "cutaneous capillaries." A full, generous diet should be allowed, and the hygienic laws strictly enforced during the whole progress of this disease.—*Cin. Lancet and Observer.*

Case of Strangulated Hernia successfully treated by Pneumatic Aspiration.

Two new cases of the above have been communicated by Dr. Chauveau, of Courtolin, to the *Tribune Médicale* of Paris. In both cases puncture of the intestine gave issue to a colored liquid and to a certain amount of gas; in both cases reduction by means of a taxis took some time to be effected (ten minutes in one instance), and required some degree of exertion. Cure took place very rapidly, and both patients were able to resume their work twenty-four hours after the pucture.—*London Lancet.*

On Vaccination. By S. W. ABBOTT, M. D., Wakefield, Mass.

The question so frequently asked, "What is the best mode of vaccinating?" leads me to issue the following extracts:

From Seaton's Monograph on Vaccination, (the best English authority.)

"The best results, on the whole, as regard size, depth, and foveation, are those which follow the plan of cross-scratching, or abrasion * * * * and this plan is in most hands eminently more successful than puncture, when dry lymph has to be employed."

"The degree of modifying power is in the exact ratio of the excellence and completeness of the vaccination, as shown by the cicatrices."—*Marson.*

"The deaths from small pox among the vaccinated bear the following ratio:

Of those having but one cicatrix, - - - - - 7.73 per cent.
Of those having four or more cicatrices, - - - 0.55 per cent."
—*Marson.*

"Vaccination by scarification cannot be better done than with a common lancet."—*Seaton.*

Guided by these authorities and my own experience, I transmit the following directions:

For Ivory Ponits, scarify the skin lightly with a sharp lancet, in at least two places (better still, four or five). Moisten the charged end of the points with a minute quantity of water, and wipe off the virus upon the abraded surfaces. Allow the scarifications to dry.

For Capillary Tubes (intended rather for warm climates, and long preservation of virus).

After withdrawing the tube from its case with great care, break or cut each end with a pair of scissors, and blow the liquid lymph upon a piece of glass. Scarify the skin as usual, and transfer the virus to the scarifications with the point of the lancet.

I would especially caution the profession against the use of spindle-shaped tubes, accompanied with directions to "stir the virus thoroughly" before using. Such tubes contain at least 90 per cent. of glycerine.

Pure virus needs no stirring to ensure its efficiency.

[See card for vaccine virus under table of contents.]

AMERICAN MEDICAL ASSOCIATION.

The Twenty-fourth Annual Session will be held in St. Louis, Mo., May 6, 1873, at 11 A. M.

The following Committees are expected to report:

On Cultivation of the Cinchona Tree.—Dr. Lemuel J. Deal, Philadelphia, Pa., Chairman.

On Measures to Prevent the Extension of Diseases of Inferior Animals to Man, and the Sanitary Measures to Arrest the Progress of such Diseases in Animals.—Dr. A. W. Stein, New York, Chairman.

On the Treatment of Fractures.—Dr. Lewis A. Sayre, New York, Chairman.

On Gunguillia, a Substitute for Quinia.—Dr. Wm. Chew Van Bibber, Baltimore, Md., Chairman.

On Gynæcology.—Dr. Montrose A. Pallen, St. Louis, Mo., Chairman.

On the Renewal of Prescriptions without Authority, and on the Relations of Physicians and Druggists.—Dr. R. J. O'Sullivan, New York, Chairman.

On Vaccination.—Dr. T. N. Wise, Covington, Ky.

On Skin Transplantation.—Dr. J. Ford Thompson, Washington, D. C., Chairman.

On some Diseases peculiar to Colorado.—Dr. John Elsner, Denver, Colorado, Chairman.

On Correspondence with State Medical Societies.—Dr. N. S. Davis, Chicago, Illinois, Chairman.

On National Health Council.—Dr. Thomas M. Logan, Sacramento, Cal., Chairman.

On Nomenclature of Diseases.—Dr. Francis Gurney Smith, Philadelphia, Penn., Chairman.

On American Medical Necrology.—Dr. J. D. Jackson, Danville, Kentucky, Chairman.

On Suggestions on Medical Education.—Dr. A. M. Pollock, Pittsburg, Penn., Chairman.

On Medical Education.—Dr. Wm. Carson, Cincinnati, Ohio, Chairman.

On Medical Literature.—Dr. Austin Flint, New York, N. Y., Chairman.

On Prize Essays.—Dr. John S. Moore, St. Louis, Mo., Chairman.

On Plan for better Arrangement of Sections, and more rigid Examination of Papers offered for Publication.—Dr. E. L. Howard, Baltimore, Md., Chairman.

On Ethics.—Dr. H. F. Askew, Wilmington, Delaware, Chairman.

On the Climatology and Epidemics of—Alabama, Dr. T. C. Osborn; Arkansas, Dr. G. W. Lawrence; California, Dr. W. H. Williams; Colorado, Dr. R G. Buckingham; Georgia, Dr. G. M. McDowell; Illinois, Dr. David Prince; Indiana, Dr. Dugan Clark; Iowa, Dr. G. M. Staples; Kansas, Dr. Tiffin Sinks; Kentucky, Dr. L. P. Yandell, Sr.; Louisiana, Dr. S. M. Bemiss; Michigan, Dr. S. H. Douglas; Minnesota, Dr. Chas. N. Hewitt; Mississippi, Dr. S. V. D. Hill; Missouri, Dr. T. B. Lester; Oregon, Dr. Horace Carpenter; Tennessee, Dr. W. K. Bowling; Texas, Dr. S. M: Welch; Wisconsin, Dr. J. K. Bartlett.

· ☞ Physicians desiring to present papers before the Association should observe the following rule:

" Papers appropriate to the several sections, in order to secure consideration and action, must be sent to the Secretary of the appropriate section at least one month before the meeting which is to act upon them. It shall be the duty of the Secretary to whom such papers are sent, to examine them with care, and, with the advice of the Chairman of his Section, to determine the time and order of their presentation, and give due notice of the same. . . . . ''

OFFICERS OF SECTIONS.

Chemistry and Materia Medica.—Drs. R. E. Rogers, Philadelphia, Pa., Chairman; Ephraim Cutter, Boston, Mass., Secretary.

Practice of Medicine and Obstetrics.—Drs. D. A. O'Donnell, Md., Chairman; Benjamin F. Dawson, New York, Secretary.

Surgery and Anatomy.—Drs. Edward Warren, Baltimore, Md., Chairman; W. F. Peck, Davenport, Iowa, Secretary.

Meteorology and Epidemics.—Drs. George Sutton, Aurora, Indiana, Chairman; Elisha Harris, New York, Secretary.

Medical Jurisprudence, Hygiene, and Physiology.—Drs. S. C. Busey, Washington, D. C., Chairman; A. B. Arnold, Baltimore, Md., Secretary.

Psychology.—Drs. Isaac Ray, Philadelphia, Pa., Chairman; John Curwen, Harrisburg, Pa., Secretary.

Secretaries of all medical organizations are requested to forward lists of their delegates, as soon as elected, to the Permanent Secretary. W. B. ATKINSON.

BOOKS AND PAMPHLETS RECEIVED.

RECTUM, DISEASES OF. By Allingham. Lindsay & Blakiston, Philadelphia.

MIND UPON THE BODY, INFLUENCE OF. By Daniel Hack Tuke, M. D,, M. R. C. P. Henry C. Lea, Philadelphia.

OVARIES, DISEASES. By T. Spencer Wells. D. Appleton & Co., New York.

SURGERY, BRYANT'S PRACTICAL. Henry C. Lea, Philadelphia.

MYRINGECTOMY. By J. S. Prout, M. D., Brooklyn, New York.

PHYSIOLOGY OF SYPHILITIC INFECTION. First and Second Parts. By Fessenden N. Otis, M. D.

ELECTRO THERAPEUTICS. Recent researches on. By Geo. M. Beard, M. D.

ORAL SURGERY. Being a consideration of the diseases of the Mouth, Jaws, and associated parts. By James E. Garretson, M. D., D. S. Philadelphia: J. B. Lippincott & Co. 1873.

DENTAL CARIES, and its causes. By Drs. Leber and Rottenstein. Translated by Thomas H. Chandler, M. D. Philadelphia: Lindsay & Blakiston. 1873.

TRANSACTIONS of the Medical Society of West Virginia. 1872.

Messrs. Lindsay & Blakiston, No. 25 South 6th Street, Philadelphia, issue circulars of " Recent English Editions of Medical Works," including works on the Rectum, Urine, Functional Diseases, Syphilis, the Kidneys, Liver, Bladder, etc.

Complete and descriptive catalogue furnished *free* upon application.

Editorial.

The *Missouri Dental Journal* comes out in a new dress, and in part under new editorship. The Dentists of St. Louis, many of them distinguished in their profession, will no doubt feel a pride in fully sustaining their *representative journal,* one of the best as we think in this country. *It should be found on the table of every general practitioner;* and should be read by those of the medical profession who practice in the country, in order that they may give timely and sound advice to their patients respecting the *preservation* and *treatment* of their teeth; and especially to direct them where to go and what to do in cases requiring special treatment. We wish the *Journal* every success.

☞*For information of Missouri get Campbell's New Atlas.*

GARDUATES OF THE MISSOURI MEDICAL COLLEGE.

Wm. Sharp,
A. Goodenough,
G. W. Elders,
G. W. Givens,
Chas. Johnson,
T. A. Davis,
J. B. Ryan,
T. H. Newland,
Gust. Wendlandt,
J. R. Dorr,
G. Fuchs,
Alvin Snyder,
J. R. Scruggs,
H. Lee Hatch,
W. C. Persons,
J. R. Hall,
R. B. Duncan,

Geo. Homan,
Jos. H. Moore,
W. M. Bell,
H. Waser.

HONORARY DEGREES.

E. M. Beach, M. D., Ill.,
T. L. Papin, M. D., St. Louis.

AD EUNDEM DEGREE.

O. W. Archibald, M. D., Iowa,
S. Thompson, M. D., Ill.,
W. A. Smith, M. D., Ill.,
R. E. Lightburne, M. D., Mo.,
J. M. Harnett, M. D., Ill.,
A. B. Shaw, M. D., Mo.,
W. A. Hardaway, M. D., Mo.,
T. E. Bramlette, M. D., Ky.

Dr. I. BAKER BROWN, the distinguished gynæcologist of London, died Feb. 3, 1878.

Meteorological Observations.

METEOROLOGICAL OBSERVATIONS AT ST. LOUIS, MO.

By A. Wislizenus, M.D.

The following observations of daily temperature in St. Louis are made with a MAXIMUM and MINIMUM thermometer (of Green, N. Y.). The daily minimum occurs generally in the night, the maximum about 3 P M. The monthly mean of the daily minimum and maxima, added and di/Ided by 2, gives a quite reliable mean of the monthly temperature.

THERMOMETER FAHRENHEIT.
JANUARY AND FEBRUARY, 1873.

Day of Month	Minimum.		Maximum.		Day of Month	Minimum.		Maximum.	
	January.	February.	January.	February.		January.	February.	January.	February.
1	32.0	19.0	28.0	14.0	18	17.0	65.5	7.0	38.5
2	47.5	22.0	31.5	—1.0	19	30.0	42.5	9.0	28.5
3	38.0	48.5	31.0	31.0	20	40.0	49.5	27.5	37.0
4	35.0	49.5	25.0	36.0	21	42.0	32.5	34.0	12.0
5	29.5	52.0	21.5	31.5	22	41.0	22.5	32.5	6.0
6	31.0	47.5	6.0	31.5	23	29.0	18.0	20.0	6.0
7	39.0	53.0	19.0	33.0	24	17.5	28.0	5.5	8.5
8	27.0	40.0	16.0	30.0	25	19.0	38.0	2.0	21.0
9	18.0	48.0	7.0	24.0	26	23.0	42.5	10.5	34.0
10	18.0	43.0	0.0	33.5	27	21.0	33.5	5.0	19.0
11	45.0	37.5	12.0	36.0	28	1.0	37.0	0.0	19.0
12	52.0	35.5	34.5	27.0	29	7.5		—14.0	
13	50.0	31.5	45.0	25.0	30	30.5		2.0	
14	38.	41.5	32.0	26.0	31	36.0		13.5	
15	5	37.0	38.0	33.0					
16	25.5	40.5	15.0	35.5	Means	30.5	39.4	16.6	25.4
17	12.0	46.5	—0.5	35.0	Monthly Means			23.5	32.4

Quantity of rain and snow:

	January.	February.
Rain	1.88	1.32
Snow	1.98	0.04
	3.86 inches.	1.36 inches.

Mortality Report.

FROM JAN. 26th, 1873, TO FEB. 22d, 1873, INCLUSIVE.

Date	White Males	White Females	Col'd Males	Col'd Females	Under 5 yrs.	5 to 10	10 to 20	20 to 30	30 to 40	40 to 50	50 to 60	60 to 70	70 to 80	80 to 90	90 to 100	Total
Saturday 1	93	85	9	3	83	18	10	32	19	6	13	4	5	...	...	190
" 8	117	78	10	5	82	18	14	33	15	24	10	7	6	2	...	210
" 15	87	75	5	4	73	12	12	23	15	21	14	8	2	1	...	171
" 22	96	76	6	5	90	19	11	21	10	11	12	4	5	3	...	183
Total,	393	314	30	17	328	67	47	109	59	62	49	23	18	6		754

Abscess 1	Diarrhœa............ 6	Intemperance........ 1	Scald............... 1
Abscess of Liver. .. 1	Difficult Labor...... 1	Leucocythæmia,.... 1	Scurvy.............. 1
Anemia 1	Disease of the Heart 6	Lockjaw 4	Suicide............. 2
Apoplexy........ ...10	Diptheria........... 4	Marasmus 13	Variola.............206
Asthma 2	Dropsy............. 8	Measles 1	
Atrophia 1	Dysentery.......... 4	Meningitis 41	Total....... 754
Bright's Disease.... 1	Eclampsia.......... 2	" cer. spin..29	
Bronchitis..........13	Epilepsy............ 1	Metritis 1	Stillborn............36
Cancer.............. 2	Erysipelas.......... 7	Metro Peritonitis... 5	
Carditis............ 1	Fever, remittent 2	Œdema 2	
Catarrh. 2	" intermittent... 3	Old Age............ 9	
Cerebritis.......... 4	" puerperalis.. 10	Paralysis 5	
Chill, Congestive. 8	Fever, typhoid... ...16	Peritonitis.......... 7	
Conges. of Brain .. 13	Gangrene........... 1	Pertussis 1	
Conges. of Lungs. 15	Gastritis........... 5	Pleuritis 2	
Consumption...... 59	Hydrocephalus...... 4	Pneumonia.... 68	
Convulsion..........38	Icterus Gravis 3	Poison, con lye..... 1	
Croup 11	Inanition......... 1	Premature birth..... 1	
Cystitis............. 1	Inflammat'n bowels.. 2	Pyemia. 1	
Debility 9	" liver .. 4	Rheumatism 4	
Delirium Tremens. 3	Injuries 2	Scarlatina...... 6	

THE SAINT LOUIS

Medical and Surgical Journal.

APRIL, 1873.

Original Communications.

ON TETANUS AND TETANOID AFFECTIONS, WITH CASES.

By B. ROEMER, M. D., St. Louis, Mo.

[Continued from page 131.]

In the case reported by Dr. Keen contraction and spasm interchanged with paralysis; an arterial hyperæmia of the spine with hyperæsthesia following a cerebral paresis. The peculiarity of a progressive paralysis of all inhibitory action leading to a permanent and post-mortem contraction of certain muscles (loc. cit., p. 130), and during life intermitting with spasmodic twitching of muscles and pain, alternate rigidity and flexibility, and convulsions under a semi-coma, places this case in juxtaposition with locomotor ataxia. The spanæmia consequent to an altered supply of blood induced a diminished trophism of the brain, and secondarily of the muscles involved. The investigations of *Kussmaul* show that spasmodic contractions and paralysis follow. The account of Dr. Bodine's case illus-

12

trates the transition of tetanus to other affections with
dissimilar morbid appearances, but similar initiatory
phenomena and causes.   Both conditions, of a mere
excitation of the spinal and inflammation of the cerebral centre, may therefore exist together, one a superinduced condition upon the other, either by direct continuity or toxæmically transplanted.   It might be,
however, assumed *a priori*, that tetanus from injuries of
the head should result only from slight contusions, in
other words, the effect of the primary injury must not
be sufficient to excite a predominant inflammation from
structural changes within the encephalon.

The definition and opinions of writers on the *pathology* of tetanus are multiplied by the theoretic or practical
deductions from each class of cases.   *Watson*, the Xen-
ophon of medical literature, regards tetanus as an irritation of the spinal cord or of its efferent nerves ; he
considers the brain not involved and assumes a certain

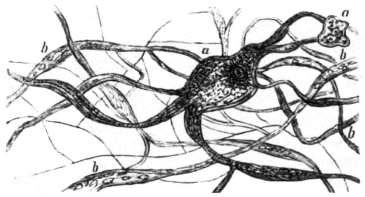

CASE VIII.   *J. B. Hartley.*—Long. section of anterior spinal cord ;
    cervical region.   Specimen hardened with chromic acid.   *a*—
    pigmentary nerve corpuscle; nuclei and ramifications; tubular
    cylinders, and capillaries traversing them.   *b*—Blood vessels
    filled with white bodies.   Hair-like fibres are seen traversing
    the field, usually attached to a nerve tube.

predisposition of the body for the most part necessary to render it susceptible of the disease. under the operation of an exciting irritation. He adds that it is a spasmodic disease, characterized by neither an increase in muscular exertion as in mania, nor by its diminution as in paralysis, but by a perversion of muscular force. *Copeland* suggested the ganglia and sympathetic nerves to be the seat and pathological cause of tetanus (*Lond. Med. Reposit.*, May, 1822), and *Swan*, following these views, stated that the ganglia after tetanus were preternaturally injected, which statement is supported by *Andral, Dupuy*, a. o.; *Meyer* and *Vetter* speak of ossific deposits (as reported by *South*, loc. supra. cit.) irritating ganglionic nerves as productive of this disease. The *French School* hold it an inflammatory affection of the spinal nerves. The inflammatory appearances insisted upon by *Larrey, Magendie, Récamier, Ollivier*, a. o., are negatived by the absence of tetanus in true inflammation of the spinal cord and its contingencies. Certain similarities between tetanus and hydrophobia have been made prominent by *Bilgner*, who calls it "*Hundskrampf*," or dog-spasm (*Chelius' Syst. Surg.*, I, p. 414), and *I. L. Bardsley* recommends a treatment like that in hydrophobia (*Cyclopæd. of Pract. Med.*, 1833), from his opinion of the pathology of tetanus. *Froriep* and *Pelletier* (*Neue Not.*, 1837, Jan., No. 1), consider a local nervous inflammation as the cause, and that the general irritability arises secondarily from it in the course of the nerve trunk. *Curling* (*op. cit.*) regards it a simple functional disturbance, the seat of which is the tractus motorius of the spinal marrow (tract. intermedio-lateralis of the grey substance). *Lawrence* (Lectures in *L. Lancet*, 1829, vol. 1) leaves the pathol-

ogy undecided, as no clearness exists in what the derangement of the spinal cord consists, and because
examinations have not shown that any derangement of
that part is characteristic of tetanus. *Wilk. King* of
Guy's Hosp. usually opened his post-mortem examinations in tetanus with these words : "We will now proceed to give you a demonstration of a case of healthy
anatomy, for there will be no *visible* morbid appearances, etc." [Italics my own.] *Richardson* (*Med. Journ.*,
1861, April, p. 523) classes tetanus among the zymotic
diseases, produced as a specific poison in the wound,
which opinion is advocated by *Roser, Wells, Thomson*,
and *Betoli*, thus approximating tetanus to hydrophobia.
Simpson also regards a peculiar blood-poison generated
in the wound or elsewhere the cause of tetanus. *C. H.
Jones* (*Clin. Observ. on Funct. Nerv. Disord.*, p. 123),
calls it a functional excitement of the spinal cord, and
gives *Heiberg's* opinion that it is an affection of the
blood localizing itself in the muscles.

   While the direct application of post-mortem appearances in tetanus has negatived a clear pathology, yet
the character of a primary disease, to which tetanus
may be a sequence, is often indicated. We recognize
in tetanus and tetanoid spasm a *progressive* and a *retrograding* manifestation. Progressive in so far as certain
diseases, characterized by a distinct and established
morbid anatomy, result at times, often as a pathogno-
monic symptom in well marked tetanic spasm, and
retrograding, because in certain cases of tetanus, perhaps impure types, we find phenomena more or less
verging towards inflammatory causes, located in the
spine and its superior nerve centre. The *middle* ground
is held by pure tetanus. Phenomena in the morbid

anatomy of progressive tetanic affections are no more indicative of the *causes*, than the evidences of hyperæmia and inflammation in retrograding tonic spasm establish the *effects* of tetanus. That there exists a certain interchange of similar symptoms based upon a dissimilar pathological condition and *vice versa*, is perhaps not difficult to show; but in how far such diseases may be deductions of one from another, their idiosyncracies and virulence gradually developing a *system* or chain of affections, is an obscure theorism and improbable of demonstration. *Brown–Séquard* has maintained that irritations emanating from a centripetal nerve may result in very different morbid conditions—insanity, hallucinations, illusions, vertigo, extasis, hysteria, chorea, catalepsy, epilepsy, hydrophobia and tetanus; but the connection of one with, and the deduction of one from another is not established. *C. H. Jones* (*op. cit.*, *Vindemiatio*, p. 344) remarks (12) in this connection, that, "a series of gradations may be traced from tonic spasm through clonic tremors and choreic agitation to actual paralysis." My present reference to cases of a spasmodic and paralytic character is made with the view of drawing attention to such a transitory concatenation, and I propose to deduct from them the following conclusions:

1. Impressions upon the peripheral nerves of unusual character, amounting to irritation or excitation, are capable of producing a train of symptoms which differ as much between themselves as in their history of existence in diseases of dissimilar origin.

In illustration of this fact, I transcribe case 114 of my diary:

"J. Dean, wounded in battle of Seven Pines, ampu-

tation of left little finger.   Resulted in nervous irritation, clonic spasmodic contractions and asthenic fever.
This case was admitted to hospital during the most
intense heat of the summer (1862), and the atmospheric
condition contributed much to the advent of febrile
symptoms.   After amputation the patient was removed
to the only vacancy in the hospital, a garret-room in
a four-story building with metallic roof, and in a few
days the alteration in his countenance, a shaking palsy,
furred and dry tongue, wiry and quick pulse, hollow
eyes, paleness, constipation, headache, etc., indicated
the amount of nervous sympathy.   A hectic fever
supervened shortly afterwards.   The treatment consisted in his removal to a cooler room, free admission
of fresh air, tonics, opiates at night, cathartics when
necessary, fomentations to the stump and whole arm,
etc., and in a few days I had the gratification to see him
convalescent."   The incubation here verged towards
tonic spasm.

I give also case 215 (S. H. B.) : "a gunshot wound
in right lumbar region, compression by a large cicatrix,
resulting in complete dysecoia.   Was returned to
hospital for treatment because of pain in his back,
neck and over the scalp, and suspected of simulating.
I found on examination the large cicatrix firmly impacted
around the lumbar vertebræ.   He complained of
sibilant noises in his ears, like in hysteria.   Local treatment did not relieve ; the disease had a rapid course of
development, it failed to oscillate, and the impaired
vision pointing to a general nervous affection, corroborated by vertigo, deafness and sinister movements of
the body, I based the symptoms upon the previous
injury.   The remarks of J. L. Gaultier (de Physiolog.

et Patholog. Irritabilitatis, p. 21) are applicable here : "Where the irritation is slight relatively to the amount of organic nervous power, or where the susceptibility is not increased, the limitation of it (*the irritation*) to its original seat may be long continued,—but where it is more considerable, organic nervous power being low, and the susceptibility, either local or general, consequently high it will extend itself or manifest its effects more or less prominently in remote situations."

2. The occurrence of one case of true tetanus under absence of inflammatory necroptic appearances invalidates their presence as causation in all cases. Multiplied microscopic examinations alone can decide on the presence or absence of inflammatory lesions in their *ultimate* existence, and having in view the want of morbid appearances in the most acute cases of tetanus and their unexpected general development in less pronounced instances, it is evident—

(a) That *microscopical* inflammatory appearances, to the naked eye devoid of all abnormality, are sufficient to account for the violence of tetanus, and that

(b) The *visible* lesions may be only a gradual expansion of those microscopic; either a morphological condition the result of structural exaltation and due to the peculiar organization of the patient, or the added effect of complications and extension.

3. Arterial hyperæmia is not the cause of tetanus, nor is venous congestion a direct or primary agent in its production.

4. Certain relations of the cerebro-spinal fluid with the central canal of the spinal cord, the arachnoid spaces and their prolongations are capable of determi-

ning the normal, exalted or depressed nerve-power; a
venous stasis of the spinal cord, and a hyperæmia of
the encephalon corresponding with an increased
relative volume of the fluid and consequent pressure,
and a congestion of the vessels of the cord with an
anæmic brain agreeing with its quantitative, local
reduction, giving as results spasm, coma, paralysis, etc.

Virchow and *Kölliker* deny that there exists a communication between the sub-arachnoid spaces and the
ventricles of the brain, and between these and the sub-
arachnoid spaces of the spinal cord, but the anatomical
preparations and experiments of *Luschka* have established this fact. There is an ebbing and flowing of the
cerebro-spinal fluid from the brain to the cord and *vice
versa*. (*Med. Times and Gaz.* 1858, Jan. 16). The
larger capillaries of the spinal cord are incased in three
tunics, the space between them and the vessels being
occupied by a clear and colorless fluid. (Robin in
Brown-Séquard's Journ. de la Phys. 1856, Oct.) The
sheath and its fluid can be traced to the smallest vessels,
and both accompany them in all their anastomoses and
bifurcations. The proportion in their diameters is in
favor of the perivascular canal, which is thus subject
to certain changes of calibre, forming under pressure
now and then a dilatation or contraction, as the force of
distension or its structural character may determine.
These minute canals are so intimately connected that
their injection is accomplished without difficulty, and
are seen to pursue in the nerve-substance a course from
without inwards and in the reverse direction. As the
cerebro-spinal fluid of the great sub-arachnoid spaces
is based and cushioned upon the venous blood of the
cord, and supports the nerve-substance of the cerebro-

spinal axis, so fulfills the fluid of the minute perivascular spaces a similar office in protecting the molecular
nerve-substance against undue pressure, obviating
friction between nerve-filaments and fasciculi, and aiding in the re-establishment of an adequate equipoise
between the transmission of blood and the hygrometric
status of the cerebro-spinal fluid. Compression,
approximation and irritation from friction result
from undue blood supply, and relaxation, irregular
constriction and elongation from want of support;
in other words, an *increase* of pressure from the
fluid in the spaces gives an encroachment upon the
elementary nerve and approximation and friction
between the component parts of a nerve-bundle; and
a *diminution* of the support leads to relaxation and
elongation of the nerve-tube with undulatory approximation of its walls and to friction of one nerve-
filament or fibre with another lying in proximity. A
tendency to locally augment the normal volume of the
cerebro-spinal fluid, either from traumatic or idiopathic
causes, has the direct effect of producing a stasis in the
arterial blood-vessels surrounding or accompanying it in
its ramifications, and a contraction of the veins in order
to balance the blood supply and the augmented pressure
from the fluid. A continuance of this mutual power
to displace leads not only to the fuller development of
the abnormality itself, but implicates also sooner or
later the entire cord. The microscopic views of the
spinal cord support this statement.

In order that the motor nerves should attain their
utmost excitation to muscular action, the inhibitory
function should be diminished to its greatest extent.
The former should receive an increased, and the latter

a decidedly reduced volume of arterial blood stimulus. I would refer here cursorily to the demonstration of a third class of nerves by *Eulenburg* and *Landois* (*Schmidt's Jahrbücher*, 1866) called the inhibiting (*Zurückhaltenden*) nerves, spoken of by Setschenow before Drs. E. and L. undertook their experiments, and the function of which is to regulate the degree of movement while under irritation, subject to exaltation, depression and paralysis. *Malkiewitz* has pointed out that in certain spasmodic effects of poisons these nerves are in a state of paralysis. The same was taught by *Pflüger*. *Lister* locates this action of inhibition in all afferent nerves according to the degree of stimulus applied, and in the absence of direct proof for the existence of Eulenburg's *Zurückhaltenden Nerven* this is sufficiently explanative. Certain peculiarities in the therapeutic action of poisons may be due to the contraction necessary for a diminished volume of blood. A dose of strychnine which kills an animal in full digestion does not act upon one during abstinence in the same length of time. Absorption alone cannot explain this, for it is more active in the favorable case. Cold acts in like manner, it requiring a larger dose of strychnine to kill a frog in winter than in summer. Remedies in general do not act upon the sick as promptly and energetically as on the well. A contraction of the arteries carries with it, if due to cardiac inaction or toxæmia, a congestion of the veins and capillaries depending on them, but this phenomenon may be so reversed as to base an arterial anæmia by contraction upon a venous hyper- or toxæmia. The minute arteries have the capacity, owing to their structure and design, to contract upon the introduction of any abnormal or non-arterial substance if brought directly in contact, or, and especially if the foreign substance comes through the veins, in antagonism with them. This contractile power assimilates them to the valvular structure of the veins and serves to hold the capillary circulation intact. The intimate connection between the circulation in the spinal cord and the fasciculous canals (theca of the vertebral substance and perivascular fluid) renders any disturbance in either of easy transmission to the whole nerve-substance by means of mechanical forces, (pressure, friction and dilatation), and without assuming the character of such structural changes as we meet in inflammation. Since functional activity, implies a certain turgescence of the structure, its exaltation may depend upon a more than usual degree of that turgescence and a greater distribution of its impressions, or it may so involve the whole of an organ, which in health is charaterized by two or more distinct and parallel functions, as to interchange and coalesce them to an abortive discharge of one or both of them, sensation, motion, trophism and inhibition. The length of time necessary to exhaust this vascular capacity is the tolerance of the organ, and the amount of vascularity determines with this tolerance the degree of subsequent inaction or rest required for a perfect and healthy renewal of the normal functional activity. Vascularity and equipoise of contraction between the fluids of the spinal cord are synonymous with action and rest, and the undue amount or unusual persistence of this vascularity leads to morbid phenomena. All organs of the body, for whose functional existence it is required to alternate the ultimate conditions of contraction and dilatation at regular intervals, have the

structural peculiarity of adapting the surrounding
tissues and formations 'to each turgescence, and the
same holds true in reference to the brain and spinal
cord. The peculiar structure of the arteries and veins,
they holding themselves in a compensating antagonism,
rests and bases itself upon the underlying cerebro-
spinal fluid in all its divisions and this parallelism is
true of the spinal cord independent of the brain. The
'cerebro-spinal opening is the dividing line beyond
which in either direction a distinct nerve centre has its
peculiar function, subject to mutual disturbances only
from more than ordinary causes. In the event of the
brain or spinal cord being under excitation, the cerebro-
spinal fluid is displaced as far and as long as the induced vascularity demands, and the subsidence of the
excitation or the replacement of the fluid to its former
level insures a state of rest,—if the former is called
disease, the latter condition must exist in *health*. The
dynamis of a normal volume of displaced fluid invading
the most minute spaces of the nerve-substance in the
cord, exalting the functional activity of motion and
sensibility, and this without inhibition because of the
coalition of the nerve filaments and fasciculi, has for
its product spasm ; and its morbid increase (spina
bifida, hydrocephalus, certain forms of mental
derangements, etc.,) results in coma, syncope and
irregular movements. Inflammatory appearances in
the cerebro-spinal axis accord with a diminished
volume of fluid, and in the reverse condition we may
suppose that an anæmia is in preponderance. Both
conditions are possible from sanguine excitation or
from undue absorption of the serosity. The uniform
and gradually augmented encroachment of the fluids in

the cord and its minute canals upon the spinal nerves without continuity upon the brain gives rise to a continued spasm, the locality and intensity of which is governed by the totality of the parts implicated. Surrounding the nerve roots and fasciculi as they pass each other in close proximity, this fluid serves to isolate and maintain them safe from mutual pressure, and their contact under an irritative compression from a relatively increased volume of fluid facilitates not only the transmission of nerve stimulus to an exalted action, but, hinders the separate current of the nerve power, motor sensitive. * The inhibition applicable to one nerve is

---

* If the volume of the cerebro-spinal fluid, as some anatomists insist, is much lessened immediately after death, the development of the rigor mortis, certain peculiar contractions of dead bodies after cholera and yellow fever, and the instantaneous rigor on battle fields from sudden and violent death, may be due to its displacement upon the spinal cord, effecting in the motor nerve-fibre the same results after death, which during life are produced in the cord itself. The progress of a dead body from relaxation to the rigor, and its subsequent return to mobility, have these important analogies : the rigidity passes from the free muscular tissues of the head to those of the neck, trunk, and extremities, in the order named; and A. G. Sommers found but one exception to this rule in two hundred dead bodies; the inferior maxilla is firmly drawn against its superior, no matter in what position death found it; and the arms and legs are contracted upon themselves; the rigor discontinues as it commenced. Tonic spam in trismus passes to the rigidity of death without intervening relaxation. The thermometric condition of the surrounding air exerts little or no influence over the advent of rigor mortis, often before the cadaveric warmth has equalized itself with the temperature, the rigidity has set in. After removal of the brain and spinal marrow, the rigor nevertheless begins. *Mende* 'asserts that in the fœtus and the stillborn infant this rigidity is not developed. The same obtains in death from hemorrhage; *instantaneous* death, however, from hemorrhage, gives an extreme rigidity, in which the last position of the body in life is retained, like after instantaneous death from brain wounds. (*Dr. Fodere* of Strasburg). Morgagni has observed a similar rigor in death from asphyxia. The likeness of this rigor to tetanus, has been noticed by *Carpenter*, and the objection of its prolonged continuation, and the succession of flexibility and true rigor mortis was anticipated by him. That these phenomena are not due to the coagulation of the blood, as *Treviranus' Orfila* and *Beclard* believed, has been demonstrated (*Sommer, Muller's Handbuch d. Physiol.* II., p. 43), nor is it indisputable that the cause of rigidity is

communicated to others lying in contact with it, and

seated in the muscles, as *Nysten* and *Rudolphi* think. The mere fact that the limbs remain rigid after division of the fasciæ and lateral ligaments of the joints, and become relaxed on division of the muscles, does not establish the cause in the muscular fibre. The divided muscle itself remains under the rigor mortis in its superior portion; beyond the division a complete flexibility exists. Of this I have satisfied myself often. Moreover a rigidity under such conditions, must be equivalent to a surviving contractibility of the muscular fibre, such as we notice during life, against which the facts militate that rigid muscles are insensible to irritation, and especially that in the preceding complete relaxation of all the muscles, no such latent contractibility can be supposed to exist. It would be impossible, satisfactorily to explain upon such grounds, why in some instances the fœtus has been known to be expelled after death of the mother, and why the finger, introduced into the pharynx of a decapitated animal, is tightly held. *Richardson's* conclusions (presented before the St. Andrew's Med. Graduates' Assoc. in London), that "the cause of rigor mortis is the coagulation of the muscular fluid—muscle fibrine—under heat as excitant," and that " rigor of the muscle and coagulation of blood are truly the last evidences of the phenomena, which in their totality we call life," are modified by the fact, that very often the rigidity is well manifest, while the blood is still fluid (p. e. after death by drowning, and prussic acid), and that textures as rich in blood vessels as the red muscle, fail in rigidity. A second objection lies in the fact that a paralyzed muscle (Busch) will tear, for instance, under a weight of sixty grm., when the same muscle, under rigor mortis, supports twelve times that weight, unimpaired. Can it be possible that the relative volume of " muscle fibrine" is changed after death, or that it is not commensurate to its muscular power? The peculiar muscular contractions of dead bodies after cholera and yellow fever, have been noticed by *Brandt* and *Brown Sequard.* (*Am. Journ. Med. Sc.*, 1856, Oct., p. 446). The muscular movements are observed only in those of strongly developed muscular force after short duration of the disease, and previous absence of decided cramp or spasm. The more rapid the attack of cholera, especially in cases of robust constitution, the smaller is the attempt of repair, and the greater the centric morbid action. Death results from the toxic abundance of an altered, and yet diminished, volume of blood by inaction of the peripheric blood vessels. The condition is a capillary hyperæmia (toxæmia), by which the supply of blood stimulus to the brain is cut off. Brown-Sequard substitutes his carbonic-acid theory. The blood being rapidly deprived of its watery portions, and without its necessary oxygen, we recognize in the absence of spasm or cramp an arterial anæmia of the spinal cord, with a stasis in the cerebral sinuses and veins. The contractions after yellow fever are noticed in the congestive type, with short paroxysm and limited pervigilium but normal incubative stage. The only metaptosis intervenes between incipient apoplexy or convulsions, and stupor. The blood under autopsy is dark, non-inflammatory, and of thick consistency. Capillary congestion, evidenced during life by petichiæ and ecchymoses, is such that extravasation is the causes which effect the increase of muscular exertion lead also to the perversion of muscular force, so that a primary and purely reflex phenomenon assumes in time a functional importance, with structural abnormalities commensurate with the continuance, power and systemic effect of the spasm produced.

[To be Continued.]

---

extensive from natural orifices, and the black vomit is but a collective emesis of exosmosed and vitiated blood. The same conditions appear, consequently, here as in cholera, and the cadaveric spasm is allied to the tonic contraction of living muscles from a diminished support to the cerebro-spinal fluid. (*Vide Valentin's Phys. d. Menschen*, II., 2, p. 366). As an adjunct to the pressure thus produced upon the nerve ramification an additional influence in the production of these contractions and of rigor mortis, is given in the shortening of muscles when cooling; but a certain degree of heat induces the reverse, a shortening upon the addition of warmth, and the peculiar position assumed by dead bodies after yellow fever and cholera may be in part the result of an increased chemico-molecular action, by which latent heat is evolved from the prior exhaustion of the primary agent, blood. The peripheric and centric nerves respond to the electric shock or current, long after death, and their activity must be supposed to be gradually diminished. *Matteucci* (in his *Fenomeni fisico-chem.* p. 118-119), and *Du Bois Raymond* (*Poggendorff's Annalen*, book LVIII, 1843, s 5 a. s.) have thought to prove this to be a muscular irritability, because muscles and single muscular fibres deprived of their nerves even to the microscopic test still possess this power to contract. This proposition involves the question of absolute dissection, and if the microscopic preparations of *Dr. Beale* are examined (*L. Lancet*, 1866, July 21), and the report of *Rouget*, supported by Krause, Waldeyer, Engelmann, Letzerich, Kühne, Conheim, Vulpian, a. o., on the ultimate termination of nerve fibres, it will become evident that the contractions of muscles or their fibres as noticed by M. and R., were due not only to nerve filaments suffered to remain, but that the contractile force was equivalent to their number and preservation. As the report of Dr. Rouget has an important bearing, I give an extract: "This nervous expansion is traversed in every direction by minute canals, establishing a connection between the numerous nuclei of the plate and communicating, probably, on the one hand with the space intermediate between the sarcolemma and the contractile fibrillæ, and on the other hand with the interstice between the matrix of the nerve-tube and the medullary layer, an arrangement which is doubtless related to the special action of certain poisonous substances upon the terminal extremity of the motor nerves of animal life."

CONCURRENT. EXANTHEMETA.

By Walter Coles, M. D.,

On the 25th of February, I was called to see Mr.
J. G., who was suffering with all the incipient symptoms of what proved to be a very severe attack of
confluent smallpox.   At the same time my attention
was directed to one of the patient's children, an infant
ten months old, who was in the fifth day of the eruptive
stage of a moderate discrete variola.   The child had
been exposed to the disease, and had never been
vaccinated, owing to a foolish prejudice on the part of
its parents.

The eruption was confluent on the nose and chin, but
on the rest of the face the pustules were quite distinct,
and on the body there were considerable areas of
healthy skin.   The child seemed to be doing very well,
and I gave it no medicine save a mild opiate to quiet
it at night, and enable its mother to get a little repose.
On the eighth day of the eruption I called at the house
and found my little patient very sick; its eyes were
red; it had a hoarse cough, and a high fever. Surprised
to find so decided *secondary fever* supervening upon a
comparatively mild attack of variola, I examined the
child carefully in a good light, and ascertained that its
little face and body were thickly broken out with a well
marked eruption of measles.   The two eruptions run
their usual course, neither apparently modifying the
other, and the child is now well.

The foregoing case is interesting in several particulars; chiefly however, in proving, as it does, that
the opinion held up to a comparatively recent date, that

no two distinct and specific disorders could progress in the system at the same time, is erroneous. John Hunter was a warm champion of this dogma. In *Hunter's Works,* edited by Palmer, vol. III. p. 4, he says: "As I reckon every operation in the body an action, whether universal or partial, it appears to me, beyond a doubt, that no two actions can take place in the same constitution, nor in the same part, at one and the same time; the operations of the body are similar, in this respect, to actions or motions of common matter. It naturally results from this principle that no two different fevers can exist in the same constitution, nor two local diseases in the same part at the same time."

It is upon just such untenable ground as the foregoing, that our homeopathic friends uphold the absurd practice by which they pretend, through a species of medical legerdemain, to drive out one disease from the system by a substitution of another.

It is unnecessary at this late day to say anything to prove that the several exanthemata are essentially distinct diseases. And it was probably a blind adherence to such doctrines as were enunciated by Hunter, that so long deluded the old physicians into the belief that they were nearly allied species, of a common genus. We have but to glance at the natural history of this class of diseases, to convince ourselves of their entire independence of each other; for we know by experience,—(a) that there is an element or material in all the human family, upon which these several diseases act and re-act in such a manner as to infinitely multiply the original germ of contagion; (b) that in a few weeks the resultant disease is eliminated

from the system ; (*c*) that in the course of the disease,
the peculiar element or material in affinity with the
contagious principle is consumed or destroyed, so
that though the patient returns to health, he is forever
after as a rule, innocuous to a like morbid poison.
This future immunity from "like morbid poison"
holds good with rare exceptions in all the exanthemata.
But the destruction of the element in the body having
its affinity for variola, in no wise affects the peculiar
pabulum in the blood upon which measles seizes, the
same may be said of scarlatina, and each other individual of the group. This process of reasoning proves
the distinctness of these diseases, and accords with
universal experience. This being the case, it is not
difficult to believe, what observation has abundantly
proven, that there is no physical incompatibility,
as Hunter would say, in the co-existence of two or
more of these diseases, and it is even strange that their
concurrence has not been more frequently met with.
Such co-existence has been noticed by many accurate
observers.

Marson (*Medico-Chirurg Trans.*, vol. XXX. p. 129)
adduces several instances not only of the co-existence
of variola and scarlatina, but of variola and rubeola,
variola and pertussis, variola and vaccinia, rubeola and
vaccinia, rubeola and pertussis, and pertussis and vaccinia.*

Bamberger, in his " *Remarques sur la variole et sur sa
combinaison avec d'autres maladies,*" has related some exceedingly interesting cases which go to prove that

---

* Consult *Cyclopædia of Practical Med.*, p. 169, transactions of a society for
improvement in medical and surgical knowledge; *Medico-Chirurg. Trans.*
London, vol. XIII, p. 163 ; *Amer. Journal Med. Science*, April, 1854.

though certain of the exanthemata may co-exist, yet each retains its distinctive characteristics, and may impart its own peculiar poison to others. That is to say, a poison having co-existent variola and· rubeola, may at the same moment impart variola to one person, and rubeola to another, or may impart both to the same person.

2346 Olive st.

EPIDEMIC CEREBRO-SPINAL MENINGITIS.

By EDWARD MONTGOMERY, M. D.

This disease, under different names, has prevailed to a considerable extent, both in this country and in Europe, since the beginning of the present century. From the descriptions given by various writers of the fourteenth, fifteenth, sixteenth and seventeenth centuries, it is probable that it visited different parts of the old world, but of this we are somewhat uncertain, because of the absence of a very minute and comprehensive clinical history of the cases, and for the lack of post-mortem examinations. "The first well-authenticated epidemic of the disease in this country occurred in 1806, from which time until 1816, it was constantly epidemic, particularly in the New England States, upon which it seemed to fasten" (*Clymer*). From 1806 until the present time, partial epidemics and sporadic cases occasionally occurred both in the old and in the new world. In 1845 and 1846 it broke out in Illinois, and was there called "Black Tongue." In 1847 it prevailed in Mississippi, Tennessee, Missouri and

Arkansas, and during our late civil war it occurred occasionally in both armies (*Clymer*). In 1846, a very
severe epidemic of it broke out in the city of Dublin,
Ireland, where it principally prevailed in the work-
houses and hospitals although there were many fatal
cases in healthy parts of the city, and where many fell
victims to its virulence whose surroundings were unex-
ceptionable.

Dr. Simon of London, a very high authority, says,
that "soldiers in barracks, the inmates of jails and
poor-houses, the inhabitants of crowded, filthy streets,
and every place where filth and bad ventilation prevail,
are its favorite resorts." But in this country we know
that it has devastated little hamlets in the prairies, fastened its unrelenting grasp on the scattered denizens of
our newly-settled districts, and prevailed for years together in the healthiest portions of Pennsylvania and
Massachusetts. "Notwithstanding its wide geographical distribution, there is no corresponding diffusion
amongst any one population during its prevalence, it,
as a rule, being limited, during an outbreak, to certain
localities, and to certain portions of the population of
such localities. The distribution of the disorder seems
to be by a series of isolated eruptions, rather than by
general spreading" (*Clymer*).

This is one of its strange peculiarities and anomalies;
it will break out in certain neighborhoods, and in certain families in such neighborhoods, without our being
able to discover any cause for such predilection. Sometimes it will prostrate a whole family at once, and again
carry off one in a large family and the rest all escape ;
in this respect differing very much from cholera, influenza, or small-pox. Like cholera and influenza it

seems to be caused by some toxic principle in the atmosphere, and by it carried to different portions of the world; but unlike those epidemics, it does not appear to spread by contagion or infection; neither will the effluvia, emanations, or excrements, of the sick propagate the disease, as I have abundant evidence of the fact; often have I witnessed the small, close chamber, where a patient was dying, crowded with the neighboring children, and yet none of them becoming infected with the disease. Another peculiarity of the disorder is its varying symptomatology. In 1847, when it prevailed in Missouri, Mississippi, Tennessee and Arkansas, the fauces, throat, and respiratory organs were implicated to such an extent that it was called "black tongue," "typhoid pneumonia," etc. In 1846, in Dublin, the cases had nearly all an extensive purpuric eruption, so that Dr. Stokes and others termed it purpuric fever; whilst in other epidemics, in other parts of the world, the type of the disease seemed of a congestive character and so suddenly fatal, that it was called the "plague," the "*Malum Egyptiacum,*" etc. And again, as in the present epidemic in this city, the spine and brain symptoms so predominate that the term cerebro-spinal meningitis seems alone to be appropriate, and to be generally employed. The term "spotted fever" has also been given to it in different parts of this country, but all these names belong to the same disease, manifesting itself under different types and forms, nearly all exhibiting the same morbid anatomy—a congestion of blood in the expanded vessels of the cerebro-spinal system, with more or less effusion and exudation of serum, semi-organized lymph or pus, and sometimes softening of portions of the brain and cord. It is true that Dr.

Woodward, chief of the U. S. Army Medical Bureau,
says that many of the cases reported by different army
surgeons, during the war, to his office, presented no
signs of inflammation or structural lesion of any kind
in the brain, cord, or membranes, and that this exemption from morbid changes in those parts, is not to be
accounted for on the supposition that death had occurred too soon for those pathological appearances to
be developed, since this freedom from structural change
was also observed in cases where death had not ensued
suddenly.   But, on the whole, it is sufficiently evident
from the signs and symptoms during life, and from the
post-mortem evidences, that the cerebro-spinal system
is the part principally involved, or at least, that it is
there wherein the disease most forcibly manifests itself.
According to Stille, Clymer, Condie, Hirsch, Wunderlich, Neimeyer, Mayne and others, the morbid anatomy of the disease consists in an expansion of the
vessels of the cerebro-spinal system, a super-abundant
quantity of blood in those vessels; this congestion and
vascularity is especially seen in the pia mater, and when
the patient has died early in the disease; an increased
amount of clear, turbid or flocculent serum in the sub-
arachnoid space, and in the ventricles; even in cases of
the briefest duration there is an exudation of thick,
pasty, semi-organized lymph, of a greenish-yellow
color on the base of the brain and medulla oblongata;
the membranes at this stage are dry, and sometimes
adherent to the brain or to each other.   The cerebro-
spinal fluid is increased, and portions of both brain and
cord are found occasionally softened.   When the disease has lasted for some time, the cerebral exudation is
soft, opaque and yellowish, two or three lines in thick-

ness, and may be compared to soft butter spread over the brain; or it may be denser, and have a pseudo-membranous look. It is found chiefly along the course of the vessels, and small in quantity, limited to, and ramifying with them, or it may be in little irregular patches of variable size scattered over the brain surface, or covering the pons or medulla oblongata or cerebellum or parts of the cerebrum, or it may completely envelop the cerebrum, cerebellum and intracranial cord. Commonly superficial it may dip down with the pia mater among the convolutions, or be found in the ventricles, or hanging and thickening, with an opaque, greenish pus, the serous fluid of the whole cavity. Purulent infiltration of the choroid plexus, and superficial softening of the walls of the ventricles have been also observed (*Clymer*).

Pus, or purulent lymph, has also been found in the spinal canal, as well as in the base of the brain, in cases which have been somewhat tedious in their course. In nearly all the cases the expanded cerebro-spinal vessels have been found full of this black colored blood, and in some cases, fibrinous clots have been found in the heart after death (*Stille*).

As before intimated, this disease presents different forms or types in different epidemics, in different countries and even in the severe epidemic, and among the same class of patients. In some cases it is ushered in without any appreciable premonitory symptoms whatever, the patient being suddenly stricken down as by some fell poison, becomes delirious, tosses about for a few hours, tries to vomit every few minutes, with sighing and slow respiration, the skin dusky, the eyes suffused and sunken, and death by coma in ten to twenty-four hours. Occasionally these fulminant, blasting, or siderant cases, as they are variously termed, are accompanied with profuse diarrhœa, vomiting, and convulsions.

The tetanic form of the disease is more tedious in its progress, and of course more amenable to treatment; it is generally ushered in with chilliness, nausea, headache, frequently a general hyperæsthesia, or pains in some, or all of the joints, sometimes sore throat, with pains in the ears; although there is some thirst, and the mouth is dry, but sparing drinks will be indulged in, the patient soon becomes much worse, there will be great jactitation, the cephalalgia will become more intense, the eyes will become suffused and injected, the face flushed, the head drawn back, the pulse quick, the bodily temperature from 100° to 103° F.; a trembling of the extremities when the patient is moved, intolerance of light, pupils contracted at first, but when exudation has taken place the pupils may be dilated or irregular, and the pulse or temperature may be abnormally reduced. In some of the cases an erythematous, eczematous, or purpuric, a morbillous or herpetic eruption may appear; but an eruption of any kind is not present in one-third of the cases, hence the misnomer of spotted or purpuric fever. There is often great deafness, apathy, and in all cases early prostration. When the case is severe the patient is terribly racked with the cephalalgia and pain in the throat and upper part of the spine from the tetanic contractions; but a few minutes' rest at a time can be indulged in, the patient suddenly waking up with piercing cries or low moans and talkative delirium, or convulsions, or complete coma, may close the terrible sufferings. In tedious cases partial paralysis sometimes occurs, and the deafness occasionally remains permanent. Sometimes, also, vision is permanently impaired, and strabismus may result from the attack.

Dr. Kempf in writing about a severe epidemic of this disease which occurred in the spring of 1863, in Dubois, Spencer and Perry counties, Illinois, describes three forms which he names respectively, cerebro-spinal asphyxia, cerebro-spinal inflammation, and cerebro-spinal irritation, the first variety, he says, carried off the patients in many instances in a few hours, and no treatment seemed to have any effect. These fulminent cases were ushered in with chills, vomiting, diarrhœa, violent head-ache, soon followed by lethargy and extreme prostration, complete apathy, stupor as if profoundly intoxicated, the eyes suffused and injected, the skin covered with dark crimson or purple spots, coma and death. The inflammatory, or tetanic form, was also ushered in with chilliness, vomiting, headache, suffused countenance, injected eyes, apathy and debility. In a short time the the head was retracted, the throat and neck painful, the petechial or purpuric spots appeared, and if not cured, delirium, convulsions, or coma, closed the scene. For these cases the treatment was bleeding, purging, plenty of calomel, veratrum viride, quinine, camphor, and opium. The doctor says he thinks bleeding and counter-irritation does harm, but the other remedies he employed seemed to save some cases. For the third variety—the cerebro-spinal irritation—morphine and quinine were all that were necessary to insure convalescence. Dr. McVey of Morgan county, Illinois, reports his treatment for the disease as it appeared in 1863 and 1864 in that section of the State: it consisted in a moderate use of aperients and alteratives, friction to the spine and extremities, large doses of opium, four or five grains of opium with six or eight drops of Fowler's Arsenical Solution every four hours, blisters to the back of the neck, and if the cases were prolonged he also gave strychnine. He says this treatment proved rather successful, but we apprehend very few physicians would venture on such a free use of opium in this disease. Dr. Brown in the same region of country, also reports his meeting with much success from similar treatment. (Transactions of Ill. Medical Society.) Dr. Liddell reports some cases treated by him in the Washington City Hospital, in 1864, in which his favorite remedy was opium, and he attempts to account for the beneficent action of this drug on the ground that it has the effect of preventing effusion from serous membranes. In one of Dr. Liddell's reported cases the patient was seized with the disease whilst taking quinine for an attack of ague, from which he was convalescing. This does not speak well for the remedial virtues of quinine in cerebro-spinal meningitis.

In the April number of the *American Journal of the Medical Sciences* for the year 1864, there is an article by Dr. Burns, on this disease as it occurred in the vicinity of Philadelphia, in which he advocates leeches, venesection, frictions, blisters, purgatives and quinine. He reports the particulars of some very alarming cases which almost miraculously recovered under this antiphlogistic treatment. If we examine the pages of the *Medical Press and Circular* of Dublin for 1867, we will find many cases exact counter parts of those of Dr. Burns which died under a stimulating treatment. Dr. Black, of Newark, Ohio, in the same journal takes the opposite ground and protests against anti-phlogistics in all cases, and affirms his belief in the efficacy of tonics only. Indeed in looking over the medical journals for 1863, '64, '65, and '66, although, epidemics prevailing in different sections of the country during those years are presented to us with great uniformity of description, the same vivid picture of the malady being almost exactly reproduced in every instance, there is much contradiction and discrepancy with regard to the treatment.

Professor Wunderlich describes the disease as it appeared in Germany in 1863, its symptomatology and morbid anatomy as given by him is a counterpart of that delineated by numerous observers in this country. His treatment consisted in local depletion in sthenic cases, ice to the head, but not to the spine as there he observed it did more harm than good. Morphine he says allayed the pain in one case and it finally recovered, but chloroform inhalations and as a liniment was also used in the same case. Iodide of potassium was given in three cases which terminated in cure, he therefore recommends it, especially in protracted cases. He says there was no evidence of the disease being contagious or infectious.

Dr. Condie in his report of the diseases of Philadelphia county for the year 1864, in the transactions of the Pennsylvania State Medical Association, treating of this malady says that for the algid form he had tried alcoholic and diffusible stimulents with quinine, and externally used liniments, sinapisms, frictions, blisters, hot baths, etc., but without being convinced of their having the least good affect on the disease. For the tetanic form he chiefly relied on opium and quinine internally, and on frictions, liniments, blisters and dry cups along the spine, especially to the upper portion. An infusion of half an ounce each of cimicifuga, wild cherry bark, serpentaria and sassafras bark in a quart of boiling water; a wine-glass of this infusion every three hours seemed also to do much good.

Dr. Githens, in his report of the cases treated by him in 1866 and 1867 in the Philadelphia Hospital, says that his principal measures consisted in ice to head, blisters to nuchæ, veratrum viridi, carbonate or muriate of ammonia, spirits of nitre, stimulants and nutrients. He was in the habit of giving thirty-six ounces of whisky, and the same amount of beef tea in the twenty-four hours. In one or two cases out of the ninety-five treated he prescribed the *secale coruntum.*

In the *Medical Press and Circular* for June, 1867, we find the disease described as it occurred in Ireland, the treatment there generally adopted was brandy, beef-tea, carbonate of ammonia, musk, ether, belladonna, turpentine, and in a few cases quinine and iron. From the reports of the cases this highly restorative treatment proved very unsuccessful. On the other hand the French physicians bled their patients and had far greater success. Niemeyer in his monograph on the disease was also in favor of abstracting blood, and giving calomel freely, the latter to say the least, is of doubtful efficacy except as a purgative.

In our city, in 1863 and '64, Dr. Ira Russell reported a number of cases in the St. Louis Medical Journal, which occurred amongst the soldiers at Benton Barracks. About fifty cases had occurred at the time of his report, one half of whom had died. The treatment was, during the period of collapse, alcoholic stimulants, capsicum and quinine, mustard-emetics, and sinapisms to the surface. Opium seemed to exert a happy influence in controlling the delirium. After the reaction pillula hydrarg. and salines have been followed by good results, but as a general rule antiphlogistic treatment has been poorly borne. Cups to spine, iodide potass. and tonics are the best remedies in the advanced periods of the disease. It is curious to observe how very seldom the *secale coruntum* or the iodide of patassium was prescribed in former times although these seem now to be the favorite remedies with many practitioners. From the numerous reports of cases which I have examined I have been also surprised at the great differences of opinion with regard to the use of quinine and blood letting. Some believe that quinine is the main remedy, whilst others affirm that it never has a curative action, but often inflicts great injury, but I believe these discrepancies can all be reconciled when we reflect on the different types of the disease in different epidemics and in different localities. With regard to cupping, leeching and purgatives the same contrariety of opinion prevails, and may be explained in the same manner, for antiphlogistics will be salutary or pernicious according to the form and type of the disease, and the constitutional stamina of the patients. As before intimated, there is a great uniformity in the different reports I have examined as to the signs, symptoms, course of the disease and its morbid anatomy. One fact stands out prominently in all the reports of the symptoms, and that is the sudden apparent prostration of the patient, I say apparent prostration for I contend that this symptom here is the result of the poisoned condition of the blood, its engorgement in the vessels of the cebro-

spinal system and the resulting functional disorders of
respiration, digestion, sanguification, etc. The great
prostration so early existing in this disease is entirely
different, especially as an indication of treatment, from
the prostration resulting from loss of blood, from any
wasting evacuation, or from prolonged bad health. In
this disease the general debility is, in part, caused by a
redundancy of certain matters in the blood, and by an
engorgement or congestion of that diseased blood in
the vessels of the cerebro-spinal system whereby the
nerves supplying the organs of respiration, circulation,
digestion, etc., are seriously involved : whereas the
debility existing from loss of blood, from profluvia,
from long continued bad health, etc., results from want
of nutritive elements and from a wasting of the tissues.
Another fact which stands prominent in this disease and
which is noted by all observers, is the expanded condition of the blood vessels of the cerebro-spinal
system, and their engorgement with abnormally fluid
dark colored blood. Very often this is the only
morbid condition found on post-mortem examination,
although in most cases there is a superabundant
exudation, sometimes fluid like pure serum, sometimes
containing floculi, and sometimes a semi-organized
plastic material like butter, and again purulent lymph
or pure pus. Now taking these prominent facts into
consideration the indications of treatment seem to be
to endeavor to prevent that stasis or local engorgement if it has not already taken place, or to remove it
if it has; to prevent exudation, or obviate and resist
its evil results if it already exists, to restore the blood
to its normal healthy condition, and to assist the natural
vital processes so as to enable the system to bear up

under the deteriorating influences of the malady. In those cases resembling pernicions intermittent or congestive fever, the algid cases of Dr. Condie, hot water baths containing salt and mustard, frictions with tincture of capsicum and camphor, and the internal use of sulpho-carbolate of sodium, sulphurous acid, sulphite of soda permanganate and chlorate of potash, applying any of these which seems to agree best with the patient. These antiseptic remedies should correct the toxæmia existing, and with that view should be given freely, and frequently and in a chemically pure form. Small quantities should be prepared each day so that they would be always fresh and unchanged. As soon as they can be administered with any prospect of happy action, iodide of potassium and the fluid extract of ergot should be given, the former to promote the absorption of the exudation, and the latter to constringe the expanded blood vessels. Quinine and a small quantity of opium will also do much good in these algid cases, the former will greatly assist the anti-toxæmic remedies, and the latter will prove beneficial in the first stage of the disease from its power in preventing exudation. Of course nutrients will be necessary, but they should be of a fluid form, such as beef essence, rich milk, cream, soft boiled eggs, etc., etc. The great difficulty in this form of the disease, is that the whole system is so completely overwhelmed by the toxic power of the malady, that no remedy has the time or the power to act, death occurring so suddenly, or the processes of organic life so completely in abeyance that no effect is produced.

In the tetanic form of the disease, those cases which seem to be of a more inflammatory nature, besides the

hot bath, in the first stage, cups or leeches to the nuchæ
and down the spine, or behind the ears will be of
decided advantage. The form of purgative I have
thought best, has been calomel and jalap, some prefer
calomel and colocynth, or calomel and aloes, from the
belief that the colocynth and aloes have the effect of
acting on the lower intestines and as derivatives from the
brain. As there is often great nausea, and consequently
pugatives administered by the mouth may not be retained, in such conditions enemata of oil and turpentine, or decoction of aloes may be given. As soon as
the bowels are evacuated the antiseptics should be freely
given, and alternating with them the fluid extract of
ergot to resist the expansion and engorgement of the
blood vessels. The tincture or fluid extract of the
calabar bean has been recommended for the same purpose, but of that I have had no experience. I would rely
on the cups and leeches, the purgatives, and the ergot of
rye, to prevent the effusion of these tetanic or inflammatory cases, as I have witnessed severe coma to ensue after
the use of opiates, but whether *propter hoc* or merely post
hoc, may be a question to be decided in the future.
Instead of the cups or leeches and purgatives in these
cases, some recommend the veratrum veridi, but from
what I have experienced in my own cases, and from
what I have read of the results of the treatment by
others, I believe this powerful arterial sedative is contraindicated in this disease. Gelseminum and digitalis
have also been highly recommended by some, but I
have no experience with them in this affection. Quinine
combined with opium in the very beginning of the
disease, and without the opium in the commencement
of convalescence, will be found a valuable remedy,

but after the effusion has taken place, and as long as we have evidence of the existence of extensive exudation this alkaloid may prove a dangerous medicine. In the very commencement of the attack opium may do good in preventing effusion, but in all other periods of the disease it is a perilous appliance. The great hyperæsthesia, cephalalgia and mental disturbance will be more safely remedied by venesection, leeches or cups, purgatives, free doses of the bromide of potassium, warm baths, and frictions with a liniment composed of chloroform and tinctures of opium, aconite root, capsicum and camphor. After exudation has taken place the iodide of potassium will be found of essential service. I have witnessed numerous cases with slow intermittent pulse, deafness, slow breathing, irregular pupils, apathy and stupor, and in some partial paralysis, which happily recovered under the use of the iodide. Of course in these cases it would be well also to blister the nape of the neck, or over the mastoids.

In young children the bromide is often substituted for the iodide of potassium; in these young patients I am very decidedly opposed to opiates in any form of the disease, as coma will assuredly soon follow their administration. As before remarked, fluid nutrients should be frequently administered, and good ventilation and the best possible hygienic and sanitary measures should be sedulously carried out wherever this fearful scourge prevails.

I have cited the treatment adopted by different physicians in different epidemics, occurring in different countries, and from the comparative clinical statistics deducable from them, I am convinced that an opium treatment, a quinine treatment, or a stimulant and

highly restorative treatment, are all incompatible with
the true pathology of the disease.   That an extreme
antiphlogistic treatment would also be pernicious, I
have not the least doubt; and I also feel convinced that
veratrum viridi, aconite, gelseminum and calabar bean,
are hazardous remedies in this protean disease.   If
opium is to be used at all it should be in the very commencement of the attack; for the only reason that I can
discover for its employment, is its reputed powers of
preventing serous exudation; and if it is given after the
exudation has occurred, it will likely imperil the life of
the patient, by encouraging the full development of the
comatose condition.   In a disease characterized as this
is, by a congestion or engorgement of the blood vessels
of the cerebro-spinal system, I cannot see the rationale
of administering quinine, unless in cases complicated
with malaria and intermittent in their character, or as
a tonic in convalescence, when the congestion and exudation are both removed.   If we carefully examine the
results of a stimulating and restorative treatment, as detailed of the different epidemics in Massachusetts, in
Pennsylvania, in Ohio, in Illinois, in Missouri and in
Ireland, we will be horrified at the great mortality.   In
these different places we can see the detailed reports of
numerous cases of the tetanic form of the disease where
the patient lives long enough to permit the action of
medicine to take place, and yet the cases nearly all died
under quinine, opium and stimulants.   From sixty to
seventy-five per cent. died in these epidemics, whereas,
the rational and scientific treatment now adopted—this
treatment which is founded on a just recognition of the
pathology and morbid anatomy of the disease—will save
at least seventy per cent. of the cases.

To epitomize what we consider a rational and scientific treatment, we would say, that in the fulminant, siderant or blasting cases, and in those cases which run a rapid course, accompanied by purpuric eruptions, in other words, the variety which has been variously named, cold plague, malum Egyptiacum, black tongue, etc., and the form denominated spotted fever or purpuric fever, putrid fever, etc., we would use hot salt and mustard baths, chlorate or permanganate of potash, sulphurous acid, sulph. carbolate of sodium, bisulphite of soda, etc., and afterwards quinine and phosphoric acid. Chemical physicians have quite recently suggested the cautious trial of the carbazotate of ammonia in these algid forms of the disease, giving one-fourth of a grain, in the form of a small pill, every four hours. In the tetanic form of the disease, we would rely on sinapisms, hot baths, leeches, cups or venesections, ice to the head, frictions, free purgation, followed by opium, or opium and quinine in the commencement of the attack, the bromide and iodide of potassium, and the fluid extract of ergot ; the bromide and ergot to be given before the exudation, and the iodide afterwards. Quinine we would use, in all cases complicated with malaria, in the beginning of the disease, or as a tonic to assist in promoting a favorable convalescence after the exudation has been removed. To essay the mitigation of toxæmia, some of the antiseptic remedies alluded to may be advantageously administered during the early periods of the malady. Of course, the best possible sanitary and hygienic measures shonld be enforced, and the patient should be supported by fluid nutrients, and tonic medicines judiciously administered after the inflammatory symptoms have abated.

1316 Olive Street.

Hospital Reports.

ST. LOUIS (SISTERS') HOSPITAL.

Clinic of Prof. E. H. GREGORY, reported by Dr. CHARLES GARCIA.

Jan. 11th, 1873.—Case of scalp wound; happened a week ago.

Remarks.—This is a lacerated injury. The blow from the flat-iron has cracked the skull. I can feel the fracture; yet it has been sewed up! The bone is denuded. It is a popular practice to close wounds in the scalp, and when you deal with a simple incised injury, all is well; but if the surfaces are lacerated, treat them as similar wounds elsewhere,—expect them to heal from the bottom; and in incised wounds, if you put in sutures, and inflammation occurs, take them out at once. There is some depression in this case; the outer table is probably driven into the diploeic structure, making an impacted fracture. Injuries to the diploeic structure are sometimes serious; large veins are found in this part, and thrombosis and consequent embolism might ensue on these injuries. Injuries about the head are frequently complicated with erysipelas. We may say such injuries are never free from danger. The treatment consists essentially in keeping the head cool and bowels open; the brain must be inactive, otherwise the head is not cool.

A guarded prognosis always important.

TUMOR.—This young man comes here at my request; he has a tumor at the bend of the arm, which he first noticed twelve months ago. The patient is a healthy-looking young man. It was first noticed above the little point we call the internal condyle; was hard at first, and not fixed; did not seem to be a part of bone; and situated between the internal condyle and artery. Has been told it was an aneurism. It has never been sore or painful. There is a sense of fluctuation or elasticity, as the most delicate touch can hardly tell the difference, and the most erudite touches have been mistaken; hence, the exploring trocar. I must feel for enlarged lymphatics in the axilla. No decided enlargement. This tumor has been of rapid growth; the sarcomas grow rapidly, but do not involve the lymphatics; on the other hand the cancers early involve these vessels.

What simple growth could reach the dimensions here seen, in twelve months?

It is not aneurismal. I feel the pulsation of the artery as it passes over the tumor; it is not circumscribed, does not implicate the joint, but it extends above and below it; its limit is not well defined, it blends with the textures. Exploration would be proper before an operation. Patient says it has been explored, and grown faster since. It is a bad plan to explore before you are prepared to remove if necessary.

Jan. 2d, 1873.—Application of plaster-of-Paris splint to fracture of both thighs and left humerus.

Gus. Conant, aged fifteen, was caught by a revolving shaft and received a fracture of both thighs, of two or three ribs on the left side, the left forearm twisted off about two inches below the elbow joint, and humerus of same side broken at middle.

The fractured femurs were encased in plaster-of-Paris. Chloroform was used.

The stump and fractured humerus were enveloped in cotton wadding, and two or three roller bandages saturated with plaster, made all firm. A piece of adhesive plaster, three inches wide and a yard long, was then passed around the chest, over the fractured ribs. As both thighs were broken,, it was thought best to provide for the Buck extension, by arranging the usual adhesive plaster loop before applying the plaster bandage.

Jan. 9th.—Plaster casts are firmly set; the one on the arm had to be cut open the whole length, on account of pain caused by excoriations from previous temporary appliances. After applying the carbolized oil to raw surfaces, the plaster cast was again adjusted.

Jan. 10th.—The plaster-of-Paris is perfectly firm, and if only one thigh were broken he might be up and around the ward today.

The case progressed well for two weeks, when tetanus supervened, and after ten days of suffering the patient died.

Chloral hydrate, calabar bean, opium, and chloroform were used freely, nor were purgatives neglected, but all to no purpose.

Reviews and Bibliographical Notices.

A PRACTICAL TREATISE ON URINARY AND RENAL DISEASES IN-
CLUDING URINARY DEPOSITS.—Illustrated by numerous cases
and engravings. By William Roberts, M. D. Fellow of the
Royal College of Physicians, London ; Physician to the
Manchester Royal Infirmary ; Lecturer on Medicine in the
Manchester School of Medicine. Second American from the
second revised and considerably enlarged London edition,
Philadelphia. Henry C. Lea, 1872, pp. 616. 8vo. preceded
by a plate of nine colors.

[For sale by the St. Louis Book & News Co.]

The first London edition as well as the American reprint of
1865, were exhausted some years since, and a second edition has
been looked for which has now come to hand. Many new
additions have been made ; two articles on suppression of
urine and on paroxysmal hæmatinuria have been added, and
some of the old engravings have been replaced by better ones,
and the list increased by twenty new ones.

The works are divided into three parts : I. The *physical and
chemical properties of the urine in health and disease*—urinary
deposits, under this we have four chapters : introduction ;
physical properties of the urine ; inorganic deposits ; and
organic deposits, all conveniently arranged under proper
sections. Part II. *Urinary Diseases*—diseases of which the
chief characteristic is an alteration of the urine ; diabetes insipidus ; diabetes mellitus ; gravel and calculus ; chylous urine.
Part III. *Organic diseases* of the *kidneys*, congestion of the kidneys ; Bright's disease ; acute Bright's disease ; chronic Bright's
disease ; suppuration in the kidneys, renal embolism ; pyelitis
and pyonephrosis ; concretions in the kidneys ; hydronephrosis ;
etc., etc.

In part I. chapter IV. sec. 7 our author gives us an account
of hæmatinuria—paroxysmal hæmatinuria (syn. intermittent
hæm.) The fact has been pointed out by Vogel, Appolzer,
and Mettenheimer that the coloring matter of the blood
(hæmatin) escaped at times with the urine (false hæmaturia)
without rupture of the capillaries ; the urine in these cases
always contains albumen, but no blood corpuscles. This con-

dition may be the result of disease, or may be artificially produced by poisonous gasses, such as arseniuretted hydrogen, by which a condition is produced known as "a dissolved state of the blood."

Dr. George Harley, as early as 1865, called attention to Hæmatinuria by the publication of two cases; since that time other cases have been published, and the author has collected, together with his own, twenty cases from which he has drawn his conclusions. "The disorder is essentially intermitting or paroxysmal in its nature. Each paroxysm begins with a feeling of cold or shivering, resembling the cold fit of ague, and terminates with discharge of a very dark bloody looking urine. The symptoms then subside, and the urine of the next micturition or the one after, is found to have resumed its natural healthy appearance." * * * "In some cases the paroxysm recurs once a day, or even twice and thrice a day. More commonly it recurs on alternate days, or twice a week, or once in ten days, or quite irregularly. The paroxysms are not followed by any hot or sweating stage. The onset of a paroxysm is usually sudden, the patient first experiences coldness of the extremities, followed by general chilliness which in most cases passes with distinct rigors, accompanied by a feeling of malaise, a disposition to stretch himself and to yawn. In most cases, a sense of weight, or a dull heavy pain is felt in the loins, sometimes extending to the umbilicus, or passing down the thighs; and there is frequently pain, or a feeling of stiffness or weakness in the lower extremities. Retraction of the testicles has been noted in several cases. Retching is a not unfrequent symptom, and vomiting was a prominent feature in one case. After these symptoms have lasted for a period varying from thirty minutes to two hours, the patient passes a quantity of dark-colored urine; the pain and general disturbance then subsides, leaving the patient apparently quite well till the next paroxysm." The urine has generally "the color of porter or of the darkest port wine." The sp. gr. "usually ranging from 1022 to 1025," and is "either acid or faintly alkaline," and "is always highly albuminous." In the chocolate colored sediment which falls after the urine has been standing for a time, Gull found numerous small crystals of hæmatine.

" Casts of tubes are also present;" and " very rarely a few stray blood-discs." The first onset "can generally be traced to some distinct exposure to cold or wet." The temperature is, during the paroxysm, generally below normal—from 96° to 97°. Of the twenty cases only four had suffered at some time from ague. The prognosis is favorable, none of the twenty having died, thus differing essentially from the structural diseases which generally furnish casts.

The *Etiology* is pretty well understood. In most of the cases the disease was clearly attributable to vicissitudes of temperature or exposure to wet. The pathology however, is very obscure. Though hæmatinuria seems to be connected in some way with ague, yet its nature is, as yet, not known. " Though related they are not identical, as in by far the greater number of cases there has been neither an aguish tendency nor any evidence of exposure to malarial influences." In the *treatment*, hygienic measures seem no less important than medicines. " In two of the reported cases the attacks seem to have passed off without any medicinal treatment, simply by exposure to cold. In one case, recorded by Dr. Dickinson, cupping over the loins, vapor baths, gallic acid, quinine, iron in various forms were tried in succession, but nothing seemed to affect the disorder; 'the hæmorrhage always ceased on the removal of the cold which caused it.' " Dr. Beal attaches much importance to giving quinine in full doses, not less than six grains. " During the paroxysm, Dr. Ritchie found the best treatment was to send the patient to bed, apply artificial heat, and administer warm stimulating drinks such as hot brandy and water. The evidence generally is strongly in favor of quinine and iron as the most effective medicinal agents." Under *diabetes* insipidus, page 203, (polydepsia, polyuria) he draws his conclusions from seventy-seven cases of this rather rare disease, five of which were under his own observation. The disease is found much more frequently in males than in females; " of the seventy-seven cases fifty-five were males, and twenty-two females." It may affect any age. "In a very large proportion no *exciting cause* whatsoever could be assigned for the disorder." The following is a list of the alleged causes in some of these cases :

Cerebral disease (tubercle, etc.) - - -	9.
Hereditary influence, - - - -	3.
Blows on the head and falls, - - -	6.
Muscular effort, - - - - - -	2.
Intemperance, - - - - -	5.
Exposure to hot sun, - - -	1.
Exposure to cold and drinking, mental emotion,	1.
Previous febrile or inflammatory disease, -	5.

"In some of the traumatic cases, the symptoms set in with maximum intensity on the very day of the accident," in others at a later date. The quantity is generally greater than in diabetes mellitus, but the specific gravity is much lower, ranging from 1003 to 1007.

The *duration* is very uncertain, and would seem to depend upon the continuance of the structural lesion; the traumatic cases generally only lasted a few weeks or months; a congenital case, however, lasted fifty-nine years, another fifty years, at the date of the record.

In ten cases of post-mortem examinations, the conditions found were similar in three, namely: "atrophied and degenerated condition of the renal substance." The others showed, in the fourth, the glandular tissue *entirely wanting*; in the fifth, multiplex abscesses were found in the kidneys; in two cases the kidneys were simply hyperæmic and somewhat enlarged, and a tumor was found in the brain; in two cases fatty degeneration of the nervous tissue of the walls of the fourth ventricle was found.

Page 217. "It may be regarded as probable, that the *immediate* anatomical cause of polyuria is a dilatation of the renal capillaries, whereby their walls are thinned and rendered favorable to increased transudation of watery fluid from the blood." The author asks the question, how this condition is brought about. There are many reasons for supposing the disease to depend largely upon some lesion of the nervous system.

"The gravity of the *prognosis* in a particular case depends on the severity of the general symptoms, and on the presence or absence of complications." Among the remedies used in the *treatment* of this disease, are nitrate of potash to diminish the thirst and diuresis, but it must be given in large doses. Vale-

rian as extract, or valerianate of zinc, has been apparently productive of good effects.   An electrical current passed through
the lumbar and hypochondrial regions has also been followed
by good results.

We like the work, and for the use of the general practitioner
can recommend it highly. It comes from the pen of an observer
and diligent worker, who describes what he has seen, as well as
what has been seen by others so far as seems to be necessary to
a clear statement of the different diseases of which he has undertaken to give an account.

The plates are generally very judiciously selected and well
executed.   The paper and type are clear and excellent.

H. Z. G.

DISEASES OF THE OVARIES.   Their Diagnosis and Treatment.
  By T. Spencer Wells. New York : D. Appleton & Co. 1878.
  pp. 478.
            [For sale by the St. Louis Book and News Co.]

Owing to the excellent arrangements made by the publishers,
this valuable work, which but lately appeared in England, is
now before the profession in America, as well as on the continent of Europe, thus widely diffusing the experience gained by
this greatest of all ovariotomists.

The American edition, a fac-simile of the English, is a hand-
some octavo volume of 478 pages, containing 397 well-executed
wood cuts.

Notwithstanding the recent appearance of the works of Atlee
and of Peasly, Wells' Diseases of the Ovaries is none the less
welcome, none the less important.   Atlee's very full, but as yet
incomplete work, the result of the personal observation of between two and three hundred cases, is mainly confined to the
subject of diagnosis.   Peaslee's is a complete and scientific treatise, but supported by a comparatively small number of cases.

The work of Spencer Wells, based upon the careful consideration of his five hundred cases of completed ovariotomy, combines the advantages of both; it is a treatise complete in all its
points, which can be put into the hands of the student; and beyond that it is a safe and valuable guide for the practitioner, as
the experience of Mr. Wells is more than twice that of even
Atlee, and his success must guarantee. It was *his* success which

has done so much to make ovariotomy an acknowledged operation on the continent of Europe, as he has proved it less dangerous than many of the capital operations, having saved three
hundred and seventy-three of the five hundred patients (14.6
p. c.), outdone only by Bradford and Keith, who, however, have
a much smaller number, probably of picked cases.

The work begins with a chapter of anatomical and physiological notes on the pelvic organs; and here Mr. Wells commits
a serious mistake in the statement he makes with regard to the
relation between the peritoneum and the ovary; an error which
it is all the more important to point out, as the weight of Mr.
Wells' authority might easily lead to the acceptance of his theory by those who have not studied the subject most carefully.
We are sorry to see that our author still clings to the old views
which were exploded by the brilliant investigations of Waldeyer, whose discoveries were soon verified by the most eminent of German workers.

Mr. Wells says that the ovary is covered by a peritoneal coat,
incomplete, "deficient at the border which is directed towards
the anterior layer of the broad ligament, where the blood vessels pass in and out of the hilus." Whereas, observation, microscopic as well as macroscopic, convinces us that the peritoneum stops abruptly near the centre of the organ, so that at
least half of the ovary projects into the abdominal cavity as a
free structure; this fact, not only "materially affects some physiological doctrines," but the author's view leads him into serious errors in this, as well as in the following chapter, on morbid anatomy and pathology of the ovaries. So in his classification of ovarian tumors he pays no attention to the very important relation of the peritoneum to the growth; and moreover,
with his view of the case, it would be difficult to explain the
development of his fourth class of extra ovarian tumors as he
does: "cysts, developed from aberrant ova attached to the peritoneal surface." It is a point we need not enter upon, as the
origin of these cysts, according to the latest and most searching
investigations, is a different one from that ascribed to them by
Mr. Wells. They spring, not from aberrant ova, but from remnants of the germinal epithelium, forming the coating of the
ovary in its extra-peritoneal part.

Though he mentions these small cysts as extra ovarian tumors, he entirely omits a class of tumors not unfrequently observed, springing from the intra-peritoneal portion of the ovary, and growing down between the layers of the broad ligament, gradually stretching the pedicle which links it to the ovary, until all but traces of it are lost, so that the cyst really becomes extra-ovarian, situated between the layers of the broad ligament, and as such they are classed, confounded with these cysts which originate there. Park's theory he justly discredits.

The very careful consideration of the pathological condition is followed by an examination of the contents of ovarian cysts, closing with an excellent statement of their microscopic and microchemical nature; our author knows nothing of the ovarian glemerulus, or the ovarian granular cell, which Atlee deems peculiar to ovarian fluids, and a sure means of diagnosis. We find bodies pictured and described which correspond to those found by Atlee, but they are not considered as characteristic and peculiar to these fluids, and justly not, for the day of the specific cell, of 'the "cancer cell," and the "tubercle cell" is passed; nor can an ovarian cyst produce a cell peculiar to it. Most valuable is the thorough discussion of the diagnosis (pp. 117–236) clear and concise, with a separate consideration of the most important states and diseases which may throw a doubt on the consideration of a case of ovarian tumor. The method of physical diagnosis by inspection and measurement, by palpation, by percussion and auscultation, is given step by step.

Interesting are the cases of hysterical tympanites cited. The note book appended is a practical statement to the physician of the author's method of procedure.

To the medical treatment of ovarian tumors, seldom more than momentarily palliative he justly gives but little consideration.

Tapping he speaks of more at length, preferring the tapping through the abdominal wall with the syphon-trocar which he considers but little dangerous, and in cases of thin walled, unilocular cysts offering a possibility of a radical cure, the tables show that tapping which is often a useful prelude to ovariotomy but little affects the mortality of the operation.

Iodine injections he thinks much more dangerous, and hardly more effective than simple tapping.

The most important part of the work is of course that devoted to the operation itself, and not only those who have seen the quiet, sure, yet rapid, hand of Spencer Wells guiding the knife with unerring precision, but all who have followed the progress of ovariotomy, who know his great ability must follow him here with implicit confidence, nor does our author attribute too much of the success to the operator, he speaks most pointedly of the cases fit for operation, the preparation of the patient, the locality for the operation, and the nurse, for upon her devolves a most important duty, above all in the after treatment.

The instruments used are simple, and few, no such variety as we have seen in the hands of French ovariotomists; but of great consequence is the anæsthetic employed, and much of his success Mr. Wells attributes to the bichloride of methylene, which he has used since his two hundred and twenty-ninth operation, administered with Dr. Junker's neat aparatus.

Though we ourselves have used chloroform almost exclusively in surgical and obstetrical operations, we became a convert to chloromethyl after we had seen it in the hands of Mr. Wells' assistants.

In the treatment of the pedicle the extra-peritoneal method and the clamp is preferred by Mr. Wells to all others, after having given them a fair trial, yet our author justly tells us that we must operate in a manner to suit each individual case, so, for a very short, broad pedicle one may occasionally be forced to adopt the intra-peritoneal treatment.

The fairness of the work is marked by the tables given of the twenty-four cases in which exploring incisions were made, and of those twenty-eight cases in which ovariotomy was commenced but not completed, and we heartily thank Mr. Wells for having put into our hands this volume,—characterised by the simple truthfulness which pervades it—based upon an experience gained in so large a number of cases in which he performed the operation with astonishing success, success not only with regard to mortality, but also with regard to the consequent good health and happiness of the patient.   G. J. E.

BOOKS AND PAMPHLETS RECEIVED.

MEDICAL AND SURGICAL HISTORY OF THE WAR OF THE REBELLION—Part First, in two volumes quarto. Surgeon General's office, Washington, D. C.

SYPHILIS—Treatment with subcutaneous sublimate injections. By Dr. G. Lewin. Philadelphia: Lindsay & Blakiston. 8vo. pp. 249. Price $2.50. For sale by the St. Louis Book & News Co., St. Louis.

RENAL, URINARY AND REPRODUCTIVE ORGANS—Functional diseases of. By D. Campell Black, M. D., L. R. C. S., Edin. Philadelphia, Lindsay & Blakiston. 8vo. pp. 300. Price $2.25. For sale by the St. Louis Book & News Co.

MENINGITIS, CEREBRO-SPINAL EPIDEMICS—By Meredith Clymer, M. D. Philadelphia: Lindsay & Blakiston. Price $1.00. For sale by the St. Louis Book & News Co.

ARCHIVES OF SCIENCE—For June and April, vol. No. 6. Published at McIndoc's Falls, Vermont, by J. M. Currier, M. D. Price $2.50 per. vol.

PROCEEDINGS OF THE AMERICAN ASSOCIATION FOR THE CURE OF INEBRIATES—For 1870 and 1871. Published by H. B. Ashmead, Philadelphia Pa.

SURGERY, ERICHSEN's NEW AMERICAN EDITION—Being a Treatise on Surgical Injuries, Diseases and Operations. Illustrated by 700 engravings. Philadelphia: Henry C. Lea. 2 vol. 8vo. pp. 780 and 981. For sale by the St. Louis Book & News Co.

ANNUAL REPORT OF THE BOARD OF HEALTH TO THE GENERAL ASSEMBLY OF LOUISIANA—With charts and Illustrations. New Orleans 1873.

HOOPING COUGH—Treatment with Quinine. By B. F. Dawson, M. D. Reprinted from the Amer. Journal of Obst. Feb. 1873. New York: Wm. Wood & Co.

TRANSACTIONS OF THE STATE MEDICAL SOCIETY OF MICHIGAN—For the year 1872. Lansing: W. S. George & Co., Printers.

TRANSACTIONS OF THE MEDICAL SOCIETY OF THE STATE OF WESTERN VIRGINIA. 1872. Wheeling; Frew, H. L. & H., Printers.

Proceedings of the St. Louis Medical Society.

At a meeting of the St. Louis Medical Society, held at their Hall, Polytechnic Building, on March 8th, 1873, it was said concerning—

CEREBRO-SPINAL MENINGITIS,

that its first recorded appearance in the United States, was in 1806, at Medfield, Mass.

Although it has usually prevailed as an epidemic, limited, or extensive, many *sporadic* cases are recorded. The symptom most characteristic of the disease, is the suddenness of the attack of indisposition in the midst of apparent good health. In a large majority of instances, without premonitory symptoms, sickness at the stomach and vomiting, with a sudden seizure of pain in the head and back; in some cases the force of the disease is chiefly expended on the brain, in others on the spinal cord, but the whole system is affected from the first. The headache is severe, and commonly occipital, extending to the nape of the neck, at the same time, pain in the joints and calves of the legs, likened to that of rheumatism, and stiffness of the jaws and neck, face suffused and eyes bloodshot, intellect dull, with remitting delirium, or *raving* delirium, has speedily supervened in some cases. In from a few hours to a day or two an eruption is observed usually, to appear first on the neck, then back, body and limbs, exceptionally on the *face*. The eruption is apparently due to congestion or extravisation of blood, causing dark red or purple spots, from the size of a pin head to that of a nickel; not raised, neither do they fade on pressure. The eruption is not constant.

It may appear after the second day or at death, and it has appeared after death. This eruption has been variously designated as purpuric, petechial, or rubeoloid.

The pulse may be quick and feeble, or little changed; likewise the breathing may be natural or slow, oppressed and sighing.

The muscles of the nape of the neck become rigid, the head thrown back, which symptom or condition, is perhaps most constant, and may extend to the muscles of the back, amounting to oposthotonos and trismus; it is usual for some twitching of the muscles to precede this condition.

The temperature has been recorded by different observers from 102° to 110° F. Numerous variations have been described by different authors, as applying to different epidemics.

The disease has prevailed in this country at all seasons of the year, but most frequently in the winter and early spring.

It has not respected age, as both the infant and octogenarian have been alike its victims; neither does it appear to have been influenced by sex, in some epidemics, women, in others, men seem to have suffered most.

The duration of the disease is short, *some* dying within twenty-four hours, and *most* within four days, who die. A slower progress is more hopeful.

It seems not to have been limited to any particular quarters or condition. The rich and poor, the well fed and poorly fed, have alike been attacked. In rural districts and city, on low lands and elevated; no point can claim exemption.

The weight of authority is decidedly against its being contagious, but due to some specific morbific agent in the atmosphere, not "malarial."

Inferior animals, dogs, pigs, and rabbits have been observed to take the disease, and die in convulsions.

Dr. Hartshorn says, "more than half of the cases have proved fatal thus far." (*Practic.*) Others estimate from 70 to 30 per cent. die, varying with the malignancy or mildness of the particular epidemic.

The inflammation of the membranes of the brain and spinal cord seems incidental to the disease, and not to constitute the disease, which in many instances destroys life prior to the establishment of inflammation, as shown by numerous post-mortems.

It would seem that the poison, the nature of which is unknown, acts primarily on the blood, impairing its vitality and integrity. Hence, the term cerebro-spinal meningitis has been objected to, as diverting the attention from the real nature of the disease to an incidental pathological condition, which is by no means constant. We prefer the name malignant purpuric fever, given to it by Dr. Stokes.

The antidote to the poison, if one exists in nature, has not yet been discovered; neither is it certain that the poison may be eliminated from the body.

The indications of treatment seem to be, to hold in check the distressing symptoms, selecting remedies on general principles, and from their known therapeutic effects in other diseases.

To equalize the circulation, the hot bath has been advised for a few moments. When the reaction is attended with much exaltation of temperature, sponging off the body with cool water and ice to the head has been approved.

Opium is king here as in many other diseases; that is, it is in better favor, and has stood the test of trial in the great variety of cases better than any other drug, being generally well borne in large doses.

Bromide of potass., we would expect good from, but the evidence so far is conflicting.

Quinine has many advocates, but the evidence concerning it, is conflicting.

The cases reported by the several gentlemen who had treated the disease recently, *varied* somewhat; a dose of calomel early in the disease was spoken well of by some who had tried it, also quinine, either by the mouth, or when not retained in the stomach, by the *rectum*, seemed to have been useful in some cases; opium, bromide of potass., chloral hydrate, cups, or leaches to the nape of the neck, hot bath to the lower part of the body, and cold to the head, to overcome the congestion and divert the action of the poison from the nerve centres, with stimulants and nutrients, to sustain the vital powers until the force of the poison is broken, exhausted, or eliminated, were acknowledged indications of first importance. The use of mercurials in so rapid a disease, and when the sources of sensation are so liable to be partially suspended, rendering the action of any medicine uncertain, was seriously questioned, that if useful at all, in the after treatment to remove the consequences or products of the primary inflammation.

15

Extracts from Current Medical Literature.

Eucalyptus Globulus in cases of Intermittent Fever.

Dr. Heller has administered the eucalyptus globulus in doses of from two to seven drachms of the tincture to 432 patients affected with intermittent fever. In 310 cases eucalyptus alone was employed. A small dose was enough to effect a cure in 202 instances, whilst only 108 required a second dose. In 122 cases the drug was employed conjointly with quinine.—*Lond. Lancet.*

Treatment of Pneumonia.—Sixty cases. Reported (by Dr. E. L. Drake, of Whitesboro, Texas), in the *Medical and Surgical Reporter.*

In cases complicated with enlarged spleen, and pleuritic pain, he gives large doses of quinia and morphia with good results. Veratrum viride was given in the early stages. Blisters and expectorants resorted to in nearly all cases. In three of the sixty cases treated, mercury was used in alterative doses; in these convalescence was slower, and typhoid symptoms more prominent. From his observation of the practice of physicians who hold mercury in favor in this disease, he believes it invites a train of typhoid symptoms. In three-fourths of his cases convalescence was fairly established in nine days, often much earlier if quinia was given in the congestive stage; seven of the sixty cases proved fatal.

Abortive Treatment of Boils and Felons.

We find quoted from the *Giorn. dell Accad. Med. di Torino* the following method of treating boils and felons, which Dr. Simon regards as almost infallible: Wherever the boil may be, and of whatever size, so long as suppuration has not commenced, rub it gently with the finger wet with camphorated alcohol, pressing especially on its centre. Do this half a minute at a time, for seven or eight times, and then cover the part with camphorated olive oil. If one operation does not produce resolution, repeat it at intervals of six hours. A felon may be bathed ten minutes in camphorated alcohol, then dried and covered with the oil. The writer has never known a felon fail to succumb to three of these operations.—*Gaz. Med. Ital.*—*N. Y. Med. Journal.*

Chloral for Toothache.

Dr. Page, in the *British Medical Journal*, recommends chloral hydrate as a local application in cases of toothache. A few grains of the solid hydrate introduced into the cavity of the tooth upon the point of a quill speedily dissolves there, and in the course of a few minutes, during which a not unpleasant warm sensation is experienced, the pain is either deadened, or more often effectually allayed. A second or third application may be resorted to if necessary.—*The Druggist's Circular and Chemical Gazette.*

Various anodynes will answer the same purpose. Among others, iodoform in one grain doses is a very efficient remedy for dental and facial neuralgia.—*Medical Cosmos.*—*Boston Med. and Surg. Journal.*

Local Uses of Tannin.

Dr. G. P. Hachenberg, *New York Medical Record*, reports several cases of the use of this remedy in prolapsus uteri, where other means had failed to afford relief. His method is as follows: A glass speculum is introduced into the vagina, so as to push the uterus into its place. Through the speculum a metallic tube or syringe, with the end containing about thirty grains of tannin, is passed. With a piston the tannin is pushed against the uterus, the syringe withdrawn, and the packing neatly and effectually completed with a dry probang, around the mouth and neck of the womb. After the packing is completed, the probang is placed against the tannin, in order to hold it, and the speculum is partially withdrawn. The packing is now fully secured, and the instrument removed.

The application of tannin holds the uterus firmly and securely in place, not by dilatation of the walls of the vagina, but by corrugating and contracting its parts. At first the application may be made weekly; finally, but once or twice a month. It not only overcomes the hypertrophy and elongation of the cervix, but even, the writer thinks, induces a slight atrophy of the parts. As a remedy for leucorrhœa, where the

seat of the inflammation is at the mouth of the womb, or within
the vagina, it actually gives speedy relief. The doctor also
reports a case of chronic ulceration of the rectum which was
cured after a few weekly packings of tannin. He has found,
moreover, that in affections of the throat, direct applications of tannin to the diseased parts give satisfactory results.
In a case of extraordinary hypertrophy of the tonsils, preparatory to the operation of extirpation, tannin mixed with tincture
of iodine to the consistency of syrup, was applied with effect
of so diminishing the hypertrophy that a surgical operation,
will, in all probability, not be necessary.

No remedy has given such satisfactory results in certain
forms of chronic ophthalmia and opacity of the cornea, as
tannin once a week placed under the eye lids—pure well
triturated tannin. An aged lady, who had chronic ophthalmia,
was relieved by one application; another, who was blind from
opacity of the cornea and chronic ophthalmia, recovered her
sight mainly from the local use of powdered tannin.—*Boston
Med. and Surg. Journal.*

On the Treatment of Enteric or Typhoid Fever.

Dr. Little remarks that the standard text-books on the treatment of this disease are not sufficiently explicit, and in fact all
is not stated that can be done in cases of typhoid fever. The
opinions that he now expresses are founded on treatment of
his own cases. Next to early confinement to bed, which perhaps
more than anything else lessens the severity and risk of the
fever, he ranks the rigid exclusion of animal broths and jellies
from the food, as tending to keep the disease mild. In this
point he finds himself at variance with the text-books, in which
such articles as beef-tea and Leibig's essence of meat are recommended. Milk should be the chief article of diet in enteric
fever. Thirsty patients sometimes object to its mawkish taste,
and in that case ice should be added, and a little lime-water in
cases where it returns curdled. Junket or renneted milk, given
before it has separated into whey, and curd, rice milk, custard,
baked custard in small quantities, rusks and hot milk, and
blanc-mange, generally afford sufficiently varied ways of giving
milk. Freshly made chicken jelly is less liable than beef-tea to
increase the abdominal symptoms, in those cases where milk

even with lime-water disagrees; but Dr. Little finds that this is a very rare occurrence, and when encountered is usually in a person chronically dyspeptic. For years he has made the administration of two or three cups of really good tea or coffee, between day-break and two in the afternoon, a regular part of the treatment in every case of fever, unless there was in the state of the nervous system some evident contra-indication. This he recommends in consequence of the well-known observations of Dr. Parkes on the effect of coffee in increasing the elimination of urea in fever; and Dr. Little finds that both it and tea lessen drowsiness and prostration, and increase the secretion of urine : once or twice in the day they may be given, poured upon a well-whisked egg, and thereby an additional means of nourishing the patient is obtained. Dr. Little considers that alcoholic stimulants in any quantity are seldom needed. Cold baths he thinks serviceable : three, or at most four, may be given in the twenty-four hours. In severe cases he has used them with great benefit, where cooing and wheezing râles exist in the chest, and where deficiency in the percussion-resonance posteriorly and muco-crepitus indicated postural stasis in the lungs, but not when there was hemorrhage from the bowels, or such pain as to justify the fear that peritonitis existed. When there is slight chilliness in the extremities after a bath, and shivering, this indicates that it should not be a prolonged one, but does not forbid its use. Twice Dr. Little has considered it unsafe to continue the baths—once because a marked shivering followed, and once because the patient was alarmed by it. In cases of the disease running a mild course, it is not necessary to have more than one bath in the day, at the height of the usual evening paroxysm of fever. By a dietary such as has been described, and the systematic employment of baths, the severity and danger of enteric fever may be greatly diminished, and the occurrence of any of the serious accidents incidental to the complaint rendered very rare, but the period of duration is not shortened. Besides these means, Dr. Little has found others beneficial under certain conditions. When during the first eight days the face is flushed, and there is headache, a high temperature, and a thickly coated tongue, and when the evacuations, three or four in the twenty-four hours, are neither very large nor very liquid, a dose of calomel, from four to six grains perceptibly lessens the heaviness of the fever. He has sometimes given the calomel a second time after an interval of a day or two, but never oftener. In enteric fever it is not uncommon to find a patient lying on his back, perceptibly impeded in his breathing, his abdomen tumid and projecting, but not markedly tender; and on inquiry it will be found either that the bowels have not acted for twelve hours, or that, though the stools are frequent, only a very little fæcal matter with wind passes each time. In these cases much relief may be obtained by giving a draught containing two drachms of castor oil with one or two of turpentine. Poultices and fomentations he has not found useful. By keeping patients rigidly to the diet mentioned, it is not found necessary to give medicines to check looseness of the bowels: when it is necessary to interfere, the most useful remedy is a pill containing one-sixth of a grain of carbolic acid, one-sixth of a grain of opium, and three grains of bismuth. Another remedy is sulphuric acid. Hemorrhage from the bowels is rare when milk diet and cold baths are employed; when it occurs, gallic acid, a scruple every second or third hour, and turpentine, were the remedies upon which he relied. Since ergotin has been shown to possess the power of arresting hemorrhage, administered hypodermically, Dr. Little has tried it in one case successfully. There is a group of nervous phenomena sometimes present in typhoid fever, for which the remedy is a full dose of quinine. For delirium and wakefulness with severe headache, cutting the hair and leeches are the remedies. Nausea and persistent retching may be relieved by an emetic of ipecacuanha or ice, or a draught containing ten grains of bicarbonate of soda, ten grains of carbonate of bismuth, and four minims of prussic acid. Scantiness of urine requires dry cupping of the loins, and the internal use of the salts of potash and spirit of nitrous ether. Indications of pulmonary congestion, which are sufficiently common in enteric fever, are best relieved by a turpentine stupe.—(*Dublin Journal of Medical Science*, Nov. 5, 1872.)—*London Practitioner.*

The use of the Poultice and Vapor of Water in Pneumonia—Cases.—"SAN RAFAEL CLINIQUE."

Pneumonia being in all climates a grave disease, and one which, however treated, results not unfrequently in death, has been treated in almost every conceivable way and success claimed by the advocates of every kind of practice.

It is not the purpose of this article to discuss the merits of the different forms of treatment, nor the pathology of the disease, but rather to call attention to an agency not in such general use as it should be, namely : moisture, and to its application to the inflamed lung, both from within and without. Surgery has for many years ceased to irritate an inflamed surface, has cast aside the old-fashioned dressings, the ointments and cerates, and now only covers the part with a wet rag; if warmth is needed, lays over it a piece of oil silk. Medicine still, we think, tries in many roundabout ways to accomplish that which simple means alone are able, if properly used, to do. If we conceive pneumonia as a local inflammation, and call surgery to our aid, she doubtless would direct us to keep the parts moist, to surcharge the air that reaches the inflamed surface with moisture, to prevent changes of temperature, to relieve the organ of labor, to give it rest, to relieve the congestion by a removal of blood, if possible, from the part inflamed by posture, by acting on the bowels with salines, and by causing the skin to act freely, and in any other way that we can without too much weakening the general system. The following cases will illustrate some of the points of treatment alluded to :

CASE I.—Called to see Miss A., *æt* 18. Her history showed me that she had a fairly healthy constitution. After exposure to cold she had been seized with her present illness, the respiration was frequent (about 35 if I remember correctly), and pulse quick and counting 130; on examining the chest I found dullness over the lower two-thirds of the left lung and fine crepitation could be heard. *Diagnosis*, pneumonia in its first stage. *Prognosis*, everything considered, favorable. Ordered a poultice of ground flax seed sufficiently large to cover the whole of one side of the chest, with oil silk stitched to its outer side, and tape to keep it even with the shoulder. The doors being closed, the room was filled with steam by putting hot bricks into a pan of water, and the clothing being removed, the poultice was applied. A blanket was next so arranged about the head of the bed that a current of vapor could be kept up which would charge the air she breathed, without itself striking against her person, the steam was generated by a spirit lamp with a large wick burning under a tripod supporting a shallow tin dish containing water, and the whole covered by a tin hood, perforated at the sides for air to enter, and connected at the top with a three-inch jointed tube. By means of an elbow the steam could readily be carried wherever needed. I then gave directions that the steam should be kept up night and day. The bowels being constipated and the tongue coated, five grains of blue mass were ordered to `be followed in the morning by a saline aperient, and to commence with a mixture of equal parts of sp. etheris nitr. and liq. ammoniæ acet. with $\frac{1}{16}$ of a grain of tartrate of potass and antimony. One teaspoonful to be táken every three hours. Soon after these arrangements had been completed, she expressed herself as feeling much more comfortable. The skin acted freely; during the night her bowels were opened, and in the morning her pulse was softer and less frequent. The thermometer also showed a lower temperature. To conclude the history of the case briefly, the moisture was kept up both within and without. The antimony and diaphoretic increased or diminished, the former never being increased over the $\frac{1}{32}$ of a grain every three hours. An expectorant of squills and nitre, to which the antimony was afterwards added, being after a time substituted. The poultices were changed every forty-eight hours, care being taken to have another one ready, and the room heated with steam. The surface of the chest was rubbed with an oiled sponge, and the fresh poultice quickly applied. Once the steam apparatus was discontinued during the night, and in the morning the patient was found excited and feverish.

She convalesced rapidly, receiving beef tea and brandy at first, with her antimony, then alone, finally only port wine and soup. She had a relapse from imprudence when nearly well, but after a time she regained her lost ground and rapidly recovered strength. The sputa in this case was tenacious, sank in water and became for a few days a prune juice color, gradually resuming a normal character.

CASE II.—Called to see B., a child two years old; found dullness or percussion over the greater portion of one lung, together with dry râles and fine crepitation; exaggerated breathing over the other; the pulse 160; respiration very rapid, 55–60; skin hot. Applied poultice and steam, surrounding the crib with a blanket. Gave small doses of ipecac. with liq. ammonia acet. and spr. nit. dul., and acted on the bowels by a dose of citrate magnesia.

CASE III.—Called to see C., a child three years old; diagnosis pneumonia; symptoms almost precisely the same as in the case of B. Treatment—vapor, the poultice, and small doses of ipecac. These two last cases recovered, each running through the disease with rapidity. In all three cases, if the steam was discontinued or ill-managed for a time, the patients suffered from it.

CASE IV.—D., *æt.* 33. A stout, healthy man; seized suddenly with a chill and sharp shooting pain in one side; dullness on percussion; a cough with tenacious expectoration, temperature 104; respiration 30; pulse 130. Applied poultice, diagnosing the case as one of pleuro-pneumonia. Room kept filled with vapor, and at a temperature of 75°; gave $\frac{1}{33}$ of a grain of antimony every three hours, afterwards an expectorant. The action of the skin assisted by a mixture of nitre and acetate of ammonia, as in the former cases. The bowels were kept open, and beef tea and brandy given at first, and after a time, port wine and ale. This case recovered rapidly.

I have given a few prominent points in three cases, simply to show that the poultice and the vapor of water *seemed* to answer a good purpose. Antimony or ipecac was used in all, and beef tea and brandy likewise. The quantities of each were small, and patients soon partook of normal food.

This treatment is by no means new. Chambers calls attention frequently to the use of the poultice, and many other writers mention the good effect of vapor. Combined as they should be in this disease, they are not in as common use as from their efficacy they deserve to be. I have, therefore, thus briefly called attention to them as having, in a *large* number of cases of simple congestion of the lungs, of pneumonia, and of pleuro-pneumonia, afforded me much satisfaction. The poultice has one disadvantage. It is almost impossible to watch with the ear the progress of the disease towards recovery. Both, if used at all, must be used continuously. Before they are discontinued, each successive poultice should be thinner than the last, and the vapor should gradually be lessened in quantity, and a small wood fire kept up in the room, if possible. Finally, the oil silk covering a piece of flannel should be applied, and worn for several weeks after recovery has taken place.

NOTE.—The room in which the vapor of water is to be used should be small, and the apparatus generating the steam arranged so as while only slightly heating the air, yet keep it surcharged with moisture, giving off a regulated quantity both night and day. The temperature of the room should be maintained at about 75° Fahr., the attendant being required to examine the thermometer every few hours, and not trust to his feelings. The apparatus above mentioned can be made by any tinner, costs little, and answers the indications perfectly. The poultice should be sufficiently large to cover the whole of the affected lung, and the cloth on which it is spread should be long enough, so that when the patient is laid on it, it can be pinned around the whole chest. Tapes should be fastened across either shoulder, the oil silk having previously been stiched on the outside of poultice. Attention is called to these *minutiæ* as the value of the poultice, like that of many other simple agencies, depends upon the proper application. The physician should examine its condition at every visit. I have found few attendants who were competent to apply it in a satisfactory manner without much drilling.

In considering these brief remarks, I would say that simple as this treatment is, yet I have learned to place great dependence on it *if properly carried out*, otherwise it is apt to do harm. I make no apology for the foregoing hints as he who calls attention to simple agencies for the cure of disease, if they be effectual, certainly does more than he who recommends medicines of great but uncertain power. The number of cases given could have been extended to some forty or more, but as in all the same treatment was adopted, nothing would have been gained without an analysis of and tabulations for which I have not the necessary data at hand.— *Western Lancet.*

Cincho-Quinine.

Contains no external agents, as sugar, licorice, starch, magnesia, etc. *It is wholly composed of the bark of alkaloids :* 1st, quinia ; 2d, cinchonia ; 3d, quinidia ; 4th, cinchonidia ; 5th, other alkaloidal principles present in barks, which have not been distinctly isolated, and the precise nature of which are not well understood. In the beautiful white amorphous scales of chinco-quinine, the whole of the active febrifuge and tonic principles of the cinchonia barks are secured without the inert, bulky lignin, gum, etc. It is believed to have these advantages over sulphate of quinine :

1st. It exerts the full therapeutic influence of sulphate of quinine, in the same doses, without oppressing the stomach or creating nausea. It does not produce cerebral distress, as sulphate of quinine is apt to do, and in the large number of cases in which it has been tried, it has been found to produce much less constitutional disturbance.

2d. *It has the great advantage of being nearly tasteless.* The bitter is very slight, and not unpleasant to the most sensitive, delicate woman or child.

3d. It is less costly than sulphate of quinine. Like the sulphate of quinine, the price will fluctuate with the rise and fall of barks, but it will always be less than the lowest market price of that salt.

4th. It meets indications not met by that salt.—*Boston Journal of Chemistry.*

Asthma.

Dr. Hale, of Kentucky, (*Chicago Medical Times*, Sept. 1872) uses the following prescription with much success, in asthmatical cases : R. Ether, sulph. ℥ iss.; Tinct. lobelia, ℥ i. ; Tinct. stramonii, Tinct. opi. āā ʒ iv. M. S. Teaspoonful every hour or two until relief is obtained.—*Canada Med. Record.*

Treatment of Effusion of Blood in the Knee by means of Aspiration.

Dr. Dieulafoy has communicated to the Société de Chirurgie of Paris a memoir recording nineteen cases of dropsy of the knee, in which puncture and aspiration had been performed sixty-five times. Not one puncture was followed by accidents of any kind. The character of the fluid varied, and was sometimes purulent or bloody. M. Dieulafoy said he had never punctured in bloody articular effusions complicating fracture of the patella.—*London Lancet.*

Editorial.

AMERICAN MEDICAL ASSOCIATION.

The Twenty-fourth Annual Session will be held in St. Louis .Mo., May 6th, 1873, at 11 o'clock A. M., in Masonic Hall, cor. of 7th and Market sts. The committees expected to report were announced in our March issue, also the officers of sections and the rules governing the presentation of papers before the Association. Secretaries of all medical organizations are requested to forward lists of their delegates as soon as elected to the permanent Secretary, W. B. Atkinson, M. D., 1400 Pine st., Philadelphia, Pa.

The Committee of Arrangements are actively employed preparing for the comfort and entertainment of Delegates, a large attendance being anticipated. We trust nothing may transpire to disappoint this expectation, we are confident no pains will be spared on the part of the committee to make this session a success.

HOTEL ARRANGEMENTS FOR DELEGATES.

Planters', on 4th st. - - - - - -	$3.00 per day.
Southern, Walnut, bet. 4th & 5th - - - -	4.50
St. James, cor. 5th & Walnut sts. - - -	3.00
Laclede, cor. 5th & Chestnut sts. - - -	3.00
Everett, on 4th st. - - - - - -	2.50
Park, (pleasant and comfortable) cor. 12th & Olive	2.00
St. Nicholas, 4th st. near Morgan, - - -	2.00
Barnum's Hotel, cor. 2nd & Walnut, - -	2.50

MEDICAL ASSOCIATION OF THE STATE OF MISSOURI.

The Seventh Annual Meeting of the Medical Association of the State of Missouri, will be held on Thursday, May 1st, 1873, at Moberly, a point so central and accessible, well supplied with hotel accommodations of the first class; and where the resident members of the profession are so clever and enthusiastic, we anticipate the largest, most enjoyable and profitable meeting the society has ever had.

We regret not to have received notice of the Annual Meeting of the *Linton District Medical Society,* in time for our March number, the only notice we have seen, was printed at Warrenton, Mo., *Feb. 28th*, and did not reach us until *after our March number was in the mail.* We hope to procure the proceedings for publication in our next issue.

ST. LOUIS MEDICAL COLLEGE AND MISSOURI DENTAL COLLEGE.

The Thirty-first Annual Commencement Exercises of the St. Louis Medical College, and the Seventh Annual Commencement of the Missouri Dental College took place at the Temple March 12th. The hall was full.

The exercises opened with prayer by Rev. Dr. Burlingham, after which Dr. Hodgen, Dean of the Faculty, introduced Mr. F. A. Clement, the Valedictorian.

DIPLOMAS.

The graduates, whose names we give below, were then called and their diplomas given them by Dr. Hodgen.

DOCTORS OF DENTAL SURGERY.

The following gentlemen received, on the recommendation of the Faculty of the Missouri Dental College, the degree of doctors of dental surgery :

David B. Campbell, R. L. Cochrane, W. C. Joslin, H. H. Keith and Russel Mace.

In his address to these graduates, Dr. Hodgen alluded to the great dentist, Dr. Tome, of London, who had achieved fame by valuable efforts.

NAMES OF GRADUATES.

The following are the names of the graduates : Thos. F. Barnard, David F. Brown, Robert W. Campbell, Joseph J. Camp, William I. Carlock, Peter F. Cassety, John R. Chatham, Anders G. Christensen, Franklin A. Clement, William A. Davidson, Jr., James L. Day, D. Smith Deadrick, Michael Engel, Julius A. Fabricius, Edward A. Gordon, Frederick W. Heitman, Warren T. Hillman, George L. Hoffman, Isaac S. Hughes, Thomas Irwin, John H. Jenks, Joseph C. Jordon, William W. Johnson, William F. Kier, Charles D. Koch, John H. Lacey, Albert C. Lonergan, Alva E. Lyle, Ransom B. Lynch, Charles F. Marshall, Richard E. Martin, William A. McCandless, John M. McCully, Abraham McFarland, John E. Moore, Joseph A. Mulhall, James H. Pleasants, John H. Ross, Edward C. T.

Royston, Louis J. J. Schifferstein, George W. Schwartz, Chandler D. Shean, Thos. J. Slaton, Ernest M. Solomon, Michael F. Spalding, Samuel S. Spicer, Samuel E. Strong, George T. Thomson, Elisha J. Thurman, James L. Tracy, Benjamin E. Van Burkeler, Charles Williams No. 1, Charles Williams No. 2, William J. Workman, Albert M. Wortman, Alexander Woods, Irwin C. Wright, Edmund R. Wright, Walter Wyman, Robert B. White.

Following the award of diplomas, Prof. L. Ch. Boisliniere delivered an admirable address.

The usual Summer Course of Lectures at the St. Louis Medical College will commence April 1st, and terminate July 1st, 1873.

We again call attention to the circular letter below; the importance of prompt and accurate replies when received, we trust will be appreciated by all.

Dr. Butler expects to have the *Missouri* circulars out in *April.*

MEDICAL REGISTER AND DIRECTORY OF THE UNITED STATES.— Work on this important publication, which was delayed by illness, is now resumed with energy, and it will be issued as soon as the vast amount of material can be collected and arranged. The *Register and Directory* will contain as complete a list of the medical men in the United States, with their professional status, as can be obtained by personal application to each, and from other sources. Also, a complete medical history of each State, including all its medical institutions, societies, etc., and all medical legislation. Nothing will be omitted that will be of possible benefit to the profession. The co-operation of medical men in every section of the country is earnestly solicited in replying to the circulars sent out, and in *giving brief outlines of the history of medical institutions, hospitals, colleges, etc., and of State, and the more important local medical organizations.*

Circulars will be sent out hereafter *by States,* and announced through the medical journals. They *have been sent* to the following States and Territories, viz: Alabama, Arizona, Arkansas, California, Colorado, Connecticut, Dakotah, Delaware, District of Columbia, Florida, and Georgia. In *March* they will be sent to Illinois, Indiana, Iowa, Kansas, Kentucky, and Louisiana, and all the remaining Territories. IMMEDIATE ANSWERS are requested, and prompt notification if circulars are not received.

Physicians are particularly requested to make as full replies as possible to the questions in the circular.

S. W. BUTLER, M. D.,
115 S. Seventh street, Philadelphia, Pa.

MISSOURI MEDICAL COLLEGE.
COMMENCEMENT EXERCISES.

Prayer by Rev. Dr. Rutherford. Address by Prof. J. S. Moore to the graduates, on delivering the diplomas.

The names of the graduates, including *ad eundems* and honorary degrees, were published in our March issue.

The Alumni society offered two prizes to the two students exhibiting the greatest proficiency in the several branches taught. The first prize was awarded to George Homer, of Quincy, Ill. The second to Gustavus Winland, of St. Louis, Mo. A third prize was awarded by the Faculty to J. R. Hall, of St. Louis, for general proficiency.

A fourth prize of a microscope, given by Prof. Curtman, was awarded to Thomas Holland, a first course student, of Platte Co., Mo. A second prize, by Prof. Curtman, was awarded to G. Winland, and a third to W. C. Lewis, of St. Louis. A sixth prize, offered by Prof. Lankford, to the student who should make the best report of the surgical classes, was awarded to Geo. T. Barr, of Quincy, Ill.

The valedictory was delivered by Prof. Lankford; subject, The Medical Profession.

After the close of these exercises, the doctors, old and young, retired to the St. James, to partake of the sumptuous banquet in waiting.

The spring and summer course will commence the first Monday in April. See card among advertisements.

TIME OF MEETING CHANGED.

Missouri Medical Society will meet on *Thursday, May 1st.* The time of meeting having been changed from April 18th, by order of the President, at the earnest solicitation of many friends. St. L., K. C. & N. R. R. commutes fare to delegates.

Mortality Report.

FROM FEB. 22d, 1873, TO MARCH 22d, 1873, INCLUS.

Date	White		Col'd		Ages											Total
	Males.	Females.	Males.	Females.	Under 5 yr.	5 to 10.	10 to 20.	20 to 30.	30 to 40.	40 to 50.	50 to 60.	60 to 70.	70 to 80.	80 to 90.	90 to 100.	
Saturday 1	157	65	8	3	76	15	18	23	20	12	12	4	3	...	...	183
" 8	112	68	1	4	72	12	20	19	21	20	11	6	2	2	...	185
" 15	114	79	6	1	88	20	12	19	24	13	13	8	2	1	...	200
" 22	76	66	0	4	70	4	9	18	17	12	6	4	6	...	...	146
Total,	429	278	15	12	306	51	49	79	82	57	42	22	13	3		714

Abortion.......... 1
Aneurism of Aorta.. 1
Alcoholism 2
Abscess 1
Abscess of Liver.... 2
Accident.......... 1
Albumenuria........ 1
Anemia............ 2
Angina............ 1
Apoplexy.......... 5
Arachnitis 2
Ascites............ 2
Asthma 1
Atrophia 1
Bright's Disease.... 2
Bronchitis 8
Cancer............ 7
Carditis 4
Catarrh........... 2
Chill............. 2
Conges. of Brain....12
Conges. of Lungs... 8
Consumption......78
Convulsions........11
Croup 11

Cystitis............ 1
Debility 11
Delirium Tremens.. 4
Diarrhœa.......... 9
Disease of the Heart 2
Diptheria.......... 7
Dropsy............ 8
Drowned........... 1
Disease of Spine.... 2
Dipsomania 1
Dysentery. 4
Enteralgia 1
Eclampsia 8
Encephalitis 2
Endocarditis 2
Enteritis 4
Erysipelas...... .. 9
Fever, petechial 1
   "   intermittent... 3
   "   puerperalis.... 3
Fever, remittent..... 2
Fever, typhoid......12
Gastro-Enteritis..... 1
Fracture Vertebra... 1
Gastritis............ 4

Hemiplegia......... 2
Hemmorrhage 5
Hepatitis 2
Hydrocephalus...... 4
Hydrophobia 1
Icterus Gravis...... 2
Inanition 2
Inflammat'n bowels.. 1
   "   liver ... 1
   "   brain... 2
Icteris............ 1
Injuries 3
Intussusseption 1
Laayngitis.......... 3
Lockjaw............ 7
Marasmus 15
Measles 2
Meningitis 25
   '   cereb-spin.84
Metro Peritonitis... 1
Occlus. of Intestines. 2
Old Age............ 3
Paralysis 6
Peritonitis.......... 7
Pertussis 5

Pneumonia 63
Pyemia............ 2
Scarlatina.......... 5
Shot Wound 1
Spina Bifida........ 1
Stomatitis.......... 2
Septicæmia 1
Suicide............. 2
Spendular Thoraci.. 1
Softening of Brain... 1
Syphilis 2
Tabes Mesenterica.. 1
Teething 1
Trachitis 1
Uterine 1
Unknown........... 1
Vulvulus 1
Variola............225
Vitium Cordis....... 2
Trismus 7
Typhus 1

Total...... 714

Stillborn............37

THE SAINT LOUIS

Medical and Surgical Journal.

MAY, 1873.

Original Communications.

ON TETANUS AND TETANOID AFFECTIONS, WITH CASES.

By B. ROEMER, M. D., St. Louis, Mo.

[Continued from page 183.]

5. Tetanic spasm has its origin in the disturbed equilibrium· between the several fluids of the spinal cord, and in its modifications and irregularities we trace the phenomena of spasm in its transitory forms. Tetanus in its progression, the true type of this disease, originates in the spinal cord and is complicated with brain symptoms only in the continuance of the exciting cause upon that organ. Retrograding tetanus, on the contrary, is a symptom of hyperæmia of the brain, which in time involves the spinal cord. The portion of the spinal cord first affected in trismus lies near to the atlas and axis. Descending to the lower cervical, dorsal and lumbar regions the spasm becomes general, symmetrical or lateral. Hyperæsthesia has reference to the medulla oblongata, and in true tetanus, an increased sensibility is consequently very early manifest. The opposite implies a congestion or softening of these parts ; loss of consciousness, dilatation of the pupils, spasm of the respiratory muscles, glottis and diaphram with deficient oxygenation of blood connect the base of brain. The lower the regions of the spinal cord in-

volved the more general, and the higher or more restricted to the atlas, the more limited are the symptoms.

6. Post-mortem appearances may be classified as follows:

I. PROGRESSIVE TETANUS.		II. RETROGRADING TETANUS.	
1. *Pure type.*	2. *Complicated.*	1. *Sympathetic.*	2. *Direct.*
No visible lesions after death. Microscopic displacements and preponderance of cerebrospinal fluid. Sometimes these appearances are fully developed and become evident to the naked eye. These lesions are confined to the spinal cord and nerve tubes.	Lesions of the spinal cord and brain from causes distinct from tetanus, and might have existed without tetanic spasm.	Lesions of the brain but not of the spinal cord. Tetanus is the result of a secondary displacing pressure, and displacement itself of the cerebral fluid.	Lesions of the brain and spinal cord. General inflammatory condition from injuries of spine, etc.
True tetanus. Hysterical tetanus.	Tetanus with secondary brain symptoms. Cerebro-spinal meningitis.	Tetanus in hydrocephalus; delirium tremens.	Certain mental derangements; cases of Drs. Rodgers and Bodine.

Further microscopic examinations will perhaps reveal also *local* changes of the nerve-ramifications and anastomoses in traumatic tetanus. These, probably, are not the direct effect of the injury, but the result of the centric disturbance which pervades a particular nerve-trunk to the wound from a spinal point opposite to the injury.

7. The proximate cause of this spinal disturbance may be traumatic and idiopathic. The former embraces an excitability in the nerves by which the circulation of blood is determined, and the latter demands in addition, a predisposition for a disturbance in the cerebro-spinal fluid from centric and not peripheric (traumatic) causes. h e predisposition may be determined by cold, mois-

ture, lowered vital powers, etc., but it should not be overlooked, that a wound leading at once to systemic irritation, fever, etc., gives seldom cases of tetanus, while wounds characterized by slight local irritation and a reflex or derived implication of the nerves give the largest number. A purely idiopathic tetanus is therefore within the category of traumatic causes, which in their minuteness may altogether escape the memory of the patient and the diagnosis of the surgeon. A given number of gun-shot or other wounds may produce a certain percentage of tetanus, just as the same number exposed to the inclemencies of temperature, etc., furnishes a certain percentage of pneumonia, pleurisy, bronchitis, diarrhœa, etc., and this ratio will be found to correspond to the predisposition of each case for one or the other. *Hunter* very justly remarks, that in tetanus "there must be a predisposition to the disease; thus madness is produced from the slightest cause when the mind is predisposed; so it is in agues and fevers, the constitution being particularly predisposed at the time to such diseases."* He errs, however, when he maintains "that those most susceptible to the disease

---

* To illustrate the general application of these views, I give Case No. 125 of my diary:

Parker, Wm. T., entered hospital under sequelæ of vuln. sclopet. (fracture of os frontis without compression of brain), received two months previous. His present condition, (August 1863, wounded June,) is one of dementia in its first stage; wound healed; seems continually in profound meditation; loss of memory; despondent; fears the steps of any one behind him, and even in the profoundest listlessness, turns quickly round if any one nears him; violent gesticulations, involuntary and during sleep; sometimes periodically spasmodic; liver torpid; urine scanty and abounding in hippuric acid; tongue dry and parched; pulse hard, not full, 90 per m., and intermitting. In the treatment I exhibited antimony, digitalis, and mercurials to ptyalism, cold water, etc. His father applied for his discharge, which was readily obtained, and from him I learned that insanity was inherited from the mother. I transcribe the following question, made by me at the time in my report: "Is the seat of this disease a *direct* se-are of sickly and weak frames and of suspicious minds, and not of strong and robust ones." The trophic and ganglionic nerves are usually involved in withholding the organic stimulus to the secretions from the liver, pancreas and the glands of Peyer, Lieberkühn, etc., and the spasm of the intestinal muscular coat contributes much to the early production and to the persistence of constipation, one of the most important levers for tetanus, and competent of sustaining the exalted polarity of the nerve-cells in the muscular fibres of the intestines. The expression of tetanus is an *intravascular auxesis* of the spinal cord; not an increase of the absolute volume of the spinal, subarachnoid and intravascular fluid, but a centralization of and a reciprocal displacing pressure from a normal quantity, with microscopic but without, to the naked eye, visible lesions in true tetanus and with morbid appearances of inflammation, partial disorganization and other structural changes in symptomatic and consecutive tetanic spasm.

In the *treatment* of tetanus two propositions should be considered as having a vital bearing upon the successful exhibition of a remedy, and as explaining in

---

quence of the injury, or had the reflex action upon the hepatic system induced and, together with the injury, located a predisposition for insanity? In other words, does the following diagram verify the pathogeny in this case?"

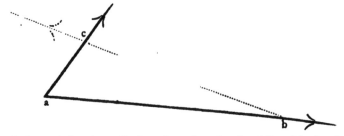

a—seat of injury. *b*—hepatic complication. *bc*—reflex action of morbid condition from *b* towards nerve centre. *ac*—idiosyncratic or hereditary tendency of latent morbidity. *c*—result.

some degree the contradictory results obtained by different practitioners,: 1. The mode of treating this disease should be directed either to the *resistance* of the system to the morbid action or to its tolerance ; and 2. The remedy should not be looked upon as fully tested and curative, unless it has been so administered as to impress upon the system its own toxic effects. As an example I quote quinine, which, in acute rheumatism scarcely ever lowers the pulse nor lessens the other symptoms without its physiological effect derived from its therapeutic virtue—deafness. I propose now to give a cursory synopsis of the treatment as reported from the most reliable sources.

I. Amputation, division of nerves, local applications, etc.

Tolland (*Pacif. Med. and Surg. J.*, 1869, Jan.), reports two cases of traumatic tetanus successfully treated by division of the injured nerves, combined with internal treatment of secondary importance. The removal of a large cystic tumor, reported by me (Case VIII), had no direct effect upon the spasm ; in Case V amputation was performed thirteen, and in Case III two days before tetanus set in ; in Case IV I amputated five days after the appearance of tetanic spasm, and in the very acute case (Case I.) amputation became necessary on the second day after tetanus, in every instance without modifying the attack or seeming to control its advent. The removal of pieces of the right lower alveola and maxilla, and the extraction of two implicated molar teeth (Case II.), four days after tetanus, had no relation to the spasm. It will be seen that, with the exception of Case VIII, no operation was undertaken with the view of influencing the tetanic spasm. In India, amputation was uniformly unsuccessful unless performed early and before centric irritation had developed itself; and in Guy's Hospital, amputation, division of the injured or implicated nerve, local applications, baths, and the free opening of the wound, exerted no control over the spasm. Gherardi amputated for tetanus three times unsuccessfully. Dr. Th. Mack (St. Catharine in Canada) likewise amputated in a compound dislocation of the elbow, resulting fatally a few hours afterwards. A division of the median nerve by Dr. Fayrer of Calcutta, combined with the internal treatment of chloroform, cannabis indica, camphor and opium by smoking gave a successful issue. The internal treatment, however, preceded the division of the nerve seven days, and the section seems to have had the greatest share in this recovery from a sub-acute tetanus. Dr. Middleton (Blockley Hosp. Phil.) reports a recovery after division of the ulnar nerve; it does not appear that any internal treatment was added. Section of nerves gave no curative results in the practice of Baron Larrey. In connection with this mode of treatment, I add that the Jamaica Med. Journals recommend long and deep incisions along each side of the spinal column until free bleeding is established, followed by cauterization of the wound with caustic potash. The treatment of Trousseau includes blood-letting and cupping along the spinal column, and Mursina was successful with the actual cautery.

II. *Mixed Treatment.*

The following table will give a brief account of cases treated with a variety of remedies; it is, of course, impossible to assign a curative agency to any one of them, nor can this plan of treatment be recommended as possessing the indications required.

Authority.	Form of Tetanus.	Remedies and their doses exhibited in the order named.	Result.
J. F. Thompson,	Sub-acute.	Warm fomentations, with laudanum and camphor; Tr. opii. and spts. ether,. e. àà gtt. xl; laudanum gtt. 25 every half hour; chloroform anæsthesia for six and one-half hours; opium and whisky.	Died.
W. Allingham, (St. Thomas Hosp.)	"	Calomel and colocynth; castor oil; enema of turpentine and castor oil; Battley's Sedat. sol. gtt., 40; chloroform gtt. x, every two hours; mercurial oint. and opium to back and neck; incision of wound X; Tr. opii. gtt x. every hour; ptyalism; blister to spine; sol. morph. mur. f ʒ ss, ether, chlor. gtt. xv at night and repeated; brandy, wine, and tr. ferri. chlor.	Recov'd.
E. E. Millholland, (Balt. Infirm.)	Acute.	Ex. cannab. ind., gr. 1 to 2 every two and 1 h.; morphia internally and hypo dermically; chloroform inhalation; injection of sol. of corroval in arm; two drops repeated three times.	Died.
Wm. Farrage, (L. R. C. P. E.)	"	Calomel grs. viii, ex. hyosciam, grs. xii in four pills, two every four hours; enema with ammonia; stimulat. linim. to spine; turpent. to abdomen, and hot fomentations: sol. morph. mur., Tr. hyosc., àà f ʒ ij., sp. ether. sulph. c. f ʒ iss, mist. camphor f ʒ iv. M., one-fourth part every two hours; enemata; ex. cannab. ind. grs. vi, ex. hyosc., assafœt. àà ʒ ss. M. 12 pills, one every hour; Tr. cannab. ind. gtt., 30 every two hours; counter-irritation to spine with Croton oil, turpent.; morphia alone and with hyosciam.	Died.
Dr. Papin, (reported by H. Z. Gill.)	Trismus nascent.	Purgatives: nourishment; blistering of spine by chloroform repeatedly; chloroform inhalations; not to complete and persistent anæsthesia.	Recov'd.
Dr. Büttner, (reported by H. Z. Gill.)	Acute.	Ung. morph., morph. one-eighth gr. quin. s. 3 grs., twice daily; magnes. sulph. as required; also from commencement Tr. gelsem. s. gtt. 20 every hour; quin. s. 5 grs. every three hours; podophyl. one fourth as cathartic; other simple remedies.	Died.
S. Job, (Newark Hosp.)	Sub-acute. (chronic.)	Enema of turpentine; opium, gr. i, with one ounce of Tr. colchic. f ʒ ij, ammonia carb. ʒ i, ether. chlor. f ʒ ij, aquæ f ʒ i. M. every two hours ?); laudan. ʒ i at night, and repeated; sponge bath with dilute vinegar; belladonna plaster to spine. This case partially relieved in two, and fully in three months.	Recov'd.

Authority.	Form of Tetanus.	Remedies and their doses exhibited in the order named.	Result.
W. H. Wickham, (King's College Hosp.)	Acute.	Cathartics; aconite in frequent and increasing doses; ex. woorara injected sub-cutaneously; brandy and quinine every four hours; cold to spine.	Died.
H. L. Burton,	Sub-acute.	Chloroform; calomel, jalap, tart. emet.; morphia full dose; castor oil, turpent., enema; hot water to abdomen; calomel, morphia; blister over whole spine; morphia one-third gr., calomel, tart. emet. every three hours.	Recov'd.
Dr. Ademollo,	Sub-acute. (chronic.)	Large doses of opium, morphine, belladonna, hyosciamus.; assafœt., camphor.	Died.
H. Steele.	Acute.	Cathartics, belladonna, and potass. brom. in full doses; ice bags to spine; inhalation of chloroform; atropia; cannabis ind.; morphia at night. The resume of remedies given by the author, includes the hypodermic injection of ex. calabar bean one-third, and 1 gr. internally, which is not apparent from the context.	Recov'd.

In an interchange of remedies it is generally impossible to attribute a passing or final amelioration of symptoms to any one; hence, cases are here given under a mixed treatment, which, in the opinion of some, may belong elsewhere.

III. *Supporting and Stimulant Treatment.*

Authority.	Form of Tetanus.	Remedies and their doses exhibited in the order named.	Result.
Dr. Williams, (England.)	Sub-acute. (chronic.)	110 bottles of port wine in forty-two days.	Recov'd.
Mr. Bott, (England.)	Sub acute.	2 gallons brandy in eight days.	Recov'd.
G. Rouse, (S. Reg. St. George's Hosp.)	Acute.	Brandy and turpent. injection; one-half ounce brandy every ten minutes.	Died.
G. Derby,	Trismus	Wine, nourishment, and *small* doses of morphia.	Recov'd.
Prof. Barnes, (St. Louis.)	Sub-abute.	Free purgation, with salts and senna; Madeira wine *ad lib.*	
Reps. Guy's Hosp.	Not stat'd.	Of the 72 cases 10 recovered, of which, in three instances, the treatment with wine, musk, and tonics, seems to predominate.	

Rush advocated wine and stimulants, generally combined with mercurials.

IV. Stimulant and Quinine Treatment.

Authority.	Form of Tetanus.	Remedies and their doses exhibited in the order named.	Result.
Hayn. Walton,	Trismus	Quin. grs. x, three times daily, with 6 ℥ Port wine or 4 ℥ brandy.	Recov'd.
Dr. Gunkle,	Sub-acute.	Morph. one-third to one-half gr. every two hours, alternated with 2 grs. of quin. in 2 ℥ whisky.	Recov'd.
P. D. Delagarde, (St. Barthol. H. Vol. II. '66.)	Sub- cute. (Chronic.)	Quinine; stimulants and supportive treatment; in 17 days.	Recov'd.
Reps. Guy's Hosp.	Not stat'd.	The 10 cases of recovery already referred to, owe their issue (Polland) to those medicines which support the system. At all events, 7 cases received quinine, and 3 wine, musk, and tonics.	

V. Ice and Applications of Cold.

Authority.	Form of Tetanus.	Remedies and their doses exhibited in the order named.	Result.
Dr. Carpenter, (N. Y. Journ. of Med. Jan. 1860)	Not stat'd.	Claims 16 successful cases out of 17 treated by the application of ice along the spine.	
W. V. B. Bogan, (Armory Square Hosp.)	"	Used ice over the spinal column and the local use of morph. to the wound.	Recov'd.

Hippocrates recommended the treatment by ice, and it has been adopted since by a number of practitioners. *Celsus*, however, considers the cold bath injurious, and *South* (Chelius' Syst. Surg., I., 420), says : " One mode of proceeding must be deprecated, viz., that of plunging the patient into a cold bath, which I once witnessed during my apprenticeship ; the result was, that the patient was immediately lifted out—dead." As a revulsive, derivative, and anæsthetic, the local application to the spine of ether spray, especially rhigolene, may promise good results from the treatment of M. Mazade

(*Lyon Medic.*, 1869, July 4), and from the experimental results of S. W. Mitchel.

V. *Hot Applications and Warm Baths.*

Dr. Hassal, Royal Free Hosp., had a case of acute tetanus, which was treated with repeated hot bath and chloroform, Hoffman Anod., etc., in very small doses The case proved fatal. The Guy's Hosp. Reports speak of baths as valueless.

VI. *Electricity.*

Dr. Althaus recommends electricity as a curative agent in tetanus, but gives no cases. (*Vide* W. Watson, Phîlos. Trans., London, 1863, and the case of S. Perry, *N. York Med. Reposit.*, vol. IV., p. 77). Dr. H. Griffin reports a traumatic tetanus, in which Dr. W. T. Owen gave ex. calab. bean ½ gr. every half hour, until 4 grs. were taken without effect ; ordered chloral hydr., 20 grs. every four hours, and flaxseed poultice with opium ; Dr. G. continued the chloral grs. xv., + morph. mur. gr. ¼ every four hours ; also chloroform inhalations; Prof. Holland, in consultation, applied the continuous galvanic current with marked success. Patient recovered (*Vide Amer. Pract.*, 1872, Feb., p. 93). Mendel also reports a successful case with galvanism, and J. W. Holland specifies the application of certain currents from 16 cups as follows: directly through masseter m. no advantage ; + electrode upon infra-orbital nerves, and — elect. over masseters and temporals relieved the pain ; the exciting of antagonistic muscles (Mendel's proceeding) gave no benefit ; — *elect. behind sterno-mast. and the + over ensiform cartilage* gave immediate relief to the diaphragmatic pain and spasm, relaxing the sterno-mastoid m., and *still more benefit* was obtained from the + pole behind angle of jaw, and the — elect. retained. The spasm of the rectus and intern. obliquus muscles relaxed under this constant current in ten minutes.

VII. Cetonides aureæ.

M. Guerin Meneville noticed before the French Academy of Science the experiments of Motschouski, a Russian Entomologist, upon this insect as producing, reduced to a powder, a profound sleep lasting some-times thirty-six hours, and which has the reputation of relieving the spasm in hydrophobia. M. has been successful in most cases and I insert this notice of the cetonides in order to renew the attention to this subject. *

VIII. Ammonia.

Dr. Charbonnier (*L. Lancet*, 1867, July 6) had a successful case after failing in seven other instances with a different treatment, from the administration of six drops of Liq. ammoniæ every half hour.

---

* The proper name of this insect is *cetonia aurea* or *aurata* (Linn.), and be-longs to the family of *Scarabæidæ*, and to the sub-family of *Cetoniini*. Their me-tasternum is porrected, the epimera very large and the elytra sinuated at the side. Prof. C. V. Riley, entomologist for the State of Missouri, has kindly furnished me for experimental purposes, the following specimina, obtained by him in this coun-try (the aurea being European): Euryomia (Cetonia) melancholica; (Lac.), E. inda; (Linn.), and E. fulgida (Fabr.), and it is probable that all Cetonides par-take of similar therapeutic properties as the C. aurea. Future results with these insects will be given, and the profession should investigate their claims to a place in the *Materia Medica*. As the name of *Cetonides aureæ* given by M. is entomo-logically incorrect, and as nearly all the cetoniæ have a bright, or golden color, it appears to me possible that M. did really not mean the cetonia aurea alone, but all cetonides which possess the characteristics *aurata*.

IX. *Hydrocyanic Acid.*

H. Ward (Gloucester) exhibited it successfully in one case every half hour and, after relief had been obtained, every four hours. Dr. T. C. Curling, gave small doses in three cases with fatal results.

X. *Oil of Turpentine.*

E. Phillips records a fatal case. J. Wilmshurst claims for the fumes of the oil of turpentine anæsthetic properties, allaying spasm and pain without impairing the heart's action. The South Sea Islanders, who are said to be especially subject to tetanus, produce for its relief an artificial irritation of the urethra and the beneficial effects of turpentine may reside in its action upon the urinary organs to induce in full or over-doses strangury and hæmaturia. It is probable that on similar grounds extensive blistering with empl. canthar. has given satisfactory results. Wm. Leigh (St. George's Hosp.) reports a recovery from the internal use of turpentine and conium suppositories. Mott gave in a successful case a teaspoonful of turpentine every fifteen minutes, and one hundred and twenty-three teaspoonsful in all.

XI. *Strychnine.*

Dr. J. W. Fell treated seven cases successfully with strychnine, in doses of $\frac{1}{16}$ to $\frac{1}{12}$ gr. in proportion with the specific twitching which he induced. He used, however, rather a mixed treatment of opium, mercury, and wine internally with the spinal application of antimony. Dr. E. Vanderpool reports nine cases of tetanus, eight traumatic and one idiopathic, treated with strychnine of which all recovered. Another case died, as he thinks

from the injudicious suspension of the remedy. The
doses used were $\frac{1}{14}$ to $\frac{1}{12}$ gr. every two hours, until
involuntary twitching of the muscles took place and
the massseters relaxed, then the same dose was continued every six hours. Prof. Haughton (Proceedings
of the Royal Irish Acad. 1856, November, and 1858,
June) and Dr. O'Reilly (St. Louis, Mo.) have successfully acted upon strychnia tetanus with its antidotal,
nicotine; and nicotine, as we shall see hereafter, is
especially engaging the medical profession on account of
its opposite action in true tetanus. The proposition
is consequently nicotine *vs.* strychnia tetanus and
tetanus proper, and strychnia *vs.* true tetanus; leaving
the third logical conclusion *a similia similibus:* strychnia
vs. strychnia tetanus. From the argument of Brown-
Séquard it follows that strychnine increases the amount
of blood in the spinal cord by paralyzing the blood-
vessels, and in cases of tetanus (characterized by congestion) it should increase that condition. Ergot
excites the muscular coats of the bloodvessels to action,
and should therefore be an opponent to strychnia tetanus
and applicable in all cases of tetanus in which the
exhibition of strychnia is forbidden. Atropia also is
allied to ergot in this respect, which (ergot) is a
standard remedy in tetanic spasm from cerebro-spinal
meningitis.

XII. Nicotine.

Morgan (*Am. Jour. Med. Sc.*, July, 1869, p. 255) gives
a recovery with this treatment: ice-bags fully and
persistently tried, mercury, camphor and opium substituted, then nicotine $\frac{1}{12}$ drop, liq. morph. five drops
and wine every three hours, in two days increased the

dose to $\frac{1}{15}$ drop every four hours, fifteen minutes after each dose slept about ten minutes, nausea ; nicotine $\frac{1}{15}$ drop.   Babington (Londonderry) gave nicotine in doses of $\frac{1}{4}$ drop, but frightful depression compelled him to desist, and Tufnell has two successful, and one fatal case with nicotine as recommended by Haughton (*Amer. Journ. M. Sc.*, Jan., 1860, p. 280) exhibiting in one case fifty-six drops in six days. Simon (Eng.) considers tobacco the best antitetanic remedy. My case No. VII. is not a fair exponent of the power of nicotine in controlling tetanic spasm, the tobacco enema and the $\frac{1}{15}$ drop of nicotine internally, preceding death only a few minutes.

XIII. Liquor Potassæ.

Dr. J. Reid (*L. Lancet*, 1861, March, p. 230) gives a recovery from subacute tetanus under this treatment : mercury with anodynes and antispasmodics in the beginning, on the 8th day, liq. potassæ with syrup of poppies and camphor water. He says, (p. 221) " to obtain a less easily excited condition of the system, also a diminution in the tonicity of the muscular fibre, and a decrease in that portion of the blood through whose agency is supplied irritability or vital activity to the nervous and muscular structures would be to gain a certain control over an exciting cause and a relaxation in the leading features of the disease." This he believed to effect by liquor potassæ.

XIV. Tartar emetic.

Dr. Conway (Neuschatel in Switzerland) had a recovery in a subacute tetanus. Continued it until excessive pain in the mouth and severe alvine evacuations were produced. (*Vide Md. and Va. Med. Journ.*, 1861, March, p. 261.) Dr. Powers details the particulars of a case in which the full effects of strychnia upon the muscular system were relieved by small doses of tartar emetic. (*Vide Med. News and Libr.*, 1857, Feb., p. 25.) Dr. E. Vanderpool records a fatal case of traumatic tetanus treated with the same in combination with anodynes, stimulants and counter-irritants, and a successful issue under venesection to relaxation, tartar emetic ⅛ gr. every two hours regularly increased in forty hours to four grs. at a dose without producing nausea.

XV. *Bromide of Potassium.*

Authority	*Form of Tetanus.*	*Remedies and their doses exhibited in the order named.*	*Result.*
H. F. Andrews.	Sub-acute.	Potass. brom. grs. 30 every two hours; slept and relieved; the bromide every three hours 20 grs.; no paroxysm after one day's treatment; bowels acted spontaneously.	Recov'd.
Dr. Brown.	"	Pot. brom. grs. 10 every two hours, with increase of dose at night; continued four days without effect.	Not stat'd
Mr. Brown. (England.)	" (chronic.)	Pot. brom. grs. 20 every two hours and reduced to three doses in twenty-four hours; yielded after seven weeks' treatment; not severe.	Recov'd.
H. K. Steele.	Acute.	The bromide preceded and followed other remedies.	Died.
G. Derby.	Sub-acute.	Pot. brom. grs. 40 every hour, treatment continued for twenty-one days; took nearly twelve ounces of the salt.	Recov'd.
Dr. Bakewell. (Trinidad.)	Acute.	Potass. brom. grs. 30 repeated only once in a few hours.	"
Mr. Hancock. (Charing Cross Hosp.)		Potass. brom. grs. 30 every four hours with 20 minims of Tr. A. belladonna.	Died.

Bromide of Potassium exerts a decided influence over epileptiform spasm, at least while its exhibition is continued. It seems applicable as an adjunct to the treatment of tetanus on account of certain physiological and therapeutical properties: it diminishes the excitability of the senso-motory nerves, of the spinal cord and encephalon, producing sleep, and while the heart is paralyzed under its full action it resists longest and is the last affected. Dr. Brown gives its effects as follows : " it mitigates the convulsive movements and spasmodic twitchings which are the result of a rapid conversion of sensory impressions into motor im-·pulses, ... it acts as an anodyne, under certain circumstances relieving hyperæsthetical sensations and promotes sleep." (*Am. Jour. M. Sc.*, 1866, Oct., p. 525.)

XVI.   Quinine.

In Guy's Hosp. twenty-five cases were treated with quinine, seven recovered, and eighteen died. (Compare cases under IV., especially Walton's successful exhibition of. quinine with port and brandy.)   Dr. H. Z. Gill gives a fatal case treated with twenty drops of tr. gelsem. semp., every hour ; symptoms at first improved ; quinia grains five every three hours was followed, etc. (*Vide supra* III.) J. M. Malone reports a recovery with quinine, and a case of a mixed treatment by D. E. Bishop received large doses of quinine with morphia and stimulants with satisfactory result.

Tonics in general have been at times productive of recoveries in tetanus.   Drs. Elliotson and Hamerton gave carbonate of iron, the sulphate of zinc has been recommended and arsenic as an alterative tonic gave a successful issue in the hands of Wm. J. Holcombe. (Cases of an arsenic treatment are recorded in the *Am. Journ. Med. Sc.*, Vol., III, Old Ser., p. 133-376.) Quinine, however, seems especially of service when tetanus supervenes in broken-down or impaired constitutions, in soldiers after fatigue, improper nourishment and exposure to malaria. The benefits from quinine are in a great measure due to its anti-zymotic properties: zymosis, not as a cause of tetanus, may be one of the may additional agents not only predisposing to nervous excitation, but especially hastening the rapid issue of tetanus. Dr. Binz observes in regard to this subject (*Experimentelle untersuch. über das Wesen der Chininwirkung*, 1868) that "quinine prevents fermentation, its power of destroying the animalcular life is superior to that of creosote, morphia, and strychnine, the permanganate of potash alone is of great power." It prevents the development of penicillium glaucum (mould as found upon organic bodies) and exerts a like antiseptic influence upon the lowest organism. The anology between fermentation and the symptoms of zymosis explains the benefits of quinine in large doses. In my cases I have usually combined quinine with other remedies, the patients being soldiers out of camp. Should internal medication become impossible from the violence of the muscular spasm of the jaws and neck, then quinine-enemata should be substituted.

[To be Continued.]

17

PATHOLOGY OF THE BLOOD.

By S. Stricker.

[*Taken from the " Medizinische Jahrbucher herausgegeben von der K. K. Gesell-schaft der Arzte, redigirt von S. Stricker, Jahrgang* 1872. *II. Heft.*"
By H. Z. Gill, M.D.]

It is now more than a year since Lostorfer of Vienna, announced to the medical world his discovery of certain bodies or forms in the blood of syphilitic subjects. On the first appearance of this intelligence, many were disposed to hail it as something new in the history of the histology of the blood, as well as in the pathology of the blood contaminated with syphilis. Important it was supposed to be in the diagnosis of that disease, as well as in determining the relative efficiency of therapeutic measures. Others were very ready to reject it as an error, and valueless, without sufficiently examining the case. Stricker, however, with his usual thoroughness, has, it appears, investigated the subject more extensively perhaps, than any one else up to this time, and we propose to give, in abstract, the substance of his contribution on the subject, the article in full being made up of the *method* of *examination* in *detail*, as well as of the important points, we have thought best to abbreviate. He proposes to himself the examination of two questions:

1. What is the nature of the corpuscles discovered by Lostorfer? and

2. Do these corpuscles only occur in the blood of syphilitic subjects, as Lostorfer has declared?

The investigation was commenced with the blood of

three syphilitic patients who were placed, successively by accident, at his disposal. In all three cases the corpuscles in question were to be seen in great abundance *after a few days of breeding.** He therefore supposed the material at hand was quite sufficient for the first question. But first of all arises a *preliminary question :* Do not the Lostorfer corpuscles also occur in fresh blood? Before answering this latter question he gives the *method.*

The glasses are to be cleansed perfectly, and when the blood is to be examined in its fresh condition with the highest powers, the preparation is made as thin as possible. A very small drop is taken, as it issues from a slight wound, by placing the middle of the thin glass on the exuding blood, and immediately it is transferred to the slide. The drop should be as near as possible to the middle of the covering glass, so that, when using the immersion lens as he always does, the edge of the preparation may be examined without danger of the water flowing over the edge of the cover, which would spoil the preparation. A little pressure may be needed to spread the drop. The appearances in fresh blood are very numerous. Of course we see the well-known morphological elements—red and white corpuscles and colorless granules. Often, however, colorless particles appear in great number, from the size of a nucleus corpuscle to the average size of the nucleus of a white blood corpuscle.

Their appearance is especially interesting when observed with very high powers. Without giving details, he says many of these corpuscles look as though they were particles from young cells, while others make an

---

* *Zuchtung*—breeding, propagation, raising, cultivation, generating.

impression as though they might form points for the formation of coagula. The latter are mostly found where the preparation is somewhat thicker, and in places free from blood corpuscles but thickly traversed with fine threads. He, hence, presumes that the threads as well as the knotted points are probably fibrin. The particles are mostly like the colorless corpuscles, multiform, but seldom round. The fine granules are always most numerous where the fibrinous net-work is thickest. They are in a large measure the optical sections (at right angles) of the fibrinous threads. In addition to these there are, in the fresh blood of many individuals, very small corpuscles, scarcely to be defined with the immersion lens No. 10, and often found in lively movement. Whether these are the Brownian molecular movements,* or belong to organisms showing vital movements, he cannot say. We must not exclude the possibility of the existence of small, low forms of organisms in the healthy circulating blood. Foreign bodies are easily distinguished by an experienced observer. There do occur, very seldom, in fresh blood, bodies mostly spherical with dark contour, of which it is difficult to say whether they are or are not foreign bodies; they are very dark when seen with very high powers (No. 15, immersion, Hartnack).

The breeding (propagation), for the purpose of examination, consists in keeping a good preparation as long as possible, with access of air. The object is attained best by keeping it in a place where it will be protected at once from dessication, and from the reception of vapor of water. The former condition, that of dessication, is not favorable of course, to the breed-

---

* Medical Record, Feb. 15, 1872, p. 84.

ing; and the latter is nearly as bad, the water causing a dilution of the blood, for the morphological elements are very sensitive to the dilution of the plasma, the corpuscles become pale from loss of coloring matter, and the plasma becomes cloudy from the presence of coloring matter; in a word, we must prevent the two unfavorable conditions. The details each must learn, in measure at least, for himself.

The preparation must be placed near where there is an exposed surface of water. A moistened piece of sponge as large as a walnut is sufficient for a glass such as chemists.use for keeping things dry. The preparations may be put on a stand or shelf within the glass together with the sponge. If labeled, several preparations from as many individuals may be put in at once. These need not be so extremely thin for the purpose of breeding. It is well to place two lines of wax across the slide for the covering glass to rest on. In completing the preparation the cover should be pressed down sufficiently to spread the *rouleaux* of corpuscles until they shall have a reticulate arrangement. In the meshes of this net-work (Plasma-Inseln) filled with plasma are the small breeding spaces (Züchtungsräume) so admirably adapted for our purpose. The blood must be small in proportion to the size of the covering glass, then it can be examined micro-chemically. In this way the particles are kept in place while being examined. When examining the preparation for several successive hours he builds a wall of filtering paper around it, and by occasionally wetting the paper, keeps the preparation moist. By this plan, modified to suit circumstances, we can also make use of the warming table while making the observations; in this way he has accomplished some very interesting results. For warming, he places a copper wire under the slide and heats it to the desired degree by means of a spirit lamp placed farther or nearer as may be necessary. If we desire land-marks in the preparation by which we may recognize the same spot, granule, or plasma-island, it may be accomplished by placing untwisted silk threads across from one wax line above described to the other, passing directly through the preparation. By this means also, a description or drawing of the preparation may be easily made.

Examination.—On the plan just described, he has followed the visible morphological elements of fresh blood through several days to their destiny, in a large number of cases. From facts as above observed, he is now enabled to say, that those bodies which he presumed to be products of coagulation, or fragmentary pieces of protoplasm, disappear, as a rule, after about twenty-four hours of breeding. For our purpose it is of no importance whether the interpretation is correct or not, for the question here is, whether these bodies are identical with those of Lostorfer, or whether the latter arise from the former. In either case it would show that the Lostofer bodies are to be found in the fresh blood as well as in the diseased. This, however, is too much. He had described every appearance in a series of plasma-islands in fresh preparations, both in form and situation, and had convinced himself perfectly that the bodies mentioned, page 252, were really present and visible though pale and with indefinite outline, while around them came within sight new, and previously invisible, corpuscles which by repeated observations became larger and larger, until they presented most beautifully those images which must be pronounced Lostofer's corpuscles.

In what manner the visible corpuscles in fresh blood disappear, he cannot decide, neither does it belong to the question.

The *preliminary* question, whether Lostofer's corpuscles are to be found in fresh blood or not, is partly answered. An additional observation will still more definitely settle the question. He found a very favorable case for observation in the syphilitic wards, in March, 1872, a case of syphilis of four months standing, badly nourished, in an individual 22 years old, who had had the primary sore followed by the exanthematous rash and iritis. Several preparations were made of the blood taken from the palmar surface of the hand; and after 24 hours the bodies in question were found just on the margin of the preparation. A second series showed the same result. In a third series, they did not appear within 36 hours, but became visible after 48 hours. Just about this time they had ceased to heat the laboratory, though the weather was still rather cold. Considering the circumstances, he was led to examine the temperature first. The next day the room was heated to 71° F., and he examined again. At the expiration of three hours the bodies were present in large numbers at the periphery. Some of them were so large as to force the conclusion, that either the bodies were present in fresh blood, and had escaped observation in spite of all his care, or their growth was so rapid as to enable it to be seen.

On the next day he took a new preparation, heated the room as before, placed a definite spot in the periphery under the microscope (immersion lens, No. 10, Hartnack), and watched it. About thirteen minutes had passed after the drawing of the blood, when it appeared to him he saw some granules in the plasma-island, which he examined, and which was otherwise perfectly clear. In the course of ten minutes more these granules had assumed such definite characters that he could now distinctly mark their situation. Simultaneously it appeared to him that numerous new granules arose to view in the same island. In the course of half an hour the first discovered corpuscles were so large that he could recognize them as the ones sought after. In an hour and a half the first granules had grown to the size of the nucleus of a pus corpuscle, while the entire island was studded with similar, though smaller granules. Beyond doubt these were the Lostorfer corpuscles; and they had arisen and grown in a clear, plasma-island under his own observation. On the next day he repeated the trial, not heating the room, but placing the slide on the *warming table* heated to 77° F. The result was the same. He repeated the observations with great care. What he had concluded from the former extended observation, was now supported by direct evidence; the *preliminary question* was answered with all certainty.

Now to the first, principal question : *What is the nature of the Lostorfer corpuscles?*

They are either organisms, or they are inorganic. From what we know of them thus far, we cannot decide in favor of either view. We know that they grow. But growth alone is not a sufficient sign to fix our verdict. Lostorfer has announced that they have buds. In this he is correct. But we have learned by careful observation that some of the buds arise not by growth, but by addition.* In quite fresh conditions most of the cor-

---

*. *Inlagerung*—annexation, addition by strata.

puscles are spherical, and appear homogenous, even when examined by a No. 10 or No. 15 immers. He succeeded in observing how a small corpuscle, when lying near a larger, approached the latter and sat upon it like a deligated head. After a little while the outlines changed in such a manner that *the sharp constrictions seen on the edge between the two, became only depressions ; these filled themselves out ; it became a conical body ; then the apex withdrew itself, and the cone became transformed into a sphere.* He could not say whether all the bodies having buds arose in this way. If he had observed one such occurence, it was enough to enable him to announce, that the completed buds proved nothing whatever in favor of the life of these forms. Lostorfer had also stated that the corpuscles sometimes produced protuberances. The author has only in a single case seen a corpuscle with a long, adherent pedicle. But he also in this one case, observed the origin of the pedicle with distinctness. It occured by three small corpuscles in a row, arising to a larger one, which three (accepting his observation), lay close to each other. The constrictions rounded themselves out, and the homogenous process, which projected from the large body, was completed. We could not decide concerning the organization, neither from the buds, nor from the processes which the corpuscles exhibited.

His observations of the origin of the buds put the growth-phenomenon, of which we formerly heard so much, in a very doubtful light. If it is once proven that smaller corpuscles coalesce with the larger ones, why may not the smaller ones grow by the annexation or apposition of still smaller ones. Still, such an inference (by *apposition*), could not be drawn from the corpuscles whose growth he observed.

He observed, at least once, that the corpuscles arose
to sight, in the field of vision, as such small forms that
they could scarcely be perceived. Still, they must be
there; and yet more, we may almost say that they were
at first beyond and outside the range of the visible, and
only became visible by growth. Why may we not say
that the corpuscles, while they grow under our sight,
do so by *apposition* of invisibly small bodies. Some
will object that we are not aware of any example of such
a process in bodies not crystaline. On the other hand,
are we acquainted with an example such as above described, an organism growing in the course of an hour
from the invisible (with No. 10 immers.) to the size of
quite a large nucleus-corpuscle?

It appears to him to be settled that from *the growth
alone, nothing can be decided* of the *nature* of *these corpuscles.* This much, however: we find ourselves in the
presence of an *entirely unknown form* or *structure.* Still
another discovery brings us nearer to the interpretation of the nature of these bodies; namely, that these
bodies have a chemical reaction, different immediately
after they have grown upon the warming table, from
what they have after they have been kept for several
days as larger granules in the breeding spaces. A short
time after they have grown up rapidly, they may be destroyed by acids and by alkalies, or even by water. When
produced by the slower process, however, they have
considerable capacity for resistance, either to acids or
to alkalies; they become shrivelled, but not destroyed.
Hence, no water should be admitted to the preparation
in the beginning of the breeding. After they are once
formed they remain, even though the blood corpuscles
are destroyed by watery vapor. These properties ad-

mit of a ready explanation, by supposing them to be organisms. We have, then, the young and the old condition, the same as we have in animal cells. In the young condition we have the relatively soft external layers; in the old, the outer layer has become hardened. If we consider they are not living, and yet are of colloid substance, the possibility still remains that the outer layers, in course of time, become hardened. He was about to close the examination of those questions with such indefinite results, but wished to make only one more trial, to know whether by heating the object still more, we might not get some practical experience. He had already tried it with the blood of another patient, and it appeared that the bodies, which had by degrees become visible, disappeared by the formation of vacuoles. To know the manner of origin of these vacuoles in its details was now desirable. When he had cautiously and gradually warmed a preparation of the blood of the patient above mentioned (syphilitic) to 100° F., a remarkable appearance presented itself. In the course of fifteen minutes a perfectly clear plasma-island became so thickly studded with fine granules, that he was compelled to suppose a precipitate had suddenly formed. A single granule in its growth could not be observed. Their number was so great, and their proximity so close, that he was unable to identify a single granule when looking from time to time. The number of visible granules gradually increased, and soon some of them were so large as to be again recognized as the bodies in question; a large number of them were also provided with an attached piece, like a head. Watching one continuously as long as possible, it was found that the two smaller and larger bodies, first approached each other, then separated. He was compelled to take a new pair at each look, for the field was full ; and he observed that often two adjacent corpuscles were united by a very fine thread. Every two such bodies when oscillating, moved as though a firm bridge of union existed between them. Occasionally this thin, structureless thread could be seen. He definitely observed how two such bodies first approached each other slowly, then separated, again approached, again separated, and finally rapidly separated from each other. The granules apparently increased in number, but they did not attain the size they had when the preparation was slowly heated to 77° F. He did not this time witness the confluence of the corpuscles. He saw in many cases the line of separation between two bodies become broader and narrower, so that two appeared as one, with broad, furrowed lines, and even these lines became respectively broader and shorter, and longer and narrower. After these phenomena were repeated the following day, under like circumstances, he concluded the first question was answered. We can explain this phenomenon of approaching and separating of two corpuscles so often repeated, only by conceding that the connecting thread between them was contractile, and that the corpuscles themselves were organisms.

Now the phenomena of growth had gained a definite signification. The former conclusions were made before these latter observations ; for, however often he had observed that two bodies united with each other, yet it was never such a confluence as is seen with two drops. Two drops may lie touching each other for some time, but as soon as the surface is broken at one point, or the mass becomes confluent at one spot, they rapidly form one drop. With these corpuscles the process was slow; the contours change slowly; the bud becomes the biscuit form, then one incision after another is smoothed out; then, for the first time, the line of separation becomes visible upon the surface; and finally, the oblong form presents itself without the line of separation; here it now tarries for a time; facetts form, and again become smooth. The final result of all this movement was the sphere; and with this there was a state of rest. He would not interpret-these changes of form as vital appearances, because the disappearence and return of definite forms could not be observed; it is certain that those morphological changes frequently occur in the protracted process of division. It was as easy to admit that two corpuscles, which suddenly pressed against each other, were united by a thread, as that they approached by mutual attraction. The two halves of a cell in the process of division, in the tissue of the frog, may be seen to push off from each other till they are limited by a thread, which even becomes invisible, and the products again move together and gradually commingle. Every histological pathologist knows that pus corpuscles, so long as the division occurs under certain conditions—so vegetate—attain no considerable size. If the conditions become unfavorable to division, they begin to grow considerably, and then begin to form permanent tissue. With all this experience, our observations on the *corpuscles* in *question* agreed — observations that they grow more considerably in a temperature of 71 to 76° F.; but in a temperature of 100° F. they increase more in number, while they attain a less size. We have, then, a considerable series of indications in favor of the view that these bodies are organisms; indications which belong to the same category, but still are not sufficient to establish the proposition.

We have here, then, organisms which develop themselves but *slowly* at a temperature of 50° F., and probably *not at all* at a really low temperature; the development is *tolerably rapid* at 71 to 76° F., and still *more rapid* at the temperature of the human body. When they have attained a certain size they remain as spheres or discs, either in a state of rest or as dead bodies; and they may be kept for days, even when the blood is destroyed by watery vapor.

These organisms multiply either by budding, or by division (Theiling). He has in no case seen an outgrowing to threads or strings. Their development is essentially favored by the proximity of a large number of blood corpuscles, and on the other hand by air bubbles; and they may generally be best found where a plasma-island is bounded on one side by an air bubble, and on the other by a thick layer of blood corpuscles. He has distinctly seen them extend from the margin, as well as from the boundary of the air, towards the centre of the preparation, though not as pushing forward. The finest granules begin simultaneously to appear in a zone, in the vicinity of an air bubble, then the entire adjoining plasma-island becomes filled with them, and later they can be seen in the next-adjoining island. Their source is either the air or the blood; if the latter be their origin, either the germs were in the circulating blood, or they arose by free generation. He does not class himself as belonging to those holding the latter view. There is no contradiction in supposing the *generatio æquivoca* as one of the possibilities. For as soon as we go so far as to declare that organisms arise out of germs, invisible by the best microscopes, we then announce something not susceptible of proof so long as the possibility of a *generatio æquivoca* is not entirely ex- cluded.

If the germs have their origin directly or indirectly in the air, we have here, probably, organisms which are well known under some other forms, probably bacteria, which finally arise in each propagating preparation. We must then further suppose that in the blood of certain persons they take on a form of development which has not become generally known. The beginning of devel- opment is first seen where the plasma borders on the air; this argues in favor of their origin from the air. The adjoining air may only favor the conditions for development. In case the newly-discovered organisms originate neither directly nor indirectly from the air, and yet do not arise by way of *generatio æquivoca*, we must then consider that in the blood of one individual may circulate *offspring* of the cells of this individual or one similar to him, which the first had received from the fluids of the genitals, or by the transference from individual to individual. The *existence* of such *offspring* of *cells*, too small to be seen by the best microscopes now used, is indeed *hypothetical*; but their *existence* can- not be excluded at present.

We turn now to the second question: *Do those corpuscles only occur in the blood of syphilitic subjects*, as Lostorfer has declared? This question he answers in advance with *no*. He examined thirteen cases in all, of general syphilis, and in these found them in nine; in two cases they were certainly not to be found; and in the last two they were so scattered as to count them among the negative, for reasons given later; nine then against four of all the cases examined. In the beginning of the examination, in ten cases of well nourished individuals, in one case of pneumonia, one with cardiac disease, four with typhoid fever, one with typhus, and ten cases with variola, not a trace of these bodies was found. In the first case of lupus they appeared in considerable numbers, and in nine other cases of lupus they were found once though not in large number; thus in ten cases they were present twice. Accordingly, as Lostorfer represented, the subject gains in probability. He found them only twice in thirty-seven cases of non-syphilis, and in both these the supposition was at least admissible that an entire difference between syphilis and lupus is not yet beyond every doubt. In the mean time a circumstance occurred which turned his attention in a new direction. The patient who furnished the favorable blood before, had quite a severe attack of hæmoptysis. While he had observed the appearances described in no other case so distinctly, the thought occurred that the imperfect nutrition, or the combination with another general affection, might come into the account. Some cases of serious chronic disease were examined; even these few preparations were quite sufficient from which to draw a conclusion. He found the corpuscles in a case of carcinoma ventriculi, and in two cases of tuberculosis in exceedingly large number, and in all three cases as early as the second day of the propagation; also they were found in moderate numbers in an advanced case of Bright's disease with emaciation and combined affection of the heart; and in one case of anæmia after variola, hence the matter appeared to be closed so far as the first conclusion was desirable. The examination of these cases authorized the statement, that *the* said *organisms* do not *occur exclusively* in *the blood* of *syphilitic persons.*

Considering, however, that he did find the corpuscles in the blood of so considerable a number of persons, some healthy, and some diseased, we cannot deny to the discovery of Lostorfer a certain importance for the pathology and especially for the doctrine of syphilis. He will not insist that those bodies do not occur in the blood of healthy persons and those suffering from acute disease. The number of cases examined was too small for such a deduction. The following may be taken as general conclusions from his observations : the morphological elements, recently become known in the blood of healthy persons and those suffering from acute diseases, occur *very often* in the blood of *syphilitic individuals, but seldom in the blood of persons who suffer from long continued chronic lesions of nutrition.* If his discoveries should accord entirely or proximately with a larger series of examinations, then we may proceed farther in the investigation of the facts. At present we cannot escape the conclusion that a very near relation exists between the bodies discovered by Lostorfer, and the appearances which we comprehend under the name of syphilis. The question will then arise, whether the germs were present in the blood, or not. If not, then the supposition of a very close relation will have little justification ; it will then become more probable that in the blood of certain persons there exists a chemical combination which exercises a favorable influence upon the organisms from without in their development. If it should appear that the germs are in the blood

18

itself, then we must *conclude* that *organisms* under certain conditions can take on *certain* peculiarities which we are inclined to ascribe to syphilitic virus. If statistics shall demonstrate that these organisms are really present in the blood of all persons suffering with severe chronic lesions of nutrition; then the last conclusion, expressed conditionally, will be justified. For there is nothing to deny that the syphilitic virus may arise in persons under conditions unknown to us, that chronic lesions of nutrition may present those conditions—and that it only attains to its peculiarities under certain conditions, probably when it passes over from individual to individual in simple or in manifold descent. The fact that these bodies were found in greater number only in syphilis, carcinoma, and tuberculosis, is certainly not against such a view: again the fact that we find in all three of these forms of disease, a series of entirely unexplained appearances must incite us, on the other hand, to a desire to follow every trace that could lead us to an explanation.

Finally this circumstance, namely, that these very numerous and careful examinations, in every other direction, of the blood of syphilitic persons, were fruitless like those of Lostorfer, this may also contribute to the farther testing of these discoveries until we arrive at a certainty respecting their nature.

PYÆMIA AS A CAUSE OF FATALITY IN OVARI-OTOMY.

By JOSEPH R. BECK, M. D., Fort Wayne, Ind.

On reading Mr. Sims' late monograph relating to pyæmia as a cause, or rather *the* cause of the fatality attending the operation of ovariotomy, I was struck with the lucidity of the explanations given by that illustrious operator; and my mind at once reverted to the first case of ovariotomy I ever attended in the capacity of consulting surgeon.

The case progressed quite favorably for a period of twenty-five days after the operation, and then suddenly died; and no post-mortem examination having been permitted, the cause of the fatal issue of the case has always been somewhat of a mystery to me, at least until now, when my mind has become entirely satisfied, by reason of the article above alluded to, that the death was due, primarily at least, to pyæmia.

I at once set about hunting up the notes of the case, made for me at the time by the attending physicians, and, after a long search, was finally enabled to put hands on a part of them, which, although not the most important, were yet sufficient to give an idea of the progress of the case, during that period which is usually regarded by operators as the most critical. It is to be very much regretted, that the notes covering the latter part of the case, were somehow lost, and cannot by the most diligent search on my part be brought to light. Nevertheless, I believe the substantial parts, both of the case before operation, and of its decline after the notes cease, can be given with sufficient accuracy from my memory to determine the analogy between it and those of the other deaths from pyæmia after the same operation.

Repeating then parts from memory, which will necessarily be brief, I will give first something of the history of the case. The patient was a maiden lady, aged about thirty-two years, whose abdomen had been slowly enlarging for more than two years prior to the time of my first visit, and whose request for relief by some operation, had been refused by several quite respectable surgeons. These facts were detailed by the family physician, in a consultation had in our office (I was at that time professionally connected with a gentleman in Southern Ohio), I think sometime tolerably early in May, 1867, inasmuch as I remember that the warm weather was discussed in connection with the operation.

After hearing the history of the case clearly set forth, I advised that she be immediately subjected to tapping, as much with a view to establish the diagnosis, as anything else. This was done on the following day, and about twenty pounds of fluid were removed. I did not see this operation by reason of other engagements, but at once advised extirpation of the cyst, upon hearing the result of the paracentesis. This advice was not acted upon, for some reason or other, until a period of perhaps two or three weeks or more had elapsed from the time of tapping. In the interim the cyst had rapidly re-filled, and had become much larger than before.

However, on the tenth of June, in the presence of, and assisted by four other medical gentlemen, I emptied and removed through an external incision extending upward five inches from the pubes, a large, unilocular ovarian cyst, which with its contents weighed (as nearly as can now be remembered) a trifle over thirty-two pounds. The pedicle was of good length, and of average thickness, and was secured in the lower angles of the incision, after the manner of Baker Brown. I saw the patient but once after the operation, ·which visit was made on the second or third day, say June 13th.

This recital includes substantially the whole of my individual connection with the case, although my partner continued to see the patient once or twice a week until she died. With this much of a prelude, I now introduce what notes I could find, and quote them *"verbatim et literatim"* as given me by the attending physician, Dr. H——. I also take occasion here to disclaim any and all share in the treatment following the operation.

NOTES.

Monday, June 10th, 11 a. m.—Operation concluded, and the patient placed in bed. Pulse 88, and feeble; gave brandy and water, and opii pulv. grs. ij.

12 m.—Pulse 80; fuller; feels very well except slight sensation of burning over the course of the incision.

1 p. m.—Pulse 92; tolerably easy; vomited once.

2 p. m.—Pulse 90; very slight nausea; took some coffee; eats ice; passed half a pint of urine; applied cold cloths to the abdomen; respiration 30 per minute; gave opii pulv. grs. ij in brandy.

3 p. m.—Pulse 86; soft and tolerably full; seems quiet.

4 p. m.—Pulse 85; resting well; not much nausea; skin moist; some desire to urinate.

5:15 p. m.—Pulse 84; nausea almost entirely gone; slight sensation of burning in stomach; desires to urinate; sleeps some; gave opii pulv. grs. iss, and hyd. chlor. mit. grs. ł.

6 p. m.—Pulse 90; complains of burning in stomach; gave ice.

7 p. m.—Pulse 88; resting well.

8 p. m.—Pulse 90; quite easy.

9 p. m.—Pulse 90; some shooting pains in abdomen; continue the opium and calomel in same doses as at 5:15.

10:30 p. m.—Pulse 88; no pain; has slept some.

Tuesday, June 11th, 12:30 a. m.—Pulse 88; rests well; no pain; respiration 28; gave opii grs. ss, and calomel grs. ł.

4 a. m.—Pulse 84; resting easily; repeat the previous dose.

7.45 a. m.—Pulse 90; quite easy; no pain; no sickness; slight soreness about edges of wound when moved; ordered opii pulv. grs. iss, and calomel grs. ł, to be given every four hours; ordered chicken broth, milk, and beef tea; passed one pint of clear urine.

11 a. m.—Pulse 88; rests easy; slept quietly; voided a small quantity of urine; vomited some greenish matter.

5 p. m.—Pulse 100; no pain; some nausea; vomited once.

7 p. m.—Pulse 100 after lifting her on lounge and using catheter; nausea abating; ordered morph. sulph., grs. ss in solution, to be taken every three hours, and calomel grs. ł to be taken every fourth hour; to have beef tea in small quanties; drew off three pints of urine; felt no pain upon being moved.

9 p. m.—Pulse 110; some nausea, with a slight griping pain.

Wednesday, June 12th, 1 a. m.—Pulse 104; respiration 23; slight nausea, but vomited only once since last note; slight hiccough; rumbling in bowels; very little thirst; slight griping pain; ordered sinapism over epigastrium.

6 a. m.—Pulse 108; very little pain or sickness.

.8 a. m.—Pulse 100; used catheter, and drew off two-thirds of a pint of rather high-colored urine; slight nausea; tongue rather heavily coated with a white fur; considerable thirst, but hiccough is not so frequent; respiration. 18; to have milk and beef tea, and continue medicine.

11 a. m.—Pulse 104; resting well; slight griping pain; skin dry but not hot; slight sickness on moving; considerable thirst; wound is healing by first intention; ordered cream and ice continued.

1:30 p. m.—Saw patient with Drs. Beck and W.; pulse 118; very slight griping; not so much nausea; skin dry but not hot; tongue moist; sweated slightly after sleeping; no irritability of bladder; occasional hiccough while awake; none during sleep; is taking beef tea, cream and ice; countenance calm, placid, and cheerful; respiration 20; extremities warm and comfortable.

6. p. m.—Pulse 120; some thirst; not much pain; right cheek is flushed; not much hiccough; slight borborygmi; tongue about the same; has taken beef tea and milk; last dose of morphia seemed to produce nausea which was relieved by sinapism; expression of countenance good; condition much more comfortable than at this time yesterday.

9 p. m.—Pulse 125; some nausea after taking cream; some hiccough yet; considerable borborygmi; tongue about the same; has taken beef tea and milk; gave

sodæ bi-carb. grs. x in water, every hour; which quieted stomach; drew off one pint of urine; wound looks
well; there is some distention of abdomen; requires
strong pressure to develop tenderness; was menstruat-
ing at time of operation, and still menstruates slightly;
skin dry, but not burning hot; tongue dry, but not.so
much thirst; to take through night calomel grs. ⅓, every three hours, and morph. sulph. every three or four
hours as indicated; to take ice frequently; slight griping pains, but no constant pain; continue cream and
beef tea; eructations becoming troublesome; continue
sodæ bi-carb. in ten grain doses.

11 p. m.—Pulse 120; respiration 20; has slept quietly since 9 P. M.; has no nausea; slight griping; thirst
moderate; tongue moist, but still furred; slightly dry
at tip; no eructations while sleeping; continues calm;
voice strong and natural; has taken some beef tea; skin
not so dry; palms of hands moist, and feet warm.

Thursday, June 13th, 12:30 a. m.—Pulse 120; vomited once; still has some nausea.

1:15 a. m.—Pulse 120 and weak; sleeping; to have
brandy and beef tea when she wakes.

5. a. m.—Pulse 125; vomited once; more nausea;
complains of burning in stomach; griping pain continues; tongue drier; deep inspiration does not produce
pain; respiration 21; drew off half a pint of high-colored urine; some headache.

8 a. m.—Pulse 120; skin moist; not so much thirst;
complains of aching in limbs; no pain from deep inspiration; eructating some greenish colored matter, and
complains of a bitter taste.

10:20 a. m.—Pulse 122; eructations continue unabated; skin moist; some headache; dozed a little; took

some beef tea and cream, but the stomach immediately rejected it.

11:30 a. m.—Pulse 120; skin cool and moist; tongue dry, and covered with a brown fur; respiration 16; abdomen considerably distended, but no pain except upon strong pressure; pedicle is intact, with slight indications of sloughing; borborygmi; has had no operation from bowels since seven hours before operation, making now seventy-seven hours since they were moved; skin quite cool; countenance good, and expression is cheerful and tranquil.

11:40 a. m.—Saw patient with Dr. W.; ordered ol. amygdal. amar. gtt. ss every hour, and morph. acet. grs. ⅓ every three hours, with calomel grs. ss, every four hours; if distention of abdominal walls should increase, with no indications of inflammatory action, give enema of ol. ricini et ol. terebinth. at six this P. M.; discontinue cream on account of acidity of stomach, and give beef tea freely.

12 m.—Gave emulsion of ol. amygdal. amar., which has been retained; patient is fanning herself, and feels quite hopeful.

1:45 p. m.—Pulse 120; skin cool and moist: has vomited twice since last visit; has some hiccough; the symptoms do not indicate inflammatory action, but rather debility; pulse feeble, and feels as if the feebleness were due to some hemorrhage; slight pain in abdomen; ordered brandy and water every hour, to be continued until the circulation becomes less frequent and more forcible; discontinue the mercurial for the present.

3:20 p. m.—Pulse 126; rather more distinct; eructated twice in the last hour and a half; some pain as before; complains of slight deafness; skin soft and moist; tongue moist.

5:25 p. m.—Pulse 128, and stronger; skin still moist; considerable hiccough; has retained brandy and beef tea for half an hour.

7 p. m.—Pulse 126; skin same; tongue unchanged; drew off half a pint of highly colored urine; vomited once, first time in three hours; gave brandy, which was at once rejected.

8:20 p. m.—Pulse 130; tongue moist; vomited; had severe hiccough; no action from enema as yet; slept some; gave three tablespoonfuls of ale, which was retained longer than the brandy.

9:25 p. m.—Pulse 125; not so much nausea; slept some; no hiccough since last note; pulse is stronger and more distinct; respiration same; eructated once, when some bile was rejected; has taken more ale; complains of some pain in abdomen.

10:15 p. m.—Repeated enema; gave sol. morph. acet.

11 p. m.—Vomited after taking beef tea; considerable pain in abdomen; pulse more frequent and weaker.

11:15 p. m.—Vomited brandy and beef tea; complains of pain; ordered anodyne.

12 m.—Vomited again; complains of an oily taste in mouth, and upon examination, found portion of enema rejected by the mouth.

Friday, June 14th, 12:30 a. m.—Vomiting more than at any time; complains of feeling chilly.

1. a. m.—Vomited again; hiccough is very persistent and distresses patient very much by producing pain and soreness in abdomen; gave sol. morph. acet. and ice, which were immediately rejected; gave ol. amygdal. amar., which followed suit.

1:15 a. m.—Gave ext. valer. fld., aq. cinnamon. āā f ʒ ss., morph. sulph. grs. ss., and repeated the dose in five ·minutes; hiccough ceased; is sleeping quietly, and is better than at any time during the night; pulse 118; respiration 20; sweating.

3 a. m.—Has slept two hours; still perspiring; pulse fuller; had another attack of hiccough, which yielded as before to valerian and morphia; pulse 116 and stronger; respiration 21; no vomiting since she commenced the valerian; tongue red, but moist.

8:10 a. m.—Is sleeping quietly; to take nothing but ice in small pieces; if hiccough returns, to take valerian every ten minutes until checked.

9 a. m.—Resting better; skin dry but not hot; pulse 120 and more distinct; patient feels weaker; has had hiccough twice since last note, but the attacks are decreasing in severity; not much tenderness of abdomen, and distention subsiding; passed two-thirds of a pint of rather dark-colored urine; no action from bowels; tongue red and rather dry; has taken nothing since one A. M. except valerian, morphia, and ice; continue the ice in small pieces.

11 a. m.—Pulse 128; skin cool and moist; commenced to hiccough, but checked it with valerian and morphia as before.

11:30 a. m.—Saw patient with Dr. W.; slight hiccough; gave ext. valer. fld., and liq. bismuth, cit. āā f ʒ ss, which instantly quieted hiccough; pulse 115; countenance cheerful; respiration 18; skin moist and cool; circulation fuller and more distinct; removed upper deep-seated suture; union by first intention, and no pus on suture; general appearance of the patient is much improved since this time yesterday morning; no nausea nor vomiting since one A. M.

1:10 p. m.—Pulse 127 ; skin cool and moist; no nausea nor vomiting ; tongue moist ; no pain ; patient quiet and tranquil ; has taken no nourishment, nor have bowels been moved ; continue bismuth and valerian, and as soon as the stomach will bear it, order some beef tea given ; respiration 18; pulse is quite full ; has not vomited for twelve hours.

2:30 p. m.—Pulse 132 ; some hiccough, which ceased upon the administration of valerian and bismuth ; feels comfortable ; slept some ; wound looks healthy ; very little distention of abdomen ; tongue red, but moist.

7:45 p. m.—Pulse 116 ; tongue dry and red ; distention decreasing; no tenderness of abdomen ; resting well ; no nausea ; hiccoughed twice slightly ; voided half a pint of urine, rather lighter in color ; has considerable thirst ; no eructation nor vomiting ; slept quietly ; continue ice.

8:45 p. m.—Pulse 130 ; firmer ; respiration 18 ; has rested well ; no hiccough ; considerable thirst ; tongue quite red, and the papillæ prominent.

Saturday, June 15th, 12:15 a. m.—Pulse 130 ; respiration 18 ; perspiring ; slept quietly ; tongue red, but not so dry ; craves some food now, for the first time since operation ; no nausea, hiccough, nor eructation ; still thirsty.

3 a. m.—Slept quietly since last note ; hiccoughed once on awaking ; no pain nor nausea ; tongue dry and very red ; pulse 130 ; patient quite cheerful.

4:15 a. m.—Pulse 130 ; respiration 18 ; feels easy ; removed her to lounge ; mouth and tongue dry and red ; to have beef tea.

5 a. m.—Still on lounge ; looks cheerful and feels well ; circulation still the same with regard to frequency, but much stronger; drew off one pint and a half of urine.

8 a. m.—Pulse 120; skin moist; resting easy; no pain, soreness, nausea, eructation, nor hiccough; patient says she feels well enough to walk to table for her meals; thirst still great; tongue red, and mouth dry; ordered three teaspoonsful of beef tea every hour.

12 m.—Pulse 130; has been removed to bed, and rested well; took beef tea three times; thinks it produces some uneasiness; therefore ordered its discontinuance, and its place supplied by a little toast and tea; tongue red and dry; has taken no ice since ten A. M.; complains of a feeling of weight in abdomen, in umbilical region.

1:20 p. m.—Somewhat restless; some fetid pus is discharging from pedicle; distention of abdomen disappearing more rapidly from left than from right side; (left ovary was removed); some disposition to eructation, which was checked by morphine and valerian."

This last entry closes all of the notes that I am able to find at this time, and I am compelled perforce to fill the remaining blank from my recollections of the case.

The patient, from the date last given, progressed very rapidly in the most favorable manner, except as to the pedicle, until the morning of the twenty-ninth of June, when, while sitting in her chair, she suddenly complained of a complete deafness in her left ear. This continued to increase until the next day, when her face and neck on the left side were observed to be somewhat swollen, and were quite painful. She also, on the day last named, had quite a marked chill; and on the morning of the second day of July, she suddenly died, apparently just after something like an abscess in the mastoid portion of the temporal bone had discharged itself internally.

I very much regret that the notes of the latter portion of the symptoms and treatment are lost; inasmuch if they could be found, the death, I am satisfied, could be shown beyond a doubt to have been caused by pyæmia.

It is also much to be regretted that no autopsy was had, as that would have in all probability demonstrated the existence of a metastatic abscess in the mastoid cells.

Nevertheless, notwithstanding the absence of some important links in the chain of symptoms, I am perfectly satisfied that Dr. Sims has described the material fact, in which the fatal issue in this case had its origin.

15 East Washington St., March 3d, 1873.

Proceedings of the St. Louis Medical Society.

INSANITY AND CRIME.

The St. Louis Medical Society held its regular meeting April 5th, at Polytechnic Building. Dr. Porter presiding.

A discussion took place on the following propositions offered by Dr. Hughes at a late meeting of the Society.

1. That all the facts of physiology warrant us in regarding the brain of man as the seat of the intellectuality, emotions, propensities and passions which constitute mind as appreciable to mind.

2. That in the physiological action of the mind and brain, the intellect and affective faculties are capable of acting, and do act, independently of each other as well as exert a mutual influence upon each other.

3. That in disease of the brain constituting insanity, the physiological relationship of the faculties of the mind is not necessarily changed, especially in partial insanity, monomania, or moral insanity; that disease of a portion of the brain may exist so as to involve the impulses, propensities, emotions or passions without necessarily changing the intellectual or reasoning faculties.

4. That disease of a portion of the brain may exist and involve particular moral or intellectual faculties without involving the whole mind either in intellectual or moral derangement.

5. That an insane man may know right from wrong and yet not have the power to resist his impulses to do either the former or the latter.

Resolved, That for the protection of science, as well as for the protection of the insane, and the security of society, we recommend a legal provision for the consignment to insane asylums of persons acquitted of capital crime on the plea of insanity.

Dr. Hughes read a paper in support of the above propositions. The following (from the *St. Louis Globe*) is a synopsis of the same.

The various forms of insanity are matters of observation purely, and not of conjecture, based upon the supposed possible or impossible metaphysical division of the faculties of the mind.

The various forms of insanity are not questions for the bar, but for practical physicians, to determine, and the latter can determine them by no manner of theorizing upon the nature of mind, which divides it into intellectual and affective faculties, the latter embracing the emotions, propensities, and passions acting at times independently of the intellect.

Lawyers cannot reason out how it is that there can be insanity without derangement of the intellect or reason; but facts are stubborn things, and the facts of science have revolutionized many of the theories of the bar. The facts in regard to insanity, which are now recognized by nearly every scientific physician accustomed to the study of mental disease, will remodel the jurisprudence of this subject, so that grades of moral action, highly exalted moral and religious enthusiasm, as well as the most debased moral depravity, will be recognized before the courts as we see them in lunatic asylums, as resulting sometimes from overmastering disease, in which the intellect seems not perceptibly involved.

Esquiroe, whose practical observations among the insane outweigh all theories upon the subject, after defining what he terms intellectual monomania, speaks of monomaniacs not deprived of the use of their reason, but having their affections and dispositions perverted. " By plausible motives, by reasonable explanations they justify the actual condition of their sentiments, and excuse the strangeness and inconsistency of their conduct." He calls this affective monomania.

Another class of cases he calls instinctive monomania.

Dr. Isaac Ray, regarded as the most eminent and practical writer of the day upon the jurisprudence of insanity, believes in the existence of moral insanity. He puts the case as follows :

"It will not be denied that the propensities and sentiments are also integral parts of our mental constitution, and no enlightened physiologist can doubt that their manifestations are dependent upon the cerebral organism. Here then we have the only essential condition of insanity, a material structure, connected with mental manifestation; and, until it is satisfactorily proved that this structure enjoys a perfect immunity from morbid action, we are bound to believe that it is liable to disease, and consequently that the affective, as well as the intellectual faculties, are subject to derangement. In fact it has always been observed that insanity as often affects the moral, as it does the intellectual perceptions. In many cases there is evinced some moral obliquity quite unnatural to the individual, a loss of his ordinary interests in the relations of father, son, husband, or brother, long before a single word escapes from his lips, sounding to folly."

Again he says : "The essential question is not whether the intellect is impaired, but whether the affective powers are so deranged as to overpower any resistance made by the intellect. It is a matter of relative power, and hence it is quite immaterial whether the result proceeds from impaired intellect or irresistible activity of the affective powers."

False training, long persisted in, may develop moral insanity, vicious indulgences long continued may do so. Crime and sin may lead to disease of brain, disease of brain may lead to criminal and sinful practices.

The difference between the man morally depraved from disease and criminally depraved is that the depravity of the former is comparatively sudden, and inconsistent with himself, while that of the latter is quite natural to him, and progressive. He goes on from bad to worse.

In conclusion Dr. Hughes said : I cannot ignore the influence of disease on the production of moral evil. I would hold the individual responsible for immorality, the result of willful and consciously entailed disease, but not for crime due solely to the resistless tyranny of a bad organization, the result of disease entailed upon him or unavoidably acquired, but I would be wary of concluding that such a disease as moral insanity existed solely from symptoms, which may be only the manifestations of a mind depraved. Disease should not be inferred, but demonstrated to exist, either in the brain itself or in its circulation, or reflected there from other portions of the nervous system, or physical organism involved in disease, or in congenital deficiencies of mere nerve element concerned in the manifestation of mind.

19

It was said by Dr. Edgar: that the several propositions introduced by Dr. Hughes for discussion, and perhaps to be adopted or rejected by a vote of the Society, suggest the occasion for expressing our views on the various points or doctrines contained in the same.

The first, that the brain is the seat or organ of intellectuality, and the fifth, which affirms that the insane may know more of right and wrong than they are able to practice, may be excluded as no longer in controversy. The declaration that disease of a portion of the brain exists in moral insanity, producing the same, without necessarily disturbing the reasoning faculties, is not so well settled but one that demands our most thoughtful consideration as affecting the guilt, or innocence, of a large portion of the perpetrators of the highest crimes against the peace and security of society.

Therefore it is well the question is presented here that we may the better understand each other, and the "vexed question" if required to testify in the courts, for no small reproach has befallen the medical profession, on account of the disagreement on this point by medical witnesses on insanity.

The organization of the race into communities, social and political, is based upon the recognized difference between right and wrong, as determined by reason and intuition.

· Responsibility depends upon the power of the individual to do or not to do, what reason and the moral sense dictate to be right or wrong. *Selfishness*, the embodiment of instinct, is ever at war with *conscience* enlightened by reason, which prompts to the cultivation of morality; properly placed with the arts, a matter of personal election and not *fate*.

The duality of man's nature consists in his passions and instincts common to animal organism on the one hand, and the soul, comprising the reason and conscience or moral sense, which are not believed to be evolved by any vital or organic process.

The dividing line of the duality is not between two attributes of the soul, the conscience and the intellect, thus disintegrating the entity of the soul by making *character* depend upon physical integrity.

To this doctrine we perceive two grave objections.

1st. If the moral sense is so independent and separate from the mind or reason, why may it not perish with the organism?

2d. If it should survive the wreck of material structure, why is it not a separate entity in the future life ? The consequence of this doctrine is to impair confidence in the immortality of the soul.

This push of modern materialism seems to us in the wrong direction, and if accepted must end in the impairment of our faith in the future life. On what evidence does it rest; has it been demonstrated by any physiologist or histologist, that the conscience has a special locality assigned to it in the brain ? Are not the premises assumed, on which this theory of moral insanity without unsoundness of mind is constructed, hence unphilosophical ?

We may not recognize *physical force*, as the origin of our moral nature, more than our intellectual, both must be regarded as parts of the entity, originally the endowment of the Creator.

The conscience, the law of right and wrong, the tribunal by which every man stands adjudged, at the same time made capable of virtue, is so identified with the mind as a part of the special endowment that it cannot be seriously affected by disease of the brain without involving the reason ; so we believe, at least.

We have admitted this faculty to be susceptible of cultivation or almost obliteration. Cultivated, it restrains and bridles self-indulgence ; neglected, we yield to the promptings of passion to the commission of immoral acts, condemned alike by the laws of God and human society.

To hold the accused guiltless on account of disease perverting the moral sense, without impairing the reason or judgment, is revolutionary and subversive of all government, divine or human, for how can you punish disease? Admit this principle of moral insanity, and every culprit in the land will take advantage of the plea, and create a doubt at least as to his having sufficient disease to effect his escape from punishment.

Pertinent to this discussion is the question of *moral depravity* and what the differentiation of it, and *moral insanity?* Would Dr. Hughes say the latter consists in a perversion of the feelings, affections, and habits, in which truth, honor, honesty, benevolence and purity have given place to dishonesty, falsehood, obscenity, passion and profound selfishness, without impairment of the reason ? If so, what of *moral depravity?* The impossibility of distinguishing between *this kind* of moral insanity, and moral depravity, cannot be ignored. Even Dr. Ray admits in his "*Contributions to Mental Pathology*" that we may be unable to see the difference and mistake one for the other, but thinks this fact ought not to weaken this doctrine of moral insanity,—we suggest that it not only weakens it, but in our judgment, practically leads to immense mischief.

The question of accountability in medical jurisprudence turns necessarily on the soundness or unsoundness of the *mind*, and not on the *morals*.

There is so much method in the homicides of these times, that the necessity arises on the part of defendants, to twist unsound *morals* into the place of unsound *mind*.

The diagnosis of moral insanity, we insist to be admitted in courts of justice must include *some unsoundness of mind* in each individual case, otherwise it must be adjudged a case of moral depravity, where the mind and judgment may be intact; only the moral sense is effaced, passion is in the ascendent, after a long schooling to vice and recklessness. A lad about twelve years old, passing my house one day this week, seeing a servant-girl washing a front window on the inside (without a word of provocation), threw a piece of coal as large as his fist at her, smashing the glass in her face, and succeeded in making his escape around the corner of the street, before the alarm was given. He had calculated his chances of escape with sagacity and judgment, as the result proved ; if arrested, he might, under the *insane impulse* doctrine, have been dismissed as the subject of disease, instead of wicked mischief, likely to culminate in murder if not overcome by timely restraints.

The American Law Review for January, page 377 says : "If a series of verdicts rendered by juries can be taken as establishing any abstract or general truth, they certainly seem to have settled the doctrine that no *sane* man can commit murder, for so violent and terrible a crime can hardly be perpetrated by one whose mind is working in a perfectly tranquil and healthy manner; the practical result is immunity of murderers." Petty larceny may be criminal, but murder and arson are *disease*, as Dr. Ordronaux suggests, the more expert in lying, stealing, cheating or murdering, a man becomes, the more indubitably is he irresponsible.

A man may know and keenly appreciate a wrong done him, without knowing it is wrong for him to do the like or worse to another. Col. Sickles, Cole, McFarland and many others claim to have been overborne by virtuous indignation at the wrong done them, while they did not know to *kill* out of pure deliberate revenge was wrong. "Reductio ad absurdum."

The progress claimed in this department of human knowledge consists in the discovery, that what heretofore has been considered *crime*, is only a symptom of disease, "that there is no such thing as *moral evil*, other than a pathological product, which ruling practically reverses all historical characters."

It has been said by the advocates of this kind of progress, that the man who gets drunk must only be held responsible for the imprudence of getting drunk; to impute to him the actions he commits when he lost his power of reasoning, is punishing as a crime a purely material action, abstraction being made of the guilty *will* of the agent. Again, his *drunkenness*, we are told, is a symptom of disease, perhaps inherited, how then hold him responsible even for the imprudence of getting drunk?

Can any one under this ruling, define where the line of self-control ceases, or irresponsibility begins? As Dr. Butler, in the *Reporter* justly says, "The tendency to view all human actions as the result of certain physical conditions very prominent at present, is one replete with danger to individual uprightness, and if carried out to its logical consequences, destructive of those invaluable landmarks which separate vice from virtue—the good from the bad." And what of *impulsive insanity*—mania transitoria, this "flash of lightning" kind of insanity, as Professor Ordronaux calls it, disease without a symptom or trace of physical consequence, no incoherence, no prodromata, no sequelæ, it lasts to fire a pistol, or thrust a knife only, revenge and the homicidal purpose are its diagnostics. An insane explosion, which leaves no consequences except the offender's lifeless remains.

Is *it* a proper object of legal evidence when no one knows where or when to look for it, and leaves no trace of existence, who from his own observation of such cases is prepared to testify in court that it is *insanity?* Drs. Woodward, Bell, Choate, Jarvis and Wharton, say they are not. But the latter suggests the alleged cases are either *imperfectly reported*, or that they do

exhibit proofs of *permanent mental lesion,* which Prof. Or-
drenaux (in the *American Journal of Insanity*) thinks the key
to the riddle of mania transitoria, *i. e.,* to say the reason is not
affected is an assumption not sustained by facts, it borrows
the name of a disease, but refuses to bear the features of one,
that it starts with an assumption and ends with an assumption,
its tendency being to emancipate crime from penal obligation,
a plea whose admission in court is against scientific truth and
public policy, as well as the sovereignty of man's moral nature.

Hence the practice of the courts is not so much at fault as the
medical witnesses in claiming an advance in mental science to
the effect that there may be moral insanity without disturbance
of the intellect, attention was called to the immediate and pressing
necessity for the establishment of an asylum for the *criminal
insane.* Under any ruling or practice of the courts in the matter
of insanity, every State should provide a special asylum (some
already have) for all criminal insane, constructed especially for
their safe keeping, as well as treatment; for a greater outrage
can hardly be practiced, than to send the insane from the
Penitentiary, and prisons, from all parts of the State, to the
same asylum where good citizens are sent; to be subject to
constant insults by this class of criminals, is an unparalleled
outrage we trust not long to be tolerated.

The sixth resolution was adopted with an amendment by Dr.
Hodgen, omitting the words relating to the "protection of
science," which he thought could take care of itself.

Reviews and Bibliographical Notices.

DENTAL CARIES AND ITS CAUSES. An investigation into the influence
of fuingi in the destruction of the teeth. By Drs. LEBER AND ROTTENSTEIN.
Translated by Thomas H. Chandler, D. M. D., with Illustrations. Philadelphia: Lindsay and Blakiston, 1873. pp. 103. Price $1.50. For sale by St.
Louis Book and News Co.

Dental science has come to be regarded of so much importance that any information respecting the origin or nature of
dental diseases must be held as valuable, for it is only by

understanding the cause and intimate nature of any disease that the best means of prevention or cure will be most effectually and rationally applied.

Caries is the most common form of disease from which the dental organs suffer, and it is an inquiry into this subject that the authors have undertaken, as set forth in the volume before us.

It is not claimed that the work shall have even the importance of a monograph, but something more modest—inquiries, observations—" giving upon the progress, the symptoms, and the consequences of caries, only the details indispensable to the exposition of the subject," and brief therapeutic deductions.

In all there are 108 pages; and two fine lithographic plates containing eleven figures.

The work proper is preceded by a résumé of investigations made, and views held, up to the time of writing, 1868. The chemical, the vital, and the parasitic theories are reviewed briefly, and in closing this chapter they remark: " In general, we can say that the chemical process plays an essential part in the production of caries; but it is a question if the organic processes enter equally for a certain share. We shall show in the course of this work that the organic process is nothing, or nearly so, and that a parasitic element plays an important part in the production of caries, but in a wholly different way from what has been described up to the present time."

The enamel cuticle, discovered by *Nasmyth*, and which is a pavement epithelium of two or three layers of large polygonal cells covering the surface of the enamel, is not regarded as taking a very important part in protecting the teeth from caries.

A fungus called *Leptothrix buccalis*, almost always found in the mucus of the mouth, is held to be the principal agent in the production and extension of dental caries. Hallier holds it to be a form of development of the fungus *penicillium glaucum;* the authors " have verified the truth of this opinion." The pressure of the *leptothrix* may be recognized by the microscope and by chemistry. The existence of the epiphyte *protococcus dentales*, described by M. Klencke, is very much doubted, and of course any part which may have been ascribed to it in the destruction of the teeth, shares the same doubt. On page 82, they say, " In our opinion the progress of caries of the enamel is this:

by the action of an acid the enamel becomes porous at some
point, and loses its normal consistence. At the same time there
is seen to appear a brown color, in consequence of the change
which has taken place in its organic structure. There is formed
at the surface a bed of *leptothrix*, which probably penetrates the
dental cuticle (Nesmyth's membrane), if it still exists, and
destroys it. Chinks and fissures are opened in the enamel,
which has become less consistent. Acid liquids and granulations of *leptothrix* penetrate these, while minute fragments
become detached, and are promptly enveloped by the elements
of *leptothrix*, which joined to the continued action of the acids
hasten the dissolution." Under *Caries* of the *Dentine* we find,
page 33, the following : " We can also divide into two periods
the action of caries in the dentine, viz., *that of the preparatory
work of the caries, and the period of destruction.*" And again, " we
observe, moreover, when the disease has progressed to a
certain degree, certain histological changes which were thought
to be the result of an active, vital action, and which can only
be attributed to the proliferation of the *leptothrix*.

In the very commencement, page 9, the authors asserted
most positively that "this process (dental caries) has nothing
in common with caries of the bones but the name. It differs
from it entirely in its nature." We were surprised at the statement, and doubted if their examinations would not show something like inflammation in the destruction of an organized
structure like the teeth. On page 56, we find : " We can have
no doubt of a vital action in an organic tissue like dentine, even
when it has reached its complete development, even if these
vital properties are but little marked. We can very well conceive that the delicate fibrils which, according to Mr. Tomes's
discovery, fill the interior of the canals, and preside, in all
probability, over the phenomena of nutrition in the dentine,
[and sensation also] may become changed by an abnormal
excitation and thicken like cellular elements irritated or
inflamed, and produce by division new elements, as M.
Neumann has established. It is evident that we must admit
changes of this nature at the outset of the diseased action, and
before the elements of the *leptothrix* have penetrated into the
dentinal canals and destroyed the fibirils which they find there."
Also page 58, " we assert that this caries comes not from such

causes (—an inflammation) although it is *impossible* to *deny with certainty* that there exist slight histological changes òf the dentine, observed at the beginning of the malady, which are not due to the action of the leptothrix.

They say, page 68, that in the formation of dental caries *two principal phenomena* manifest themselves, viz., "*the action of acids*, and the *rapid development of a parasitic plant*, the *leptothrix buccalis.*

On the action of acids they say farther, page 75, "If the action of acids alone could occasion caries of the teeth, it should be easy to demonstrate the phenomena out of the mouth. It is not so. Acids cause, it is true, a portion of the alterations of caries, but its totality differs essentially from the effects which they produce."

On the nature of the acids, page 94, they say, " As far as we know, the veritable nature of the acids found in the mouth has not yet been demonstrated by any direct experiment; nevertheless, it is generally thought to be lactic acid, and this opinion has the greatest probabilities in its favor."

Therapeutic indications. " Dr. Bowditch, in examining forty persons of different professions, and living different kinds of life, found in almost all vegetable and animal parasites. Those only were found to be free who cleaned their teeth several times a day, and at least once with soap. * * * The means ordinarily employed to clean the teeth had no effect upon these parasites, whilst soap appeared to destroy them." page 96.

Alkaline solutions are recommended. " With great care even malformed teeth may be preserved from caries. In cleaning the teeth such brushes should be used as are not too hard, and which, by a slight pressure, can be made to enter the spaces between the teeth. We may advise as useful for this purpose, the employment of soap, which, by imparting a slight alkaline quality to the, water, neutralizes the acids and hinders the employment of fungi." If necessary, powders which are not too gritty should be added. A solution of the permanganate of potassa is also recommended as beneficial to the mouth, and as a means of preventing fermentation.

The work is gotten up in good style.

ODD HOURS OF A PHYSICIAN. By JOHN DARBY, Philadelphia : J. B. Lippincott & Co. 12 mo. 256 pp.

The interesting little volume with the above title was sent us some time since by the author. We confess to have been greatly entertained in reading it, and we hope we are wiser in considering the rich truths it contains. Surely "John Darby" has not spent his odd hours in vain. Indeed the work contains material for recreation, instruction, entertainment and thought for both the professional and non-professional readers. The author will accept our thanks for the same. Some of our friends have expressed themselves as delighted with the work. The following is the table of contents: Antecedents ; Success ; Spending ; Principles ; Law ; Correlation ; The Philosopher's Stone ; To-Day ; Living ; Wise and Otherwise ; Utopia ; In the Country ; Addendum.

Editorial.

AMERICAN MEDICAL ASSOCIATION.

The Twenty-fourth Annual Session will be held in St. Louis May 6th, 1878, at 11 o'clock A. M., in Masonic Hall, corner of 7th and Market sts. The committees expected to report were announced in our March issue, also the officers of sections and the rules governing the presentation of papers before the Association. Secretaries of all medical organizations are requested to forward lists of their delegates as soon as elected, to the permanent Secretary, W. B. Atkinson, M. D., No. 1400 Pine street, Philadelphia.

ASSOCIATION OF AMERICAN MEDICAL EDITORS.

In accordance with a resolution adopted at the last meeting, this Association will hold its next annual meeting in St. Louis, on the evening of Monday, May 5th, commencing promptly at eight o'clock. Accommodations have been secured for the meeting in the Polytechnic Building, corner Chestnut and 7th streets, where members and delegates will please assemble.

All editors and assistant editors of regular Medical Journals, who have not already done so, are invited to attend and connect themselves with this Association. F. H. Davis, M. D., Sec'y.

MEDICAL ASSOCIATION OF THE STATE OF MISSOURI.

The 7th Annual Meeting of the Med. Association of the State of Missouri, will be held on Thursday, May 1, 1878, at Moberly.

Meteorological Observations.

METEOROLOGICAL OBSERVATIONS AT ST. LOUIS, MO.

BY A. WISLIZENUS, M.D.

The following observations of daily temperature in St. Louis are made with a MAXIMUM and MINIMUM thermometer (of Green, N. Y.). The daily minimum occurs generally in the night, the maximum about 3 P. M. The monthly mean of the daily minimum and maximum, added and divided by 2, gives a quite reliable mean of the monthly temperature.

THERMOMETER FAHRENHEIT.

MARCH, 1873.

Day of Month.	Minimum.	Maximum.	Day of Month.	Minimum.	Maximum.
1	30.5	36.0	18	50.0	59.0
2	28.0	35.0	19	39.5	65.0
3	11.0	26.0	20	28.0	40.0
4	8.0	27.0	21	30.0	46.5
5	23.0	49.0	22	29.5	56.0
6	34.5	65.0	23	42.0	51.5
7	49.5	61.5	24	37.5	41.5
8	36.0	64.0	25	24.0	32.5
9	41.0	56.0	26	15.0	32.5
10	34.5	69.0	27	25.0	50.0
11	37.0	51.0	28	41.5	65.5
12	27.0	42.0	29	37.5	60.0
13	33.0	62.0	30	43.0	65.0
14	41.5	72.0	31	36.0	64.5
15	50.0	69.0			
16	31.5	52.5	Means	32.2	52.5
17	34.5	63.0	Monthly Mean 42.8		

Quantity of rain and melted snow :

Rain 1.47
Snow 0.45

1.92 inches.

E. BREY, Linguist and Instructor in the Classical, Biblical and modern languages, especially the German. Teaching rooms, 118 North Third street; 1319 Franklin avenue; 12 South Fifteenth street; (Haydn Conservatory of Music.) He is the originator of a NEW SYSTEM of teaching languages thoroughly and rapidly, which, consisting of translating not only verbatim, but also by ROOTS and AFFIXES greatly assists the memory, and is perfecting in ENGLISH.

Etymological queries on MEDICAL or general terms, as well as geographical or personal NAMES will be answered, more or less satisfactorily, by the above.

Mortality Report.

FROM MARCH 22d, 1873, TO APRIL 19th, 1873, INCLUS.

Date	White. Males.	Females.	Col'd. Males.	Females.	Under 5 yrs.	5 to 10	10 to 20	20 to 30	30 to 40	40 to 50	50 to 60	60 to 70	70 to 80	80 to 90	90 to 100	Total.
Saturday	29 102	68	2	1	75	12	14	19	20	9	14	7	2	1	...	173
"	5 83	56	3	2	61	16	5	14	12	12	14	3	4	2	...	144
"	12 85	60	6	6	54	18	17	15	15	20	4	4	4	5	...	157
"	19 95	69	1	1	77	15	11	20	14	15	7	3	2	2	...	160
Total,	365	253	15	10	267	61	47	68	61	56	39	17	12	10		640

Asphyxia... 1	Disease of the Heart 10	Inanition 5
Abscess of Liver... 1	Diptheria 7	Inflammat'n Lungs 2
Accident............ 1	Dropsy 5	Intemperance....... 2
Albumenuria 2	Dysentery. 2	Laryngitis........... 3
Anemia 2	Eclampsia 2	Lockjaw............ 3
Angina............. 2	Encephalitis 1	Marasmus 15
Apoplexy........... 4	Enteritis 1	Measles 1
Bronchitis 9	Epilepsy 1	Meningitis 15
Cancer............. 5	Erysipelas.......... 6	" cereb-spin.138
Carditis 1	Fever, Cong ... 4	Metro Peritonitis. 1
Cerebritis.......... 3	" intermittent... 3	Morbus Coxarius .. 1
Cholera Morbus.... 3	" puerperalis.. 10	" Maculosis 1
Cirrhosis 8	" remittent 1	Peri Carditis 2
Congestion .' ... 1	Fever, typhoid..... 12	Parotitis........ 1
Conges. of Brain ... 8	Fracture 1	Metritis 1
Conges. of Lungs. 5	Gangrene........... 1	Œdema 1
Consumption...... 59	Gastritis 3	Old Age........... 4
Convulsions.........29	Hernia 1	Paralysis 26
Croup. 2	Hemiplegia........ 1	Peritonitis....... 4
Cyanosis....... . 3	Hepatitis 6	Pertussis....... 2
Debility 7	Hydrocephalus...... 1	Pleuritis... .... , 1
Delirium Tremens 1	Icterus Gravis 1	Pneumonia 73

Poison, Pyemia. ... 1
Pyemia.............. 4
Rheumatism........ 1
Rubeola... 8
Splenitis 1
Syncope............ 1
Scrofula............. 2
Stomatitis........... 1
Septicæmia 1
Suicide............. 2
Teething 1
Trismus............ 3
Tumor of Neck..... 1
Ulcer (of Leg) 1
Variola 63
Total....... 640
Stillborn............ 7

Obituary.

Dr. George Johnson, an eminent physician of this city, died April 15th, in the fifty-sixth year of his age.

Baron Justus Von Liebig, died at Munich, on Friday, April 18th, in the seventy-first year of his age.

Dr. Hugh Lennox Hodge, Em. Professor of Obstetrics in the University of Pennsylvania, died in Philadelphia, March 1st, after a short illness.

Dr. Uriah G. Bigelow, of Albany, died February 24th, in the fifty-third year of his age.

Prof. John Torry, M. D., of Columbia College, N. Y., died of pneumonia, February 26th, in New York.

THE SAINT LOUIS

Medical and Surgical Journal.

JUNE, 1873

Original Communications.

*ON TETANUS AND TETANOID AFFECTIONS,
WITH CASES.*

By R. ROEMER, M. D., St. Louis, Mo.

[Continued from page 249]

XVII. *Sulphuric Ether.*

W. V. B. Bogan had one recovery and one death from injections of this remedy. The case of E. W. Theobald had twelve successive inhalations, the lacerated hand having been amputated, and from the fifth day also large doses of opium being used; recovered. Dr. Tibaldi (Italy) records a successful case which he bled ten times, eight times in five days as much as twenty ounces of blood at once, applied one hundred leaches to painful parts, and loins rubbed repeatedly with sulph. ether of which one ounce over back and neck allayed the spasm.

19

XVIII.   Chloroform.

Dr. Poland in the Guy's Hosp. Reports gives the opinion, that in most of the cases in which chloroform was exhibited the disease was aggravated.   Dr. G. H. B. Macleod abandoned chloroform in favor of opium, in one case the chloroform "was persevered in with the result of losing the patient."   Dr. J. F. Thompson after trying other remedies kept up the influence of chl. for six and a half hours with fatal result ; the force of the spasm and its frequency were diminished but prostration increased.   T. Sp. Wells treated a case unsuccessfully with opium and ether, then woorara and lastly with chloroform, the influence of which was fully sustained for forty-eight hours.   Also the case of Curling reported by Busch died, in which, after chloric ether and laudanum, chloroform to complete anæsthesia was persisted in.   W. C. Van Bibber exhibited it exclusively in a fatal case, and Jas. L. Ord had a recovery from trismus with tr. opii., chloroformi àà f ℥ iv. M. a teaspoonfull every hour and applications of same with flannel to hand and arm.   J. Ford Hassall lost his case under a treatment with hot baths and enemata, chloroform gtt. v and Hoffmann Anod. gtt. xx every four hours and chloroform anæsthesia for eight hours.   H. Steele's fatal case had chloroform inhalations which affected the respiration dangerously.   In my Case VI the internal and anæsthetic exhibition of it failed to control the spasm, in Case VII the inhalations gave violent spasm of the glottis and a labored and spasmodic inspiration, and in Case VIII, the operation being commenced under chloroform with symptoms of

Trismus only, tetanus was developed while under anæsthesia, nor did the subsequent local and internal use of it have any ameliorating effects. The fatal case of M. Labbé had opium and afterwards chloroform; several members of the Association of Physicians (France) concurred in the opinion of danger from giving chloroform in tetanus. Fayrer's case was successful after division of the median nerve, chloroform having been given for seven days, also cannabis ind., camphor and opium. H. Z. Gill (St. Louis) reports a fatal case in care of Prof. Gregory treated with the hypodermic injection of morphia, croton oil and enemata, full chloroform anæsthesia, cannabis indica (one trial, patient could not swallow) and atropine hypodermically. Also two additional deaths (cases of Prof. Gregory and Dr. Frazer) under cannabis ind. and chloroform, and a fatal trismus nascentium (case of Dr. Papin) under chloroform,—this last case however was irregularly managed in Dr. P.'s absence. Dr. Hinkle gives a successful instance of traumatic tetanus in the management of which chloroform, cannabis indica, etc., were employed, but it is probable that it was a hysteric tetanus. M. Aran adverts (in *Bullet. Général de Thérapie*, 1860, March) to spasmodic cramp, tetanie or intermittent tetanus, in which the local use of chloroform is recommended. These spasms are exceedingly liable to relapse, yet each application gave immediate relief. Wm. Corson reports a successful case in which the symptoms were modified and in the end entirely arrested by the repeated inhalation of chloroform. H. Z. Gill recommends anæsthesia with chloroform alternated in intervals of rest with opium.

Anæsthesia is a product of the brain; the vapor of the agent employed impressing its virtues directly upon the nerve-centre. Its exhibition in tetanus may thus court the progressive cerebral symptoms from the spinal cord by which its failure as a curative remedy would be explained. The two nerve-centres being co-ordinated in their controlling influence over the organism it follows, that the cessation of anæsthesia is the beginning of renewed tetanic spasm. The existence of one is the succumbing but not the annihilation of the other. The more vital and sensitive influence of the encephalon forcibly brought under anæsthesia overpowers the spasm, but its own existence forbids a total destruction of the opponent. M. Chassaignac notices the cyanotic condition of the blood after chloroform, and that its inhalation is in a certain degree always accompanied by partial asphyxia. This should be duly considered and have its||full weight in the therapeutic exhibition of chloroform for the relief of a disease, which is characterized by a death from asphyxia. In partial proof of my views heretofore expressed, chloroform, exhibited under certain conditions, may be a direct cause for the continuance of the tetanic spasm, and it would follow that in complicated tetanus, where the tendency points to such an existing cause, its use is absolutely contra-indicated. In the primary cerebral disease with true hyperæmia and arachnoid inflammation, and in the prototype of nervous exhaustion and brain atrophy, delirium tremens, the inhalation of chloroform is attended with different results: in the last often beneficial and curative, and in the first almost uniformly injurious and destructive. The cases of delirium tremens treated by Chamberlain show that the inhalation of chloroform to full anæsthesia gives "opisthotonos, laryngismus, general spasm, stertor, etc. In delirum tremens of sthenic inflammatory character, the action of chloroform is almost parallel with the morbid tendency, while in that of a nervous erethism it may prove and has proved its opponent. In tetanus, the supervention of anæsthesia monopolizes the encephalon, through which as the superior nerve-centre, the spinal cord is placed *hors de combat*, and that without any agency of its own,—the disease is only masked. With the freedom of the brain from the overpowering anæsthetic, the spinal cord manifests its independent action, and this the more rapidly, because the encephalon has by anæsthesia lost in a certain measure its inhibitory power and its resisting capacity to the progress of the disease. The want of *immediate* consequences in a majority of cases, the faculty of allaying pain and spasm, and the occurrence of sleep now and then have combined to place chloroform in the false position of a permanent and positive remed*'* in tetanus, while the best results ever to be expected from it lie in its usefulness in mild cases to prevent the derivative effects of the disease upon the system at large, in reducing the exhaustion of the nervous and muscular force, and in thus rendering the equalizing and restorative endeavors of nature and the necessary therapeutic action of other remedies possible.

XIX. Chloral Hydrate.

A. G. Lawrence had a successful case of subacute tetanus following myelitis with this remedy in half drachm doses every three hours, three doses relieving the spasm. Widerhofer had a recovery in trismus neonatorum, giving one to two grains at the onset of each

convulsion, and reports five other successful cases out of
ten or twelve (?) treated in like manner; he adminis-
ters it in two to four grains' doses by the rectum if the
infant cannot take it by the mouth.   Dr. Dufour (*Gaz.
des Hôpit.* No. 65, 1870) gives two speedily fatal cases in
which the chloral had no time to act, and a third, a
chronic tetanus, which recovered, the chloral being
given in 30 grs. doses; 100 grs. were taken daily for 6
days and 240 grs. on the seventh were required to
induce sleep.   Morphia was found useless.   A. Ballan-
tine's case of acute traumatic tetanus received 60 grains
of chloral, which produced sleep in five minutes; 3½
drachms were used in 24 hours, and the treatment continued for 20 days with success.   H. Leach lost a case of
idiop. tetanus with chloral ℨ i every 3 hours and chloroform anæsthesia.   H. Griffin's case has been noticed
already under electricity, and the recovery from acute
tetanus under the treatment of Mr. Branfoot followed
the exhibition of 30 grs. of chloral every 4 hours, after
4 days increased to 60 grs., with 15 grs. every 2 hours
afterward, which again were increased to 25 grs. as the
spasm yielded or became worse.   His patient had also
opium gr. i every three hours in the onset of the disease and wine *ad lib.*

Anhydrous chloral was discovered by Liebig more
than 35 years ago; this in contact with water gives the
chloral hydrate.   With caustic soda it is decomposed,
chloroform and formate of soda being the chief results.
This decomposition explains the physiological effects of
chloral in the system.   Although Demarquay denies
this decomposition and action upon the nerves from the
resulting chloroform, yet the subsequent researches of
Richardson (*vide* also the experiments of MM. Per-

sonne and Roussin in *L'Union Med.*, 1869, Nov. 30 and Dec. 2.) who obtained by distillation chloroform from the blood after the exhibition of chloral, prove the correctness of Liebriech's position. Chloral hydrate replaces opium in many respects, and is admissable in cases where opium is contra-indicated. Its action as a hypnotic and sedative is reliable and does not lead to torpidity of the bowels, etc., on the contrary, it seems to stimulate them to action. The sleep induced by it, especially if resulting from repeated and moderate doses, is often so profound and accompanied by so thorough a relaxation, that great. care should be exercised in its exhibition—the accumulative effects of repeated doses, in other words, must be guarded against. One case in my practice, after three doses of 15 grains each, and 3 hours apart (in spasm of the intestines with great pain) resulted in a persistent stupor verging to collapse, and only after 10 hours did the patient slowly recover from the effects of an accumulated dose. Hence chloral should be given in adequate doses without hasty or expectant repetition. Its physiological action is directed first upon the ganglionic cells of the brain, then upon the spinal cord, and lastly upon the ganglions of the heart, and chloral hydrate seems especially indicated in true tetanus, one circumstantial reason being its capacity, so desirable in the treatment of violent cases, to lower the temperature of the body from 6 to 8 degrees. Liebreich thinks chloral the antagonist of strychnia, their physiological effects neutralizing each other. It may be of further interest to the treatment of tetanus, to combine opium or morphia with it, because the full and prompt effects of both are obtained with smaller doses, and in cases of pre-existing feeble heart's action,

care should be exercised in the use of chloral in full
doses, but opium and chloral (or the bromide of potassium, opium and chloral) might be advantageously combined.

XX. Conium.

The report of St. George's Hosp. for 1867 gives
one fatal case, subacute tetanus, treated with suppositories of ex. conii grs. v every four hours and a recovery, also subacute, from spts. turpentine ʒ ss (and
repeated) and suppositories of the extract three times
daily. Fergusson (King's College Hosp.) reports a
fatal case of trismus under ex. conii grs. iii every two
hours, gradually increased to six and seven grains, and
Radcliffe stated before the Royal Med. and Chir. Soc.
1859, No. 22, that several cases of tetanic spasm had
given way to conium administered by the stomach ; he
believes it of very certain action and a better agent
than woorara.   Harley, however, claims to have proven
by experiment that the extract of conium is a very
uncertain preparation. Conium diminishes the irritability of the cord, has no purely cerebral effect and
does not interfere with the sensory functions.   Its
peculiarity is that it has a greater action during rest
than motion.   Its full effect is sleep and it replaces
opium in the corpora striata, smaller nervous centres
and in the whole motor heart.   Gradually increased
doses until the full energy of the remedy is obtained
(in a reliable preparation) would, therefore, fulfill certain
indications in the treatment of tetanus.

XXI. *Belladonna. Atropia.*

Authority.	Form of Tetanus.	Remedies and their doses exhibited in the order named.	Result.
Dr Dupuy, (Gaz. Méd. Lyons)	Sub-acute.	Ex. and t. belladonna in double doses without effect; sol. sulph. atrop. 25 drops injected in sub-cutaneous tissues of lumbar region; in ¼ hour symptoms of poisoning, which were relieved; second injection with same results.	Recov'd.
J. Job.	"	Mixed treatment, one of the last remedies was a plaster of belladonna to spine.	"
W. Leigh, (St. George's Hosp.)	"	Hypodermic injections of atropia 1-40 gr. morphia 1-4 gr., and atropia 1-30 gr. morphia 1-3 gr.	"
Same.	"	.Same treatment.	Died.
C. R. Greenleaf.	Acute.	Belladonna was used as a prominent remedy.	"
A. M. Brown.	"	Same.	"
Jas. Moore.	Sub-acute.	Morphine; ex. belladonna gr. 3, every 4 hours, and enemata of turpentine.	Recov'd.
Same.	"	Indian hemp; opium; belladonna, etc.	"
Ademollo.	"	Mixed treatment with belladonna.	Died.
H. K. Steele.	"	Same with belladonna and atropia.	Recov'd.
Mr. Hancock.	"	Tr. belladonna gtt. 20, with bromide of potassium.	Died.

Trousseau ranks belladonna as the most constantly efficacious pain-calming remedy. Botkin and Michéa hold that it destroys the excitability of the motor nerves especially, next of the sensory nerves and of the cerebral hemispheres afterwards. Perhaps the views of Simon (Lectures on Pathology, p. 219) should be regarded; he recommends an extended external application of a solution of atropia or belladonna. The peripheral nerve-surface is so paralyzed by it as to render reflex movements impossible. Its exhibition should be governed by these rules: in cases where the pneumogastric nerve evidences a paralyzed heart's action, *small* doses may be combined with the anti-tetanic drug; it acts thus as a cardiac stimulant; large doses under such a condition would only hasten the fatal issue. (Harley believes atropia to be physiologically

the antagonist of the calabar bean and opium.) Ergotine for a similar reason may be combined in the
treatment of tetanus with the anti-tetanic relied upon,
it stimulating the action of the heart, so that for
instance after the exhibition of a cardiac poison, upas
antiar, corroval, vao in full doses, etc., the danger to
the benefits, derived or expected, resulting from incipient
or premonitory paralysis of the heart's muscles, may
be obviated by the addition of belladonna, atropia, or
ergot.   From a case reported by Wilks in *Med. Times*
and *Gaz.*, 1864, Jan. 16, digitalis may be included as a
tonic for the heart's action.   Acting through the
pneumogastric nerve as local poisons their secondary
effects upon the excito-motor functions of the cord,
which they increase, are restricted or negatived in the
small doses required and by the continuance of the
more powerful primary anti-tetanic agent.

XXII.   *Aconitum.*

Flower of Middlesex Hosp. reports a subacute case
which recovered under Fleming's tr. of aconite gtt.
iii to v every three hours, and morphia and acon-
itine hypodermically.   My case No. IX gave under
the continued use of aconite in full doses, both
internally and locally, no improvement.   Wm. A.
Wickham gave in a fatal case aconite in frequent and
increasing doses.   De Morgan of Middlesex Hosp.
reports a successful issue from excising the cicatrix,
and administering strychnine $\frac{1}{16}$ and afterwards $\frac{1}{10}$ gr.
every two hours, which he changed to tr. aconit. rad.
gtt. v to viii every two hours, with beef tea, brandy
and turpentine enemata.   The successful case of
chronic tetanus by Sedgwick took tr. aconit. gtt. v to

vii and x every four hours, he laid the wound
open, removed a piece of woolen cloth, gave brandy
six to ten ounces per diem, changed to chlorodyne gtt.
xx every four hours with tr. sumbul. gtt. xx (because
of flatulence) but reinstated the aconite. Prof.
Wunderlich gives two successful instances which were
treated with tr. aconit. gtt. xv to lx per diem ; (his
tincture is less than one fourth of the strength of
that according to U. S. P.) one case recovered in twelve
and the other in thirteen days.

The internal use of aconite is attended with the same
depression and paralysis of the cardiac action as after
corroval, vao, a. o., and the remarks under atropia
apply also here. As an external application combined
with the internal use of other remedies it deserves
further trial in subduing hyperæsthesia and pain.

XXIII. *Opium. Morphia.*

Authority.	Form of Tetanus.	Remedies and their doses exhibited in the order named.	Result.
Macleod, (Crimean war.)	Acute.	Croton oil gtt. i, acet. morph. grs. 2 to 1 every hour with camphor. Opium as much as 15 grs.	Died.
Same.	"	Chloroform. Seeing the "utter futility of chloroform,"......he determined "to abandon it and trust to opium."	"
H. Turner.	Sub-acute.	Relied on opium as the "sheet-anchor"	Recov'd.
Same.	"	" " " "	"
Same.	"	" " " "	"
W. Allingham.	"	Chloroform with relief, etc.; finally opium freely, and stimulants.	"
S Jones, (St. Thomas Hosp.)	Acute.	Calomel and colocynth; blister to spine; Battley's sedat. sol. f ʒss.	Died.
T. Peck, (St. George's Hosp.)	Sub-acute.	Calomel grs. 3 every 4 hours, with morph. acet. gr. 1 ; hypodermic injection of morphia gr. ¼, and repeated in four hours.	"
E. E. Millholland.	Acute.	In a mixed treatment, morphia was used internally and hypodermically.	"
Wm. Farrage.	"	Hydrochlor. of morphia with other remedies in combination and succession.	"

Authority.	Form of Tetanus.	Remedies and their doses exhibited in the order named.	Result.
M. Stanley, (St. Barthol. Hosp.)	Acute.	Aperients, anodynes and opiates.	Died.
S. Job, (Newark Hosp.)	"	Opium treatment, fatal in 24 hours.	"
Same.	"	" " " 48 "	"
Same.	"	" " " 48 "	"
Same.	Sub-acute.	Opium treatment; (trismus only seems to have been developed)	Recov'd.
Jno. Rodgers.	Acute.	Opium grs. 5, camphor grs. 12, in 4 pills, one every 2 hours.	Died.
E. W. Theobald.	"	Inhalation of ether; after 5th day large doses of opium.	Recov'd.
Prof. Frick.	"	Opium and camphor; average daily quantity for 9 days: 80 grs. of opium and 160 grs. of camphor; total, 700 grs. of opium and 1400 of camphor.	"
S. T. Knight.	Trismus nascent.	By a mistake 8 teaspoonsful of a liniment containing 10 drops of laudanum to the teaspoon were given in 24 hours.	"
H. L. Burton,	Sub-acute. (Chronic.)	Calomel and morphia gr. ⅓, and repeated.	"
J. C. Nott.	Trismus.	Morphia gr. ½, hypodermically twice daily.	"
T. S. Wells.	Acute.	Opium and ether; woorara and chloroform.	Died.
J. L. Ord.	Trismus.	Tr. opii, chloroform, āā ℥ iv; a teaspoonful every hour.	Recov'd.
J. F. Thompson.	Acute.	Opiates, etc.; tr. opii gtt. 25, every h.	Died.
W. V. B. Bogan.	Sub-acute.	Local application of ice; morphia.	Recov'd.
E. Hodges.	" (chronic.)	Morphia in powder locally, and in sol. with tr. hyosciam., calomel, tartar emetic, wine, etc.	"
Case V.	Sub acute.	Opium grs. 3, every 2 to 3 hours; ex. cannab. indic. gr. 1 every hour.	"
Case VI.	"	Chloroform ineffectual; morphia gr. 1 injected in triceps m., repeated 3 times in 2 hours.	"
Case VII.	Acute.	Morphia endermically with other remedies.	Died.
Case VIII.	"	Morphia grs. 2 endermically; chloroform, opiates and morphia.	"
C. R. Greeleaf.	"	Calabar bean with morphia; 54 grains opium in 4½ hours.	Recov'd.
Jas. Moore.	Sub-acute.	Indian hemp; opium grs. 2 every h.; wine, and turpentine enemata.	"
Same.	"	Morphia alone; and ex. belladonna grs. 3; every 4 hours.	"
Same	Trismus.	Indian hemp, actively; opium, belladonna, etc.	"
Same.	Idiopath.	Indian hemp and opium.	
Gunkle.	Sub-acute.	Morphia gr. ¼ to ½ every 2 hours; quinine and whisky.	"
M. Labbé.	Acute.	Opium and chloroform.	Died.

Author	Form of Tetanus.	Remedies and their doses exhibited in the order named.	Result.
Dr. Ademoilo.	Sub-acute.	Large doses of opium, morphia, bella-donna, etc.	Recov'd.
H. K. Steele.	Acute.	Morphine in a mixed treatment.	Died.
G. Derby.	Trismus.	Small doses of morphia, etc.	Recov'd.
H. K. Toland.	Sub-acute.	Morphia gr. 1 over wound every 6 h., tr. cannabis indic. gtt. 20 every 2 hours; after 2 weeks the morph. locally at longer intervals.	"
Northern Hosp. (Liverpool.)	Acute.	Morphine subcutaneously.	Died.
Tyndale and Bryson.	"	Hypodermic injections of morphia, and occasional application of chloroform to spine.	"
H. Z. Gill.	"	Morphia hypodermically; chloroform, etc.	"
Same.	"	Same treatment, with addition of tr. cannabis indic.	"
Morgan.	Sub-acute.	Camphor and opium without benefit; nicotine.	Recov'd.
St. George's Hosp.	"	Atropine 1-40 to 1-30, with morphia 1-4 to 1 3 gr. subcutaneously.	"
Same.	"	Same treatment.	
Prof. Busch.	Acute.	Curare; morphia.	
Same.	"	Morphia gr. ¼ hypodermically, every two hours.	"

The reports from the French hospitals in the Crimean war speak favorably of the effects of opium. This statement, however, must be considerably modified, because of their intermixture of trismus and sub-acute with acute tetanus. Baron Larrey also recommended opium and camphor, and Romberg relies on opium and surgical adjuncts.

The undoubted physiological actions of opium are that of an anodyne, hypnotic and soporific; its *modus operandi*, however, is but little understood. Entitled still to the foremost rank among anti-tetanic remedies, I will only advert to two cases illustrative of its action: the case of acute traumatic tetanus reported by Dr. Van Bibber, is a type of this disease; the judicious but unflinching increase of the remedy without regard to the quantity given, but with reference to the effects obtained and to the tolerance of the system remaining should mark the exhibition of all therapeutic agents in so rapid and fatal a' disease as tetanus. The disproportion between the effects of the remedy and the tolerance of the body under a continuance of spasm is the guide for a quantitative treatment and the difference between the quantity given and its absolute effects on the one hand and its relative effects on the other, form the measure of the amount of nervous excitation to be remedied. The second case to which I wish to allude is that reported by Drs, Tyndale and Bryson, * (compare also a parallel case in *Am. Journ. Med. Sc.*, 1866, July, p. 130) of which, however, I have only these *data:* "a man aged 35 years was admitted with tetanus, which prevented his speaking and swallowing; had much pain in the neck and jaws with risus sardonicus fully developed. The attack followed a blow on the head ten days previously. Treatment: hypodermic injections of morphia with chloroform to spine. Result: death in five or six days." The majority of chronic brain affections met with in the daily practice are due to local injury of more or less grave import, a fall or a blow upon the head, a sudden shake, etc., not necessarily resulting in fracture, laceration or extravasation, but rather accompanied with a molecular disturbance of the brain-mass in and upon itself. A peculiar sensation, swimming before the eye, a pricking of pins in the extremities, etc., constitute usually the whole account given by the patient of his then condition. In grave consequences, such as tetanus in the above case, the disturbance is evidently transplanted or extended upon the spinal cord

---

(* *Cinn. Lancet and Obs.*, 1869, Sep., p. 556.)

perhaps owing to certain systemic peculiarities, and the product of morbidity from that source is really the disease itself   For should it be presumed that tetanus in this instance could not have been of a retrogressive character, the primary and preceding degree of inflammatory action would allow of no doubt.   On the contrary, however, the symptoms of tetanus in this case must be looked upon as depending on a cerebral anæmia or arterial contraction.   To produce the required narcotic effect of opium during the nervous excitement of such character would demand the full toxic dose. The agent called for seems to have been belladonna and active local irritants.   The state of the cerebral mass, instead of being preceded by signs of active inflammation, is sometimes, and usually after injuries like the above, (blows and slight injuries,) accompanied by a peculiar morbid action, neither inflammatory as understood by arterial hyperæmia, nor by atrophy from waste of substance and deficient blood-supply. The appearances have been termed a sub-acute inflammation, and its transient effects upon the parts primarily involved being characterized by few autoptic lesions, and altogether overbalanced by the superinduced spinal symptoms, have led to a disregard of its importance in the disease treated.   (Compare the cases of Drs. Bodine and Keen above given.)   Battley's solution of opium given by S. Jones (St. Thomas' Hosp.) is devoid of all reliance as an opiate;   it being in addition a nostrum, its employment becomes highly improper in any case, most especially in a disease like tetanus.

The hypodermic injection of morphine is liable to failure, as indeed, are all other remedies similarly exhibited.   Wells failed in two instances, in the first the spasm remaining unaffected, and in the second, in which the spasm was never violent and ceased altogether during sleep, a soporific effect of only two hours was the result. It must, however, be taken in consideration that nearly all therapeutic agents (Herman) especially curare and the poisons of serpents, act inadequately if introduced into the stomach or under the skin. No proportion, consequently, can be said to exist between an internal and endermic dose of a remedy. The following facts in regard to a hypodermic treatment I would here make prominent:

1. Remedies without avail internally, act decidedly if so injected.

2. Hypnotics act at once, if the quantity used be sufficient and the exitation to be overcome is moderate.

3. They act after a lapse of time if the second indication is increased; local pain, however, ceases generally much sooner.

4. They fail to act with small quantities used and much cerebral excitement, pain and spasm to be overcome.

5. Hypodermic injections are especially useful in tetanus from the difficulties interfering with deglutition.

6. The vehicle used in the injection should be as non-irritative as possible: water, glycerine, dry powder, acetic acid diluted, alcohol, etc., are solvents preferred in the order named.

7. Serious consequences sometimes arise from subcutaneous injections, but the usual and most common local effects are disproportionately counterbalanced by the benefits derived.

According to Ch. Hunter, late House-surgeon to St. George's Hospital, chloroform may be safely injected with prompt hypnotic and anodyne effects. Like chloral, it produces narcotism, lasting many hours, not succeeded as after its anæsthesia, by inhalation, by any stage of excitement. A further confirmation of such results would entitle chloroform anew to trials as an anti-tetanic. I will add that hypodermic injections sometimes fail to act on repetition, as in neuralgic pains which are not often as promptly relieved by a second as they were from the first injection. This circumstance has led me to consider a certain nerve locality in a paralyzed state, at least, in so far as the absorption of further injections is concerned, which is impaired or suspended. ' In my sixth case the three consecutive injections were made not only with an increased quantity but upon parts remote from each other.

[To be Continued.]

THEORETIC CONSIDERATIONS IN RELATION TO THE TREATMENT OF SHOCK.

By DAVID PRINCE, M. D., Jacksonville, Illinois.

There are four conditions incident to injury in which the nervous function is more or less depressed.

1. Shock of sudden development.

2. Exhaustion of slow production.

3. Syncope in which the nervous influence is first cause and then consequence of diminution of the force of the circulation of the blood.

4. Concussion in which vibration of the brain or the nerves interferes temporarily with their function.

Shock may be mechanical or electrical, or a depression from the sudden local depression of temperature, as in the introduction of ice or cold water into the stomach—ice in the uterus (employed in post partem hemorrhage) or any sudden change more rapid than is compatible with the physiological processes.

We know the nature of shock from the symptoms of depression or suspension of nerve-force. This is not dependent upon any lasting injury to the nerves, which generate or which communicate nerve-force, because the most alarming shock may be recovered from in a few hours so that the patient is as well as before the accident which caused the shock.

It being assumed that shock is the suspension of the function of the organ which produces the nerve-force, it becomes a question, whether any measures other than rest, can be resorted to with the prospect of aiding the restoration of this function. If all cases recovered, we might safely leave the case to rest and natural recuperation; but too many die without reaction, or with so slow a reaction as to be attended with chemical changes of the blood inimical to life.

The class of measures (aside from the conditions of rest) which has been uniformly employed, is that of stimulants. It is for a stimulating effect that heat is employed to counteract the lack of heat production incident to the failure of nerve-force. The only caution in this application is against an over-dose, *i. e.*, against raising the temperature above the natural grade. Heat thus applied, supplies primarily an aid to the chemical or physiological change of particles in the nerve ·which is indispensable to the generation of nerve-force.

Alcohol as a stimulant in shock or exhaustion, *i. e.*, in a dose short of its narcotic effect, may for the present consideration be assumed to increase the production of nerve-force by aiding in setting to work those intimate changes in the process of nutrition which is essential to the generation of this force. In the normal condition, the aid afforded by this stimulant induces an over-action and is therefore injurious: or the other theory of alcoholic stimulation may be assumed, which is, that the presence of the agent in the fluids and tissues retards disintegration, having thus a conservative effect in low or declining conditions of nutrition and consequent function. In shock which comes on suddenly, and in exhaustion which comes on slowly, the spark of life is liable to be lost by the preponderance of the disassimilation of the molecular constitution, and the consequent extinction of the assimilating changes. An agent whose direct effect is to preserve the fluids and tissues after life has departed, may be supposed to have this effect when life threatens to depart.

The theory which is here considered forbids the administration of alcohol in such quantity as to produce very marked phenomena. The tumultuous innervation denominated over-action, may be produced by over-stimulation by alcohol.

Opium is another agent which may be claimed as a stimulant directly aiding depressed nerve-nutrition or diminishing exhausting disassimilation. The temporary employment of stimulating doses for the temporary sustenance of nerve-depression, is in accordance with the commonly received ideas of the action of this medicine. If any caution is necessary, it is against giving ·doses which are narcotic in their effects. Tea, coffee, and

other euphrenics employed as beverages, need no caution as to over-dosing.

The stimulants thus far mentioned, heat, alcohol,
opium, tea and coffee, are supposed to act primarily and
temporarily in conserving nerve-force.

There are other stimulants whose manifestations are
in actions which are directly exhaustive. The chief of
them is the interrupted electric current. Temporary
excitation of the nerves, and of the muscles which they
supply, by this agent, is followed by diminished irritability. It is not known whether a weak continuous
current has this effect, but faradization to a demonstra-
tive degree, certainly exhausts irritability. The stimulation afforded by this agent is therefore like that of
exercise of muscles—cutaneous nutrition and action of
the mind secured by questions in a loud voice. All
these stimulants are such by calling forth functional
activity in the use of a supply of nerve-force already in
existence. In shock, this supply is reduced to the minimum compatible with life and cannot, therefore, safely
be drawn upon. Stimulants of this class are applicable
in syncope, a condition in which fundamental failure is
in the circulating system which needs to be aroused by
any stimulant, regardless of any very careful consideration of nervous depression.

In shock and exhaustion, it is unphilosophical to
reject those stimulants which act directly upon the seat
of nutrition, conserving or increasing vital power; on
account of the known effect of faradization, counter-
irritation, and muscular exercise in exhausting to a still
further extent nervous irritability, which is already
depressed.

In the abnegation of nervous function from concussion, the condition of the nerves involved is like that of a muscle contused or over-strained, in which the chief fear is subsequent inflammatory action.

Rest is here obviously the only condition necessary to be enforced. Stimulants of both kinds are out of place, and with the establishment of inflammatory action the pressure of blood must be diminished, by lessening the volume of the circulation by bleeding, by diminishing the force and frequency of the heart's contraction by digitalis or veratrium, or by lessening the size of the capillaries by posture and cold.

The condition of concussion has no resemblance to that of shock except in the diminution of nervous functions. One is mechanical and the other is vital. The recovery from one is always slow, while from the other, the recovery in cases of the most alarming depression, is often complete in a few hours. The shock from a blow upon the abdomen or the introduction of ice into the stomach is often most extreme and sometimes instantly fatal, but the speedy recovery shows that no lasting injury is inflicted.

To conclude, there are two classes of stimulants, the conservative and the exhaustive. Those of the first should be given in shock, and in exhaustion those of the latter should be avoided. In syncope, the latter are applicable and necessary on account of their speedy action; the former are inapplicable on account of the time required for their action unless the exhaustion is combined with the syncope. In concussion no stimulant is necessary, because the lesion is mechanical, and if not speedily fatal, the danger is in subsequent inflammatory action.

THE EFFECTS OF A FRIGHT.

By WALTER COLES, M. D.

We have frequently heard of persons being " frightened out of their wits,' but the following example presents the strangest case of the kind we have ever met with. On the evening of the 1st of May, we were summoned in haste to the residence of a gentleman near by, to see a boy about fourteen years of age, who was laboring under the effects of a sudden and severe fright. It seems that the gentleman of the house and his wife had gone out to spend the evening, leaving the patient, a hired white boy, with another servant boy a little older, and several of his own young sons in the house. These boys plotted a practical joke against the patient, by dressing up the effigy of a man in coat, hat, etc., and leaning it against the back kitchen door leading into the yard, in the meanwhile, one of the other boys ran around the house and rapped at the back door, which the patient was sent to open. Immediately prior to this, we should remark that the boy seemed apparently well, and in good spirits, having been romping with his playmates. He went with alacrity to the door expecting perhaps to admit one of the servants, when suddenly on opening it, the figure of a man fell in on him. The poor little fellow gave a sudden scream, and staggering back, fell on the floor insensible. When we saw him he was rolling on the floor, trembling in the most violent manner. The pupils were slightly dilated, face somewhat flushed, or perhaps natural, the pulse weak but frequent. The heart palpitated most tumultuously, but not apparently influencing the pulse. There was total loss of conciousness, while every few seconds the face would partake of an expression of the utmost terror, and the arms and hands become extended as in an effort to avoid some frightful object; at these times his screams were sometimes loud and piercing. At first this terrible vision seemed constantly before him, but in the course of an hour, there were intervals of repose, lasting from ten to sixty seconds, but no return to consciousness, though the eyes were open and natural in expression. Suddenly however, the dreadful phantom would again appear, and throw him into a tremor whilst with outstretched arms, terrified face, and sometimes a flood of tears, he attempted to shun his fancied danger. Under the influence of liberal doses of bromide of potassium, the patient gradually became more composed, and finally relapsed into an uneasy slumber, lasting six hours, from which he awoke fully conscious, though with a confused recollection of the cause of his troubles the night previous. He was also nervous, and inclined to hesitate and stammer in replying to questions. The bromide being continued, all these symptoms rapidly subsided.

In both a pathological and physiological point of view, this case is one of some interest; for, on careful inquiry into the previous history of this boy, we are satisfied that he has not been subject to epilepsy; neither did his symptoms point to an epileptiform seizure. There was neither convulsion, stertor and frothing at the mouth, nor the characteristic drowsiness and stupor, that usually follow epilepsy. It was certainly not hysteria, and the only explanation we can give of his condition, is, that he was the subject of temporary functional *mental palsy*, the result of the sudden and profound impression produced by the fright. So great was the shock, and so vivid and terrible was the impression made by the supposed man at the door, that the apparition overshadowed and paralyzed every other faculty of the mind, and held it for the time being under the dominance of this purely subjective vision, until sleep, nature's restorer, induced an equilibrium between the sensory and intellectual ganglia of the brain. As the impression upon the former became obliterated, the functions of the latter resumed their normal sway.

CASE OF AN ACEPHALOUS MONSTER.

By Geo. W. N. Elders, M. D., Cedar Hill, Mo.

I shall not pretend to enter into the literature of monstrosities, nor indeed collate the cases of that class, to which the following belongs, but content myself with as accurate a description as possible of one of those strange freaks of nature by which a conception perfect in the beginning, was changed during gestation into a monster by defective development.

May 2d, 1873, I was called about 10½ o'clock, a. m., to see a Mrs. L—— in her fourth confinement. She had been in labor about four hours when the fœtus was expelled, about twenty minutes before my arrival. On examination I found a well-formed 'and well-nourished child, except the deficient development of the encephalon, and bony cavity of the cranium ; the child weighed about six pounds. I will describe the singular deformity as it presented itself to my view.

There was an entire absence of the calvarium from a line commencing with the globe of the eye on either side, and passing back on a level with the top of the ears.

There were no bony arches over the eyes, which were kept closed and had the appearance of two large oval tumors, there being, as I supposed, considerable adipose tissue under the upper lids. This gave the appearance of considerable depression over the root of the nose.

The edge or margin of this plane was not abrupt, but a sort of fleshy roll on a level with the tops of the ears, and extending around the occiput a little above the inferior curved line of the occipital bone. By making pretty firm pressure upon the border, I could feel the solid bony base of the partially developed temporal and occipital bones. Inside of the latter was probably contained a small cerebellum, upon the center of this flat was a soft mass convoluted and of a dark veinous hue. This mass was elevated about half an inch above the plane, and was one inch and a half in diameter, and was circular ; the covering of this mass had the appearance of a serous membrane.

Between this mass and the rim or edge, there is a marked depression which seemed to have a more solid base, immediately around the circumference of this substance were a few hairs, all that were to be seen anywhere on the child.

The child was a female and well-developed otherwise, was still born, and all our attempts to resuscitate it were ineffectual.   It was living up to the moment of birth.

The mother's health has always been good and free from any hereditary taint.   The husband is a hard drinker, but otherwise a man of good constitution.

Query.—What was the cause of the arrest of development in the cranium, and of the cranial cavity—will some one please suggest?

NOVEL CASE OF SNEEZING.

In a letter from Dr. Y. A. Winn, of Libertyville, Mo., he says, I will mention a very singular case, (singular to me at least) a gentleman informs me that when prompted to sexual commerce, he is seized immediately prior to the act, with a fit of violent sneezing, not unfrequently even the *thought* of coition, produces this effect. Query—How would you prescribe in such a case? May the sneezing be excited by some pathological condition of the nervous system in which the excitation of the schneidinan membrane is due to some complicated reflex nervous action? The gentleman being married we are at a loss for a satisfactory remedy. Fortunately his wife has never *apparently* noticed this peculiarity. If she should, and he did much sneezing in the presence of other ladies, even *sneezing* might be a sufficient ground for divorce.

The *London Med. Record* is responsible for the following on sneezing :

"The custom of invoking a blessing upon persons who sneeze, is, says Dr. Seguin, in a recent article on sneezing, a most interesting one. Several old medical · authors state that the custom dates back from the time of a severe epidemic (in which sneezing was a bad sign) during the pontificate of Gregory the Great. Brand, however, and the author of an article in ' *Rees's Clyclopædia*,' state that the phrase 'God bless you,' as addressed to persons having sneezed is much more ancient, being old in the days of Aristotle. The Greeks appear to have traced it back to the mythical days of Prometheus, who is reported to have blessed · his man ·of clay when he sneezed. In Brand the rabbinical account is given, that the phrase originated in the alleged fact that it was only through Jacob's struggle with the angel that sneezing ceased to be an act fatal to man. In many countries, sneezing has been the subject of congratulations and of hopeful augury. In Mesopotamia and some African towns, the populace is reported to have shouted when the monarchs sneezed. Sometimes, moreover, it is very important not to sneeze; and Dr. Seguin has discovered what has been discovered before, but is insufficiently known, that sneezing may be prevented by forcibly rubbing the skin below and on either side of the nose. And on this observation of himself, and of Marshall Hall, Diday, and the world generally before them, he bases an exceedingly interesting study of the physiology of sneezing in health and disease."

Proceedings.

AMERICAN MEDICAL ASSOCIATION.

Notwithstanding the daily papers have given quite full accounts of the doings of the Association, it may be expected, and properly, that we should record the more important acts, though we have been partially anticipated by the daily secular press.

The Twenty-fourth session of the American Medical Association convened in the Masonic Hall, St, Louis, on the 6th of May, at 11 o'clock A. M. The officers of the Association being present and over three hundred and fifty delegates registered, the ex-president, Dr. D. W. Yandell, of Louisville, called the Association to order, and called on the Rev. Dr. Niccolls to open the meeting with prayer; following which Dr. John S. Moore, of St. Louis, delivered the address of welcome to the members of the Association. Dr. Yandell introduced the President of the Association, Dr. Thos. M. Logan, of Sacramento, Cal. Dr. J. B. Johnson, Chairman of Committee of Arrangements, presented the report of the Committee, announcing the order of exercises, etc. In conclusion Dr. Johnson moved that the names of those who desired to be accredited as delegates, but against whose reception protests had been filed, be referred to the Committee on Ethics. The motion was carried and the president nominated as such committee, Drs. N. S. Davis, E. L. Howard, H. F. Askew, D. W. Yandell and J. M. Toner.

The President's address was then delivered, for which a vote of thanks was returned by the Association, and it was referred to the Committee on Publication.

Dr. Atkins offered a paper on the education of the medical senses, by Dr. Seguin, of New York. Referred to the section on obstetrics; also, a paper on the seminal cell, referred to same section. The roll of special committees appointed at the last meeting was called, and progress reported. At request some of the committees were granted continuance, and the reports of others were made special orders during the session. A number of papers, on various topics were presented and referred to the appropriate sections. The report of Dr. Pollack, on "Suggestions on Medical Education," was made the special order for 11 o'clock on Thursday. The delegations from the various States were requested to appoint a committee of one from each State, to meet in caucus after the Association adjourned for the day, and nominate the standing committees and officers for the ensuing year.

The Association then adjourned till 9.30 in the morning.

MEETINGS OF SECTIONS.

In the afternoon the convention sat by sections, devoted to the consideration of the various branches of medical practice, and proceeded to discussions and reading of essays on topics pertinent to the several departments below named.

SURGERY.—The meeting was convened at 3 o'clock. In the absence of the president, Dr. Warren, Dr. Lankford was elected to the chair; Dr. W. F. Peck, of Davenport, Iowa, acted as secretary.

Dr. Andrews invited the attention of the profession to the use of drainage tubes in cases of pyæmia, in connection with abscesses in the chest.

Dr. Gouley, of New York, complimented the use of Chassignoc's drainage tube, preferring it to the pneumatic respirator.

The subject was further discussed by Dr. Hughes, who referred to a novel method pursued by Dr. Stone, of New Orleans, in treating abscesses in the chest—taking out a piece of rib, and thereby furnishing an opportunity for permanent drainage—and remarks were also made by Dr. Godbery, of Mississippi, Dr. Andrews, and by Dr. Johnson, of Chicago.

The subject of consecutive dislocation of the elbow was brought up by Dr. Moore, of New York, and discussed by Dr. Allen, of Louisiana, and Dr. Andrews.

Dr. Gouley, of New York, introduced a new instrument employed in arresting hemorrhage in cases where the peritoneum is divided, in cases of stone in the bladder and stricture of the urethra.

Other subjects were brought up, and the discussion continued until nearly 4 o'clock.

PRACTICE OF MEDICINE AND OBSTETRICS.—The section met at 3 o'clock in Grand Mason's room, Dr. O'Donnell, of Baltimore, in the chair, and Dr. W. Clark, secretary pro tem.

The subject of treatment of puerperal convulsions was first discussed.

Dr. Hasham, of Delaware, advocated the old remedy of the lancet, expressing the opinion that chloral and its substitutes were quite inefficient.

Dr. Catlin, of Connecticut, thought the lancet effective in apoplectic cases, but chloral, stramonium, bromide, etc., in anæmic cases.

Dr. Helm reported a case where a patient lost 252 ounces of blood, and recovered.

Dr. Montgomery, of St. Louis, advocated the lancet in apoplectic cases.

Dr. Seguin, of New York, read an interesting essay on "Education of the Medical Senses," which was referred to the Committee on Publication.

Some points brought forward were discussed by Dr. Hasham.

A vote of thanks was returned to Dr. Seguin for the essay.

Dr. Smith, of Iowa, called the attention of the section to the importance of placing the woman about to be delivered in the best position to facilitate the labor by the aid of gravitation ; in every case where delay occurs and the oblique position of the child is apparent, he maintained that by attention to the position of the woman and by so placing her as to aid the uterus by causing the weight of the fœtus to rest fairly and uniformily on the parieties of the passage, that the labor would be greatly facilitated, *e. g.*, if the head impinged on the left border of the superior strait he would place the patient on her left side, thus tilting the fundus of the uterus to a more central position or line horizontal with the axis of the strait, etc.

MATERIA MEDICA AND CHEMISTRY.—In a room opposite that occupied by the section on obstetrics and practice of medicine, was an interesting exposition of materia medica, chemicals, apparatus, etc.

The following list of exhibitors and productions were among the most prominent: Pharmaceutical goods—Wm. H. Crawford. Chemical and pharmaceutical preparations—Larkins and Scheffer. A collection from the cabinet of the St. Louis

College of Pharmacy, illustrating *materia medica* and pharmacy. Manufactured goods—A. A. Mellier & Co. Pharmaceutical preparations manufactured by W. J. M. Gordon, of Cincinnati; exhibited by Howell, Hopkins & Thurber. Valentine's preparation of meat juice. Chemicals of Missouri manufacture—G. Mallinkrodt & Co. Sugar-coated pills—Wm. R. Warner & Co., Philadelphia; pepsin powder, prepared by E. Scheffer & Co., Louisville; gelatine coated pills, McKesson & Robbins, New York; dental and surgical instruments, A. M. Leslie & Co.; chemical apparatus, Theodore Kalb; supporters, bandages, etc., Mrs. E. J. Harding; trusses, braces, etc., Chas. Schleiffarth; and electrical instruments, galvanic and faradic batteries, by the Galvano-Faradic Manufacturing Company, New York.

SECOND DAY'S PROCEEDINGS.

At 9½ o'clock the Association met, the President, Dr. Logan, being in the chair. A list of additional delegates was read. Committees on Nominations, organization of sections, new officers, section meetings, etc., submitted the following report:

Place of next meeting, Detroit, Michigan.

President, Dr. J. M. Toner, District of Columbia. Vice Presidents, W. Y. Gadbury, Miss.; J. M. Keller, Ky.; W. C. Husted, New York; L. F. Warner, Mass. Treasurer, Dr. Caspar Wister. Librarian, Wm. Lee. Committee on Library, Doctors Johnson and Elliott. Assistant Secretary, Dr. T. A. McGraw, Michigan. Committee of Arrangements—W. Brodie, chairman; James A. Brown, Morse Stewart, J. F. Noyes, E. W. Jenks, Henry F. Lyster, D. O. Farrand and Eugene Smith. Committee on Prize Essays—Doctors G. K. Johnson, A. Sager, H. Hitchcock, Mich., E. Andrews, Ill., E. S. Gaillard, Ky. Committee on Publication—F. G. Smith, W. B. Atkinson, D. M. Chester, Penn., Wm. Lee, District of Columbia, Caspar Wister, Penn., H. F. Askew, Del., Alfred Stille, Penn.

Dr. N. S. Davis submitted the following amendment to the constitution or plan of organization, to be acted upon at the next annual session.

It is proposed to strike out the second paragraph of Article II, commencing with "The delegates" and ending with "of pairs," and insert the following:

"The delegates shall receive their appointment from permanently organized State medical societies, and such county and district medical societies as are recognized by representation in their respective State societies, and from the medical societies of the army and navy of the United States of America."

Also strike out all of the fourth paragraph of same Art. II, beginning with "each local society" and ending with "one delegate," and insert the following: "Each State, county and district medical society entitled to representation, shall have the privilege of sending to the Association one delegate for every ten of its regular resident members, and one for each additional fraction of more than half that number. The medical staffs of the army and navy shall be entitled to four delegates each."

The Secretary read the following appointments made by the President to represent the American Medical Association to the British Medical Association: Drs. F. G. Smith, C. Wister, J. S. Cohen, of Philadelphia, Dr. E. Warren, of Baltimore, Dr. C. L. Ives, of New Haven, Dr. Edward Montgomery, of St. Louis, and Drs. F. Barker, E. Seguin and J. C. Hutchinson, of New York.

The Secretary stated that commissions for these gentlemen would be made out at once.

MEETING OF THE SECTIONS.

The different sections into which the convention is subdivided. to consider separately the different branches of medical science, met at 8 o'clock, and were all well attended.

PRACTICE OF MEDICINE AND OBSTETRICS.—The chair was occupied by Dr. O'Donnell, of Baltimore; Dr. E. W. Gray, of Bloomington, Illinois, acting as Secretary.

In response to the President's call, no papers were presented, and on motion of Dr. Gray a request was made that all papers belonging to the section be placed in the hands of its officers.

Dr. Todd, of Kansas City, addressed the section on the subject of physiological anomalies in the configuration of the bony and soft walls of the pelvis as a cause of retardation in labor.

The points of the paper were reviewed by Dr. Hollister, of Illinois, who also made some remarks on secondary hemorrhage after delivery.

The hour having arrived, Dr. Drisdell, of Philadelphia, read his paper on the microscopical appearance of ovarian cysts, in the course of which he announced the discovery of a new cell which he denominated the ovarian granular cell. The paper was very favorably received, and it was referred to the Committee on Publication.

Dr. Howard presented a memorial paper by an absent member, on medical education, which was referred to a special sub-committee, consisting of Drs. Howard, Pallen and Todd.

General remarks of a practical character were made by Dr. Garric, of New York, and others, continuing until nearly 5 o'clock.

THIRD DAY'S PROCEEDINGS.

The Association was called to order by the President. An addition to list of delegates read.

Passing the report on the nomenclature of disease, that of the committee on ethics, on salary of permanent secretary, national sanitary bureau, suggestions on medical education, and United States Marine Hospital service, we come to the

SECTION REPORTS.

The committee appointed to devise and recommend some plan for securing a more complete report of the doings in the several sections, submitted through Dr. Davis the following resolutions, which were adopted:

Resolved, That the Committee of Arrangements for each annual meeting of the Association are instructed to secure the services of a sufficient number of phonographic reporters to have one in attendance on the regular sessions of each of the sections in the afternoon, as well as during the general morning sessions. That the reports thus obtained be printed the same evening on slips or proof-sheets in sufficient number to supply all the members of the Association in attendance, early the following morning.

The second resolution prescribes the method of providing for the expenses hereby incurred. The third resolution provides for the selection and revision of the most valuable parts of the proceedings, and their transmission to the Secretary for publication within twenty days after the adjournment of the Association.

21

MEETING OF THE SECTIONS.

The afternoon session, occupied in the sittings of the sections, was largely attended, although many of the delegates devoted the time to sight-seeing, visiting, etc.

SURGICAL SECTION.—The chair was occupied by Dr. Fisher, of Illinois; Dr. Peck, of Iowa, Secretary.

A case of tumor of the face was introduced by Dr. Kirk, of Illinois, for the purpose of having a diagnosis pronounced by the section.

Dr. Moore, of New York, brought up the subject of fracture of the epiphysis of the humerus at the shoulder, which was discussed at considerable length by a number of members.

Dr. Kirk, of Illinois, presented for diagnosis a case of peculiar tumor of the left inguinal region.

Dr. Crawford, of Pennsylvania, said there was a spirit in his State very injurious to the profession, and he desired to bring it before the profession to see whether the same spirit existed throughout the country. He then proceeded to state that he had been prosecuted in the Pennsylvania courts for malpractice for leaving a little boy who had broken his leg, with that limb an inch shorter than it ought to be. He said that the boy had exercised his limb at his own notion, and without his (the doctor's) consent, but he thought the suit showed a wrong feeling toward the profession. He thought this revengeful feeling on the part of the public should be discouraged, and he urged the section to work to that end.

The section didn't agree with him, and squelched the thing as far as possible.

PRACTICE OF MEDICINE AND OBSTETRICS.—In the absence of the President, Dr. Bell, of Brooklyn, was called to the chair; Dr. Gray being Secretary.

An interesting paper on yellow fever, written by Dr. Matchett, was presented by Dr. Wallace, in which the author maintained the proposition that the fever named is miasmatic, self-producing, and non-contagious, and that quarantine is of no effect.

Dr. Bell, of Brooklyn, who had resigned the chair to the President, Dr. O'Donnell, of Baltimore, disputed the proposition put forward, and gave several striking examples in proof of his position. He would as soon believe in the spontaneous generation of a grain of corn as that of yellow fever, which he believed was portable, although not necessarily contagious, and would lie dormant like a grain of wheat, although for what length of time he would not undertake to say. He did not wish to see a paper published in the transactions of the convention, which did not come up within twenty-years of the accepted knowledge on the subject.

Dr. Wallace, of Texas, who read the paper, disclaimed the doctrines of the author.

Dr. Gillman, of St. Louis, agreed substantially with the remarks of Dr. Bell, and moved that the paper be re-committed to its author.

Dr. Davis, of Chicago, said the general law of infection was that the infected air contains the germs of the disease, and may be carried from one place to another, and if the condition of the air was suitable, it would propagate. Yellow fever was infectious, but perhaps not properly contagious. He favored the motion of Dr. Gillman.

The subject of cerebro-spinal meningitis was brought up by Dr. Morris, of Baltimore, who held it to be produced by a poison generated in certain localities.

Dr. Davis, of Chicago, said the disease prevailed most in uncleanly localities. It originated from, or was aggravated by local causes. One class presented many symptoms in common with typhus; another seemed closely allied with erysipelas, and a third stood closely to malarial fever. The central point of its pathology was the impairment of the vital energies, with a tendency to concentrate irritation on the cerebro-spinal cord.

Dr. Spottswood, of Indiana, presented a few points gathered in his experience, and was followed by a number of others, until the adjournment of the section.

FOURTH DAY'S PROCEEDINGS.

Attendance was light—many delegates having left for their homes. Passing the report of the Committee on Medical Ethics, as unimportant, we come to the farewell address by the President.

" *Gentlemen :* Our labors are now brought to a close. Our official relations herewith close. While thanking you for the kindness and courtesy extended to me, I avail myself of this opportunity to acknowledge the great compliment tendered, not, to myself alone, but to that far distant land I represent, on the Western confines of this glorious Republic. [Applause.] In the name, therefore, of California and of Oregon, I return you my best thanks for the kind consideration received at your hands, not only on this occasion, but for the distinction of the presidency bestowed upon me last year, in the very cradle of American medicine. Proud and thankful as I am for this favor, I am still more thankful for it, when I reflect upon the indirect influence it has exercised upon the profession of the Pacific Coast, for which the compliment was obviously intended. Not for any individual merits of my own, but for the common efforts of our medical men in giving you a grateful welcome, was the post of honor awarded to California. Prior to your advent there, the medical mind was in a state of inertia—the profession in a chaotic condition. The State Medical Society was in the fourteenth year of a Rip Van Winkle sleep. But no sooner were the clarion notes of your coming sounded. than a new spirit was awakened, and from their sheltering privacy, in all parts of California, volunteers poured in and threw themselves into the movement which was to regenerate the prostrated glory of their calling. [Applause.] How well they have succeeded, let their works and not my words tell. I have only to say that such were the high character and acknowledged merits of the papers read at the first annual meeting of their renaissance, that the Legislature made forthwith an appropriation for their annual publication. Thus recognized and indorsed by the State, the Society has continued to advance to a higher and higher plane at each successive meeting. So complete has been our success in elevating the profession in California, that at the last meeting, some four weeks ago, we were not only honored, for the first time in the medical history of our State, with a bounteous reception from the Governor, but also the President of the University left the seat of learning, one hundred and twenty miles distant from the capital, to address us on the subject of medical education and, with our honored Governor, graced our festive board. Appreciated as we now are by the State, we will continue our endeavors to add a luster to the high trusts that have been so generously confided to us, and to render ourselves more and more worthy of the next visit you may in your judgment think fit to accord to California. Grant that it may be soon. I now declare the twenty-fourth annual session of the American Medical Association adjourned.

The Association then adjourned to meet on the first Tuesday in June, 1874, at Detroit, Mich.

This incomplete report is compiled partly from personal observation and partly from what appeared in the daily papers, and may be of interest as indicating the *proposed* methods of this body in future. When the doings of each section shall be correctly and fully reported by a competent expert under pay, valuable results may be expected; and a new interest in the organization be awakened. The officers did their part admirably, harmony marked the proceedings; and undoubted good was accomplished.

In view of the rings, cliques, ambitions, and jealousy believed to exist here in the family of doctors, we think they behaved admirably in the presence of their invited guests, who seemed to consider us a "happy family," from their stand point.

THE MEDICAL EDITORS' NATIONAL ASSOCIATION.

The Medical Editors' National Association convened in Polytechnic Hall, at 8 o'clock, p. m., May 5th, and was called to order by the President, Theophilus Parvin, one of the editors of the *American Practitioner*.

After the transaction of the ordinary preliminary business, the President delivered his oration, which proved to be a most interesting and instructive entertainment, occupying the remainder of the evening. For which, a vote of thanks was tendered, and the manuscript asked for publication, and appeared in the columns of the *St. Louis Globe*, in their issue of the 8th of May.

The second meeting of the Association was appointed for the following evening at 7 o'clock, at the parlors of the Southern Hotel, when the following officers were elected for the ensuing year: President—Dr. W. K. Boling, of Nashville, Tenn. Vice-President—Dr. W. S. Edgar, St. Louis. Secretary—Dr. F. H. Davis, Chicago. Committee on Prize Essays for 1874—Drs. N.

S. Davis, Chicago, J. P. Logan, Atlanta, and J. M. Toner, Washington.

The Association adjourned *sine die.*

AMERICAN PUBLIC HEALTH ASSOCIATION.

The first annual meeting of this Association was held in Cincinnati, May 1st, 1873.

The meeting was called to order by the President, Dr. Stephen Smith, of New York. Dr. E. H. Jones, of New York, was elected Secretary *pro tem.* After an interesting session of three days, they adjourned to meet on the second Wednesday of September next, at Providence, Rhode Island.

THE MISSOURI STATE MEDICAL ASSOCIATION.

The Missouri State Medical Association convened at Moberly, on the 1st of May, and continued in session three days, with the usual number of delegates in attendance. The minutes of the meeting we have failed to secure, but presume an authentic copy with the papers read will soon be furnished the Committee on Publication, and the wishes of the Association in their publication be promptly carried out.

Reviews and Bibliographical Notices.

THE MEDICAL AND SURGICAL HISTORY OF THE REBELLION. (1861-65.) Prepared in accordance with acts of Congress, under the direction of Surgeon General, Joseph K. Barnes, United States Army. Part 1, Vol. I, Medical History; Vol. 2, Surgical History. 4to. pp. 1184 and 819. Washington: Government Printing Office.

Part 1. Of the Medical and Surgical History of the War of the Rebellion, is composed of two volumes. The first, (Medical) is prepared by J. J. Woodward, Assistant Surgeon,* U. S.

---

* We almost blush to write Assistant Surgeon as the rank of one of his age, ability and worth.

Army. It is composed of a preface of nine pages, by Surgeon General, Barnes; an introduction of thirty-four pages by Dr. Woodward. One hundred and twelve tables with index, comprising seven hundred and twenty-six pages; two hundred and eighty-nine reports, extracts from reports and letters from surgeons, of the various battles, campaigns, sieges, etc., etc., in the form of an *appendix*, comprising three hundred and fifty-three pages with table of contents.

Soon after the commencement of the war it was found desirable to modify the form of *reports of sick and wounded*, and a form was adopted based upon that devised by Dr. Wm. Farr, of London, there being some changes made from his, by a medical board, in the latter part of July, 1862, composed of Surgeons L. A. Edwards, U. S. Army, and J. H. Brinton, U. S. V., and Assistant Surgeons J. J. Woodward, and M. J. Asch, U. S. A. The introduction is replete with interesting matter, and every medical man should study it carefully. Any one can see in a few minutes what a vast amount of labor and care has been expended in collecting information from every source, comparing with the Adjutant General's department, the Quartermaster's, the Provost Marshal General's department, and Commissioner of Pensions' reports, in order to reach the exact figures as nearly as possible. Reducing the enlistments to a *standard of three years*, there is, by the report of the Adjutant General, of February, 1869, the number of "2,073,112 *white enlisted men.*" "The total number of commissions issued to white officers was 83,935, and the total number of colored enlistments, 178,895." This is the calculation for the period of the war.

The nearest approximation that can be reached (the lowest) number of deaths will be found in the following table:

	Regulars.	White Volunteers.	Colored Volunteers.	Total
Killed in battle	1,355	41,369	1,514	44,238
Died of wounds and injuries	1,174	46,271	1,760	49,205
Suicide, homicide and execution	27	442	57	526
Total violent deaths	2,556	88,082	3,331	93,969
Deaths from disease	3,009	153,995	29,212	186,216
Unknown causes	150	23,188	837	24,184
Total	5,724	265,265	33,380	304,369

" From this view it will be seen that of 280,185 deaths from *known causes*, the proportion of violent deaths to the whole number was one out of every three deaths."

From the outbreak of the war to June 30, 1865, the annual average of deaths of *white volunteers* was " 65,178, or 88 per 1,000 of average aggregate mean strength. Sub-dividing this ratio between violent deaths and deaths from disease in accordance to the proportion of these classes already indicated, we shall have an annual ratio of 33 violent deaths, and 55 deaths from disease per 1,000 of average aggregate strength." In the regular army there was an annual death-rate of only 59 per 1,000 of strength, which would give an annual ratio of 27 violent deaths and 32 deaths from disease per 1,0Q0 of strength. There is a difference of 6 per 1,000 of violent deaths and 23 per 1,000 of deaths from disease of annual death-rate against the white volunteers, or in favor of the regular army. This remarkable difference, we apprehend, was largely due to the imperfect examination of volunteer recruits.

There were discharged on surgeon's certificate of disability, as set forth in a letter of the Adjutant General to the Surgeon General dated October 25, 1870, the following :

Enlisted men of the regular Army....... 6,541
Enlisted men .of the volunteer army.... 269,197
Enlisted men of colored troops...9,807
Total 285,545

From tables C and CXI, we learn that there were "37,794 deaths of white, and 6,764 of colored troops due to the several forms of diarrhœa and dysentery, which must therefore, be regarded as the most important causes of the mortality from disease in our armies." Of the several forms of camp fever, these tables "attribute 35,965 deaths of white, and 5,233 of colored troops."

Pneumonia is next in importance, " of which 14,788 deaths of whites, and 5,233 of colored troops are reported." * * * *
" The largest number of discharges among white troops were : consumption, 20,403 ; diarrhœa and dysentery, 17,889 ; debility, 14,500 ; rheumatism, 11,779 ; heart-disease, 10,636. Among the colored troops the chief causes of discharge were : rheumatism, 874 ; consumption, 592 ; debility, 540 ; and diarrhœa and dysentery, 359."

" The report of the Adjutant General, of February, 1869,

sets forth also 26,168 deaths, included in the whole number (304,369) as having occurred among those of our men who were prisoners in the hands of the enemy."

The reports, etc., in the appendix, to this volume are very interesting in many of the details.

The particulars of some of the more important subjects set forth in this volume must receive a more extended consideration in the next (Medical) volume.

The second volume (surgical) Part I. prepared by Geo. A. Otis, Assistant Surgeon U. S. Army, is composed of the prefatory note by Surgeon General Barnes ; an introduction by Dr. Otis ; a chronological table of engagements and battles fought during the period of four years, from April, 1861, to April, 1865. The surgical history proper follows in five chapters including respectively, first chapter, wounds and injuries of the head; second, those of the face; third those of the neck; fourth, injury of the spinal column ; fifth, wounds and injuries of the chest. Other injuries of the trunk, of the extremities with amputations and excisions are treated in the second surgical volume, which will soon appear. The third surgical volume will contain the consideration of gunshot wounds in general, together with their complications ; " also the materia chirurgica, the transportation and field supplies of the wounded."

As quoted, in the first volume from the Adjutant General's report, the number of those killed in action embraced " not less than 44,238 ;" according to the alphabetical registers of the Surgeon General's office, 35,408 ; according to the chronological summary, 59,860." I will give you one instance of the comparatively large amount of material on hand from which to make a report. Dr. Longmore, in speaking of the British system of reports as being the best of all, criticises rather severely our reports as set forth in circular No. 6. S. G. O., when comparing it with " the chronological summary, compiled by the faithful and indefatigable chief clerk of the surgical division, Mr. Frederick R. Sparks, indicates the following losses : Union troops, killed, 59,860 ; wounded, 280,040 ; missing, 184,791 : Confederate troops, killed, 51,425 ; wounded, 227,871 ; missing, 384,281. The last aggregate includes the armies surrendered. Allowing for many exaggerations and omissions, the errors appear to balance remarkably, and the results to correspond with statistics derived from entirely different sources." Perfected histories of the Crimean and Italian wars made by Dr. Mathew, and M. Chenu years after the wars had closed. Yet Dr. Mathew reports only *twenty-six* cases of trephining, and M Chenu nine; while in our list there are *two hundred and twenty* cases recorded.

The work when completed, will be an inexhaustible mine of information, unequaled in military surgery; and a monument of which every one should feel a just pride who has contributed in labor or influence in collecting the facts, arranging or publishing them; or who aided in maintaining the Government which has so liberally furnished the means for giving to medical science this imperishable Medical and Surgical History.

It should be in every public library, and should be donated to every medical officer who served faithfully in the war.

This brief notice would not be excusable if we should fail to mention the nineteen medical officers killed in battle; thirteen killed by partisan troops, guerillas, or by rioters; the eight who died in consequence of wounds, and nine of accidents; and the seventy-three who were wounded in action.

We cannot attempt an analysis of the work, space does not permit.

FAMILY THERMOMETRY.—A Manual of Thermometry, for mothers, nurses, hospitals, etc., and all who have charge of the sick and of the young. By Edward Seguin, M. D., New York: G. P. Putman & Sons. pp. 72. 12 mo. Price 75 cts.
[For sale by the St. Louis Book & News Co.]

This *Manual of Thermometry*, intended especially for the family, but also for all who have charge of the sick, is addressed in the form of a letter to a mother, Madam R——P——. The work contemplates the education of women in the use of the thermometer to ascertain when a deviation from health exists, as well as the degree and importance of the deviation; and at the same time to indicate to them hygienic and remedial measures which may be judiciously applied to restore the temperature to the *norme* or healthy standard. The author does not propose to teach the names and nature of diseases, but to put into the hands of those who have more or less the constant care of the young, and the sick, means which will enable them to appreciate the existence or absence of real danger, and to aid them to assist the physician in determining the actual state.

The instrument used is a delicate thermometer having a scale of ten degrees above the *norme*—zero or health-point (0 = H), which corresponds to "the general norme of the Caucasian race—98.6°F., equal to 29.6°R., or to 87° centigrade," and running seven degrees below the same zero. The author desires to establish "the mathematical law upon which family thermometry is founded and remains unshaken viz: The distance which separates a patient from health is proportioned to the sum of the degrees which separate the index from zero, and the time that the deviations from the norme have lasted."

This is "an effort to enlighten those most interested in the subject." *The work is a step in the right direction;* and we shall gladly hail the time when information such as is here proposed shall take the place of much of the ignorance that now exists.

A SYSTEM OF ORAL SURGERY: being a consideration of the Diseases and Surgery of the Mouth, Jaws, and Associate Parts. By James E. Garretson, M. D., D. D. S., Oral surgeon to the Medical Department of the University of Pennsylvania; author of Diseases and Surgery of the Mouth, Jaws, and Associate parts; etc., etc. Illustrated with numerous steel plates and wood cuts. Philadelphia : J. B. Lippincott & Co., 1873. pp. 1091.
[For Sale by the St Louis Book & News Co.]

In the preface to this, the *Second Edition* of Dr. Garretson's work on Oral Surgery, the author tells us *his highest ambition is to bridge the gap* existing between general *surgery and dentistry.*

This volume of nearly eleven hundred pages, not including a number of the plates, is divided quite judiciously into fifty-one chapters. The field covered is very extensive, and it is evident the author has at times found it difficult to decide at what point to stop and yet not omit what might be more or less essential to a complete knowledge of the immediate subject under consideration. It is evident he recognizes the necessity of a thorough knowledge of the general principles of medicine in order properly to treat any special branch or local deviation. The first three chapters are devoted to the consideration of the anatomy of the head, face, and especially the fifth pair of nerves. Most of the figures in this portion of the work are well executed.

A large part of the volume belongs almost exclusively, and very properly, to dentistry. The chapter on neuralgia comprises about fifty pages, containing many interesting cases and much valuable information for the general practitioner as well as for the specialist. As we quoted largely from this part of the former edition in this Journal (June, 1872), we will not now repeat what was there said. On page 752 he quotes from Dr. Buzzard of the favorable effect of electricity in *ten cases*, of sixteen treated, there *was very great* and *well-marked relief*, in *two moderate relief*, and in *four* there was *very slight relief*.

The author, on the subject of palatine defects, gives a method of treating *fissure* of the *hard palate* in the infant by compression on the sides of the jaws to bring the bones together in the median line having, previously freshened the opposing sides of the fissure. Indeed, he proposes two methods, one in which the correction is made *instantly*, and in the other it is made slowly. "The first of these procedures is applicable to such cases as present but a limited separation of the bones; the latter, when the fissure has considerable width." This method seems to have been proposed before, but we are not prepared to recommend it. The usual treatment is the operation of *uranoplasty*, or the use of *obturators*. We regard the work as a valuable addition to our works on the surgery of the mouth; and it is also important in the advice given for the general practitioner, containing, as it does, a vast fund of information collected from many authorities, and from extensive observation and experience by the author. The publishers have done their work well.

BOOKS AND PAMPHLETS RECEIVED.

HIP JOINT ANCHYLOSIS.—A case of 14 years' duration; successful operation for the formation of false joint. By A. G. Beebe, M. D., Chicago, Ill.

BURNS & SCALDS—Their treatment with cases. By Joseph E. Montgomery, M. D., San Francisco, Cal.

CHEMICAL ANALYSIS.—A guide to the examination of medical chemicals, and for the detection of impurities and adulterations. By Frederick Hoffman, P. H. D. New York: D. Appleton & Co. (For sale by the St. Louis Book & News Co.) 8 vo. pp. 393.

CIVIL MAL-PRACTICE.—By M. A. McClelland, M. D. Chicago: W. B. Keen & Co. Price $2.00.

HAND-BOOK OF PHYSIOLOGICAL LABORATORY.—By E. Kline, M. D., J. Burden Sanderson, M. D., F. R. S., Michael Foster, M. D., F. R. S., and T. Lander Brunton, M. D. etc. Edited by J. Burden Sanderson. 2 vol. with 133 plates containing 353 illustrations. Philadelphia: Lindsay and Blakiston. (For sale by the St. Louis Book & News Co.).

HAND-BOOK OF MEDICAL ELECTRICITY.—By Herbert Tibbits, M. D., L. R. C. P., London, with 64 illustrations. Philadelphia: Lindsay & Blakiston. Price $2.00. (For sale by the St. Louis Book & News Co).

OVARIOTOMY.—By J. Marion Sims, M. D. Pamphlet of 85 pages. New York: D. Appleton & Co.

ABNORMAL RE-ACTION OF THE ACOUSTIC NERVE in Chlorosis and Bright's Disease. By Wm. B. Neftel, M. D. New York: J. B. Lippincott & Co.

BELLEVUE HOSPITAL MEDICAL COLLEGE—The first Decennial Catalogue of the Trustees, Faculty, Officers and Alumnia, from 1861 to 1871. By F. A. Castle, M. D. New York: D. Appleton & Co., 551 Broadway.

PRACTICAL HISTOLOGY IN VIENNA, AND THE MICROSCOPICAL STUDY OF BLOOD AND EPITHELIUM. By James Tyson, M. D. Philadelphia: J. Lippincott & Co.

LITHOTOMY.—By Paul F. Eve, M. D. Nashville: Robits & Purvis.

PROPRIETORY OR ADVERTISED NOSTRUMS.—By Ely Van De Walker, M. D. New York: D. Appleton & Co.

"RING"—New York City Origin, and Fall. By S. J. Tilden, N. Y.

EUSTACHIAN TUBE—The Function of, in relation to the Renewal and Density of the Air in the Tympanic Cavity and to the concavity of the Membrana Tympani. By Thos. F. Rumbold, M. D., St. Louis.

CONIUM IN THE TREATMENT OF INSANITY.—By Daniel H. Kitchen, M. D. (From the *American Journal of Insanity* for April, 1878).

THIRD ANNUAL REPORT OF THE SUPERINTENDENT OF PUBLIC SCHOOLS, Jacksonville, Illinois, 1870. By Israel Wilkinson.

Extracts from Current Medical Literature.

Drainage Tubing.

M. Giacopetti calls attention to the value of rubber tubing in the treatment of certain affections of the bones, in the *Bul. Gén. de Thér. Méd. et. Chir.* May 30, 1872,

He states, that the most eminent surgeons in France and England consider its use as highly advantageous in cases of chronic suppuration of the joints, in caries, necrosis, etc. The tubing is made of vulcanized rubber, and is thin, flexible, non-irritating, and is ordinarily of the diameter of a No. 4 English catheter. It can be readily fenestrated with scissors at suitable points, in order that the purulent matters may escape without difficulty. It also allows the surface of the diseased bone to be syringed with disinfectant or stimulating injections. The tubing can be introduced through the fistulous openings, first enlarging them, if necessary, with a knife, trocar or trephine. Since the use of this tubing was first proposed by M. Chassaignac, it has been largely employed in Europe, and of late, to a considerable extent, in this country, in treating deep-seated abscesses and sinuses in the soft tissues, and its great utility has been recognized by nearly every practitioner that has once tried it.

Its action is illustrated in dealing with mammary abscesses when they remain long open and pockets form deep in the gland. By piercing the bottom of these and drawing the tubing down till it penetrates the skin, the pus is drained away, and the opening soon closes, from above downward, until the tubing is finally expelled.

Chromic Acid.

In the same journal, of the date of July 15, M. Isambert publishes a paper on the use of chromic acid in the treatment of ulceration of the gums, soft palate, and pharynx, whether of strumous or of syphilitic origin. He also applies a concentrated solution of the acid (one part to eight, or even of twice this strength), with the aid of the laryngoscopic mirror, to the epithelial vegetations sometimes met with in the vicinity of the arytenoid cartilages and the vocal cords, not oftener, however, than once in eight days, till the little growths disappear. More largely diluted, he finds it effectual in treating the ulcerations of the larynx dependent on phthisis and in œdema of the glottis occurring in this disease. He has observed that its styptic action rendered the respiration easier, and so deferred, at least, if it did not do away with the necessity for a tracheotomy. The same result can be claimed in syphilitic contraction of the larynx as, by its use, time is gained and the patient can be put upon the appropriate specific treatment.

Regarding tumors of the larynx, as mucous and epithelial polypi, and, more especially, cancerous growths, it is certain that the action of chromic acid alone, is insufficient. In cases of cancer, its application should be withheld, as it is exceedingly painful.

Plants in Sleeping-Rooms.

"The quantity of carbonic acid absorbed by day in direct light is vastly greater than that exhaled during the night. According to Corenwinder's experiments, fiften to twenty minutes of direct sunlight enable colza, the pea, the raspberry, the bean, and sunflower to absord as much carbonic acid as they exhale during a whole night.

"Boussingault found, as the average of a number of experiments, that a square metre of oleander leaves decomposed in sunlight 1.108 litres of carbonic acid per hour; in the dark the same surface of leaf exhaled .07 litre (each litre is equal to about $2\frac{1}{4}$ pints) of this gas."—[Prof. Johnson's How Crops Feed, page 45.]

In this last case, therefore, the plant absorbed nearly sixteen times as much carbonic acid in the daylight as it evolved in the same time during the night; while the more active plants would decompose more carbonic acid in half an hour of sunlight than they would exhale during a whole night. The single fact, therefore, that plants do exhale carbonic acid by night does not prove that they will be injurious, on the whole, either in living rooms or in sleeping chambers. The balance may be in favor of their healthfulness, instead of their being injurious. During the day they are constantly giving off oxygen as well as absorbing carbonic acid, and the small exhalation of carbonic acid during the night may still leave a large margin on the side of health.

Not to leave this matter in the condition of mere conjecture, I have gathered and analyzed specimens of air from a room where the influence of growing plants would be exhibited in a greatly exaggarated form. Thus instead of taking the air from a room containing a few plants, I gathered it from the College green-house, where more than 6,000 plants are growing. I gathered the air before sunrise on the mornings of April 16th and 17th ; the room had been closed for more than twelve hours, and if the plants exhaled carbonic acid to an injurious extent, the analysis of air from such a room would certainly disclose this fact. The three specimens of air gathered on the morning of April 16th, from different parts of the room, gave 4.11, 4.00, and 4.00 parts of carbonic acid in 10,000 of air of an average of 4.03 in 10,000. The two specimens of air gathered on April 17th gave 3.80 and 3.80 parts of carbonic acid in 10,000, or an average on the whole of 8.94 parts of carbonic acid in 10,000 of air; while the out-door air contains four parts in 10,000. It will thus be seen that the air in the green-house was better than "pure country air.' This deficiency of carbonic acid was doubtless due to the absorption of carbonic acid and consequent accumulation of oxygen during daylight, since the windows of the green-house were closed day and night on account of the cool weather.

To ascertain whether the air of the green-house had more carbonic acid by night than by day, I gathered two specimens of air in different parts of the house, at two o'clock P. M.. April

17th. These gave 1.40 and 1.38 parts of carbonic acid in 10,000, or an average of 1.39 parts, showing that the night air contained more carbonic acid than did the air of day.

Now, if a room in which were more than 6,000 plants, while containing more carbonic acid by night than by day, contains less carbonic acid than any sleeping-room on this continent, we may safely conclude that one or two dozen plants in a room will not exhale enough carbonic acid by night to injure the sleepers.

It is so easy to be deceived by a name! I lately saw an article showing the beneficial and curative influence of flowers in the sick room. Instances were related where persons were cured by the sight and smell of flowers, and without question their influence is good. Yet flowers exhale this same carbonic acid, both by day and by night! The flowers by their agreeable odor and delicate perfume, impart an air of cheerfulness to the sick chamber which will assist in the recovery from lingering disease, notwithstanding the small amount of carbonic acid which they constantly exhale.

The presence or absence of carbonic acid is not the only question in regard to the healthfulness of plants in a room. The state of moisture in the air of the room may become an important question, especially in the case of persons afflicted with rheumatic or pulmonary complaints. But I will not take up that subject.

Very respectfully your obedient servant,

R. C. Kedzie.

—*Lansing State Republican.*

The Pulse in Childhood.

Mere irregularity of pulse is of absolutely no value as a means of diagnosis. In any febrile attack the pulse of a young child may become irregular; indeed, in many cases the mere quickening of the heart's action seems to lessen the regularity of its contractions. But while a *quick* irregular pulse is of little consequence, a *slow* irregular pulse carries a far different meaning, and, if suspicions of tubercular meningitis have been already excited, will go far to convert those suspicions into certainty.—*Smith—Med. Times and Gaz.*, April 26, 1873—*The Clinic.*

22

Temperature as an Indication of Fœtal Life.

According to Cohnstein, the temperature of the uterus is a more certain indication of the life or death of the fœtus than either its movements or the beating of its heart. The fœtus has a higher temperature than the mother, and imparts it to the uterus; so that this organ is warmer than the axilla, or even than the vagina. If the child die, the temperature of the uterus falls to the level of that of the other parts of the body, and even, Cohnstein says, below this, as the dead fœtus abstracts heat from it. This fall of temperature becomes perceptible two or three hours after the death of the fœtus, and may be ascertained by introducing a curved thermometer a little way beyond the inner os uteri. In this way, also, the diagnosis between intra-uterine and extra-uterine pregnancy may be assisted.—*Brit. Med. Journ.*, April 27, 1873—*The Clinic.*

Digestion of Starch in Infancy.

(*Gaz. Med. Ital.*, November, 1872)—It has been known that the saliva of newly-born animals has not the power of transforming starch into sugar. A recent experimenter has taken the pancreas from kittens and puppies, and has ascertained that the pancreatic juice in these animals when young is, like the saliva, incapable of converting starch into sugar. The bearing of this fact on the practice of giving starchy food to very young infants is obvious.—*New York Med. Jour.*

Carbolic Acid in Intermittent Fever.

M. Ferriète, at a recent meeting of the Academy of Sciences of Paris, related Salisbury's views on the palmellæ of intermittent fever, and Calvert's researches with carbolic acid, and put down as the results of his own investigations that carbolic acid destroys vibrions and mildew, sulphate of quinine mildew only, and that both substances elucidate the question of the etiology of intermittent and typhoid, and constitute rational means of medication in such sorts of disease.—*London Lancet.*

Radical Cure of Fistula Ani without the Use of the Knife.

This proceeding, advocated by Dr. Hute, of America, consists in the use of an injection of a solution of iodine in ether. The ethereal tincture is more exciting than the alcoholic tincture, and the ether, evaporating rapidly, leaves the walls of the fistula in contact with the pure iodine. There is scarcely any reaction, and the patient need not stay in bed.—*Ibid.*

Cholera.

The Indian Army Sanitary Commission states that "in fully developed *cholera*, verging towards, or already in, collapse, medicines were simply of no use." Recovery often follows collapse; but Indian medical experience prove that this recovery is rendered hopeless when *strong medicines*, such as large quantities of brandy and opium, are used. Such remedies are dangerous; yet, by carefully alleviating the symptoms by mild remedies— of which one of the best is simple cold water—by mild nourishment, and kind nursing, in a strictly recumbent position, many cases will recover which would, under different treatment, prove fatal.—*Ibid.*

Treatment of Cerebral Exhaustion.

In his Croonian Lectures lately delivered, Dr. Radcliffe, after describing the principal symptoms of cerebral exhaustion as failure of memory, depression of spirits, increased or diminished sleepiness, unusual irritability, a continued craving for food or stimulating drinks, lessened locomotive power, lessened control over the bladder, diminished sexual activity, inequalities of circulation, an aged aspect, disposition to tears, yawning, occasional faintness, epileptiform symptoms, or transitory hemiplegia, or coma, proceeds to consider its prevention and treatment. In diet, he thinks that the present system of urging persons at all weakly, especially children, to eat as much as they can, may have not a little to do in causing the development of many nervous diseases. He is equally opposed to persistence in "training diet" and to Bantingism, believing that the nerve-tissues as well as others may be effectually starved by excluding the hydro-carbons from the food. He further thinks that too much stress is ordinarily laid upon the importance of much walking exercise; much walking, in fact, seeming to be no insignificant cause of the breakdown in the patient's health, and little or no progress is made until he begins to economise his strength in this direction. He is also disposed to maintain that rest from head-work may be too much insisted upon in cerebral exhaustion. He is satisfied he has often met with patients with jaded brains who have certainly let their minds lie fallow too long. Mere distraction is not enough. What is wanted generally, even at the beginning, is not that work should be given up altogether even for a short time, but that it should be moderated in amount or change. He is of opinion that the wakefulness may be much better combated by attention to the position of the head in sleep than by narcotics. Sleep in bed is, as a rule, sounder with a low pillow than with a high one. On the contrary, if there be undue sleepiness the head should be kept high.—(*British Med. Jour..*)—*Pract.*

How to Employ Disinfectants.

The following are the plans employed by Dr. A. Ernest Sansom, reported in the *British Medical Journal*, October 5, 1872.

1. *Sulphurous Acid.*—If the chamber to be disinfected is (*a*) *uninhabited*, all articles capable of being bleached should be removed; orifices communicating with the external air should be closed, and crevices pasted over with paper. A vessel containing burning sulphur should then be introduced and the door closed. For the sake of safety from the chance of fire by the overflow of the molten sulphur, it should be kindled upon an iron plate, and floated upon a large vessel containing water. It is convenient to place glowing embers on the plate, and then dust over them flowers of sulphur. If the room is (*b*) *inhabited* the sulphurous acid must be disengaged in less proportion. Dr. Hjaltelin, who has employed it in small-pox wards, considers that its power of exciting bronchial irritation has been exaggerated, and that patients may be accustomed to it in a high degree. It may be employed in the manner before described; the flame of the burning sulphur being extinguished by submersion of the iron plate in the water, if the fumes become too powerful. Or, as employed by Dr. A. W. Foot, flowers of sulphur may be dropped upon a heated shovel, and carried about the room. The generation of the gas should be repeated three or four times in the day. It is certain, however that some people feel it difficult to tolerate the sulphur fumes.

2. *Iodine* may be used as an air-disinfectant in a very simple manner—first suggested, I believe by Dr. B. W. Richardson. Solid iodine is merely exposed in glass or porcelain vessels in

different parts of the room. The iodine vapor is given off at ordinary temperatures. This is a very efficient mode of attaining a constant disinfection.

3. *Carbolic Acid.*—To employ this agent when the room is (*a*) *unoccupied*—communication with the external air being closed—a quantity of the crude acid should be poured into a strongly heated metal cup, or upon hot bricks, and left to vaporize. Subsequently, the floors, ceiling, and, if practicable, the walls, should be irrigated or sprayed with an aqueous solution ; and the floor scrubbed with carbolic acid or coal-tar soap. Or Savory and Moore's excellent vaporizer may be employed, whereby large volumes of carbolic acid vapor will be disengaged. If the chamber is (*b*) *occupied* by the sick, the vaporizer just mentioned, which is so constructed that the liquified acid falls drop by drop upon a heated plate, should be put in action at intervals twice or thrice in the day. The objectionable odor of the carbolic acid may be greatly masked by its admixture with oil of wild thyme. It is obvious that this method gives off the carbolic acid too powerfully for continuous use. The agent, however, is so volatile as to render itself readily available for maintaining a constant antiseptic atmosphere. It has frequently been used in combination with inert powders for strewing about the room, or has been sprinkled upon cloths or other absorbent materials which have afforded surfaces for its volatilization. These measures, however, have their inconveniences and even dangers; for the strong acid is irritant and caustic, and may inflict serious injury on those who inadvertently touch it. To obviate the difficulty, I have requested Messrs. Savory and Moore to construct for me an instrument consisting of a piece of canvas in the form of an endless band stretched between two rollers, and dipping into a tin trough to be charged with the acid. By turning a handle at the top, the roller is drawn through the trough, and thus moistened in its whole extent. After it has become partially dry from evaporation, a turn of the handle lifts up a fresh moistened surface. I have used this in several cases, and have found it to act most satisfactorily. I believe, from the data we possess, that in carbolic acid we have the most efficient and the most manageable of all agents for the disinfection of air.—*Half-Yearly Compendium.*—*Pacific Med. and Surg. Jour.*

NEW JOURNALS.

Before us is the first number of the *Obstetrical Journal* of Great Britain and Ireland; including Midwifery and the Diseases of women and children. Edited by James H. Aveling, M. D., and Alfred Wittshire, M. D., with an American supplement edited by Wm. F. Jenks, M. D. To be issued monthly, (beginning with April.) Price $5 per annum, single numbers fifty cents. Henry C. Lea, Philadelphia.

This promises to be a valuable acquisition to our periodical medical literature judging from the number before us, which is fully up, both in art and substance, to the requirements of the times, and the just expectations of those acquainted with the reputation of both Editors and Publisher. May it receive promptly the needful *material support*.

We cheerfully place the *Sanitarian* on the list of our exchanges, attractive in appearance, and valuable in substance. The second number (May) comes embellished with a map of the city of New York, showing the localities of the *water, saturated soil, and defective drainage*. Issued monthly, edited by A. N. Bell, M. D. Annual subscription $3, single copies 30 cts. A. S. Barnes & Co., New York.

Also we have recently added on this subject *The Hygiene*, a fortnightly published by G. P. Putnam & Sons, Price $2. And a third, *The Journal of Physical and Mental Hygiene*. Edited by S. T. H. Helsby, and Thomas J. Mays, Williamsport, Penn. Price $2, issued monthly.

Prospectus for the *New Orleans Medical* and *Surgical Jour*. To be issued on the first day of each *alternate* month, beginning with the first day of July, 1873, each number to contain 150 pages of reading matter. Subscription price $5. Edited by S. M. Bemis, M. D.

Also a novelty in *Wilson's Herald of Health*, and *Atlanta Business Review*, edited by Jno. Stainback Wilson, M. D., Atlanta, Georgia.

Meteorological Observations.

METEOROLOGICAL OBSERVATIONS AT ST. LOUIS, MO.

BY A. WISLIZENUS, M. D.

The following observations of daily temperature in St. Louis are made with a MAXIMUM and MINIMUM thermometer (of Green, N. Y.). The daily minimum occurs generally in the night, the maximum about 3 P. M. The monthly mean of the daily minimum and maxima, added and divided by 2, gives a quite reliable mean of the monthly temperature.

THERMOMETER FAHRENHEIT.

APRIL, 1873.

Day of Month.	Minimum.	Maximum.	Day of Month.	Minimum.	Maximum.
1	43.5	53.0	18	39.5	55.0
2	35.0	60.0	19	41.0	66.0
3	46.5	77.0	20	42.0	74.0
4	63.0	86.0	21	41.0	71.5
5	66.0	87.5	22	45.0	61.0
6	62.0	86.0	23	33.0	49.5
7	41.0	45.0	24	38.0	52.0
8	35.0	42.5	25	35.0	49.0
9	34.5	47.5	26	34.0	63.0
10	34.0	64.0	27	43.5	63.0
11	41.0	53.0	28	48.5	56.5
12	34.5	57.0	29	43.5	67.0
13	41.0	68.0	30	50.5	63.5
14	54.0	66.5	31		
15	37.5	48.0			
16	36.5	43.5	Means	42.5	60.7
17	34.5	47.0	Monthly Mean 51.6		

Quantity of rain : 5.22 inches.

E. BREY, Linguist and Instructor in the Classical, Biblical and modern languages, especially the German. Teaching rooms, 118 North Third street ; 1319 Franklin avenue; 12 South Fifteenth street ; (Haydn Conservatory of Music.) He is the originator of a NEW SYSTEM of teaching languages thoroughly and rapidly, which, consisting of translating not only verbatim, but also by ROOTS and AFFIXES greatly assists the memory, and is perfecting in ENGLISH.

Etymological queries on MEDICAL or general terms, as well as geographical or personal NAMES will be answered, more or less satisfactorily, by the above.

Mortality Report.

FROM APRIL 19th, 1873, TO MAY 24th, 1873, INCLUS.

DATE	White. Males.	Females.	Col'd. Males.	Females.	Under 5 yrs.	5 to 10	10 to 20.	20 to 30.	30 to 40.	40 to 50.	50 to 60.	60 to 70.	70 to 80.	80 to 90	90 to 100	TOTAL.
Saturday 26	78	45	4	5	54	10	11	12	11	11	9	7	5	1	1	132
" 3	67	55	3	5	57	10	8	18	12	8	7	6	4		...	130
" 10	60	47	8	2	59	5	10	10	12	6	8	4	1	2	...	117
" 10	79	50	6	9	68	8	10	19	11	12	6	6	3	1	...	144
" 24	59	46	3	1	49	6	7	13	15	7	3	2	7		...	109
Total.	343	243	24	22	287	39	46	72	61	44	33	25	20	4	1	632

Albuminuria......... 3	Cystitis 2	Hepatitis 5	Premature Birth.... 4
Angina , 1	Debility............ 6	Hydrocephalus...... 2	Rheumatism....... 3
Apoplexy.......... 6	Diarrhœa 5	Inanition 4	Scrofula........... 1
Asphyxia 1	Disease of the Heart 9	Inflammat'n Brain 3	Septicæmia .. . 1
Asthma , . 1	Dropsy . . 5	" Bowels. 2	Suicide 1
Bright's Disease . 3	Dysentery 3	Laryngitis........ 4	Syphilis 1
Bronchitis .. 16	Eclampsia , 1	Lockjaw........... 2	Teething 1
Cancer.. , .. 6	Enteritis 7	Marasmus 18	Variola.. 41
Carditis , .. 4	Erysipelas 6	Measles 11	
Cholera Morbus.... 3	Embolism .. 1	Meningitis...... 16	Total....... 632
Conges. of Brain . 14	Endocarditis. 1	" cereb-spin. 122	
Conges of Lungs 6	Fever, Cong. 5	Old Age 9	Stillborn............45
Consumption. 70	" intermittent .. 1	Paralysis 1	
Convulsions. 36	Fever, typhoid. 8	Peritonitis 9	
Croup 4	Fracture of Skull.. . 1	Pertussis 8	
Cyanosis 2	Hemorrhage . 2	Pneumonia 60	

FOR CHOLERA.

The following Recipe was employed with good results by Dr. Hartshorn, of Philadelphia, for the first stage of Cholera, *i. e.*, for the premonitory diarrhœa :

   R Chloroform, -   f ʒiss.
    Tr. Opii, - -   ʒiss.
    Spts. Camphor,   ʒiss.
    Arom. spts. Ammonia, ʒiss.
    Oil Cinnamon, - gtt. viij
    Creosote, -   gtt. iij
    Spts. Vini Gallici, - ʒij.

  M. Dose from ten to twenty drops in a spoonful of ice water every five, ten, twenty or thirty minutes, as required.

THE SAINT LOUIS
Medical and Surgical Journal.
JULY, 1873.

Original Communications.

THE INCREASING FREQUENCY OF ASTHENOPIA; ITS ETIOLOGY AND TREATMENT.

By Charles S. Bull, A. M., M. D., St. Louis·

Scarcely a day passes that ophthalmic surgeons, the world over, do not meet with one or more patients, who complain of rapidly increasing dimness of vision, sharp shooting pains in the eyes, and lachrymation, whenever they attempt to use their eyes for a length of time on small objects or at a short distance from them. This train of symptoms, though always constant, may vary in reciprocal intensity, sometimes the pain being the subject of greatest complaint, while on other occasions the patients do not speak of pain, but complain greatly of the dimness of sight. But in all such cases of asthenopia, this train of symptoms is certain before long to be complete. As time elapses, if the work be continued, and hence the cause not removed, other symp-

toms manifest themselves. The ocular conjunctiva becomes congested, particularly upon the nasal side of the
cornea, along the course of the internal rectus muscle,
and long leashes of vessels are seen running from the
caruncle and external canthus towards the cornea. The
palpebral conjunctiva next becomes involved, and mucus
·or even muco-pus is secreted, and in the early morning
the patients find some little difficulty in opening the
lids, just as in catarrhal conjunctivitis. About this
period, the patients begin to complain of the light, and
the photophobia is sometimes so marked, that they
instinctively remain in the dark and can with difficulty
be induced to open the eyes. Another symptom which
is usually very characteristic comes on generally somewhat earlier in the course of the affection, viz : an insufficiency of the internal rectus muscle of one or both
eyes, though never, I believe, to an equal degree. This
is shown in an inability to converge for a certain nearpoint, varying in every case. Usually this symptom
does not go so far as to produce diplopia, or at least if
it does, the double vision is merely transient. But
occasionally this diplopia is exceedingly annoying, particularly as it is crossed diplopia, owing to the divergence of one or both eyes, and then the patient's condition is truly deplorable. But this muscular insufficiency
is not always situated in the internal rectus, for I have
recently seen two cases in which the external rectus had
become very much weakened, and though there was no
convergent squint, but apparent divergence of the optic
axes, yet an examination with prisms revealed homonymous diplopia. In nearly all of these cases of asthenopia, there exists some error of refraction, which, uncorrected, has been the cause of all the trouble. This

cause is almost aways a hypermetropic form of the eye-ball, though occasionally the refraction has been found to be myopic. But in some cases, and these are not very rare, the eyes have been found to be emmetropic, and here we must look for the cause in some inherent weakness in the muscles of convergence. In these latter cases, the whole system will usually be found broken down from over-work, lack of the necessary food and sleep, and exposure to bad air, over-crowded rooms and no ventilation. Of course most of the cases of asthenopia which we see, occur among the poorer classes ; among seamstresses and bookkeepers especially. The former commence their work very early in the morning, continue at it with but few short interruptions all day and far into the night, usually by the light of a flickering oil lamp or worse by candle-light. The latter class generally write all day and many of them by night, in offices which are almost always badly-lighted, and in some cases gas must be employed all day. Another thing to be taken into account in the causation of asthenopia, is the habit of stooping over their work that these people acquire, which causes a fulness of the blood-vessels in these parts, and, though at first of transient duration, soon becomes almost a permanent condition. The mere stooping posture is very apt to shut off considerable light from the person, and thus the patient is constantly working doubly to his disadvantage. This combination of defective illumination and faulty construction of desks and benches is a very important factor in the causation and rapid increase of myopia, as has been abundantly proven by Cohn and Erismann in their reports upon the careful examination of the eyes of school children in Germany.

In the case of seamstresses, there seems to be something in the rapid darting motion of the needle of the sewing machine, which particularly induces these symptoms of asthenopia, especially the photophobia; at least cases of asthenopia are much more frequently met with among women who sew by machine than among those who sew by hand.

One of the most annoying obstacles to the satisfactory examination and treatment of such cases is the irregular or inconstant condition of equilibrium of the muscles. In some cases an examination will reveal a dynamic condition very different from what it was twenty-four hours previously, and a third examination will give a totally different result from either. These oscillatory movements puzzle one exceedingly and keep the surgeon very much in the dark as to the actual condition of the antagonistic muscles. In such cases we should never be in a hurry to form either a diagnosis or prognosis, and very often an ophthalmoscopic examination will aid us materially, when without it we would have failed. A careful examination with the ophthalmoscope of these cases of asthenopia teaches us a great deal, for though all are alike in the main features of the fundus oculi, yet each case will be found to have some one distinguishing feature. Of course the pupil should be dilated and the accommodation completely paralyzed with a solution of the sulphate of atropia, as a preliminary step. The next step is to satisfy ourselves of the refraction of the eye, whether it be emmetropic, hypermetropic or myopic, and if abnormal, to what degree. We should then turn our attention to the optic disk, and if the case be one in which the asthenopic symptoms have existed fof some time, the following appearances may be noticed. The color of the papilla is changed, and instead of its being of a delicate rosy hue throughout, it will be found very much congested; the congestion being generally most marked on the nasal side of the disk, though not always. The papilla may even be somewhat swollen from transudation of serum through the walls of the vessels. The branches of the central retinal vein are engorged and tortuous and a pulsation may usually be detected in the ascending or descending main branches, and occasionally in both. If the congestion is very marked and the veins very much engorged, this pulsation can be followed for some distance beyond the margin of the optic disk, and in extreme cases may be traced as far as the equator of the eye. The arteries are usually not much altered in appearance; if anything, they are slightly increased in calibre. The retinal vessels stand out usually very distinctly, but sometimes the retina is more or less infiltrated with serum and then the details of the fundus are somewhat obscured.

The appearances in and around the macula lutea are of great importance and vary very much in different eyes. The most common condition is an irregular, ruffled or ragged appearance of the hexagonal pigment cells of the choroid, or retina more properly speaking, in which the bases of the rods and cones are embedded. This gives a slightly hazy, out-of-focus look to the region, and is soon followed by an atrophy or disappearance of some of these pigment cells, which leaves spaces or interstices between those cells which yet remain intact. The next step is a minute, punctate, dotted appearance of this region, the dots being of a yellow color and extending in all directions from the

macula lutea, but especially towards the optic disk.
The space between the papilla and yellow spot is soon
thickly strewn with these minute dots, which are probably exudations from the walls of the capillaries, but of
what nature I am unable to decide. Occasionally an
eye will be met with in which the whole fundus is strewn
with the spots of exudation. This condition has received the name of "choroiditis asthenopica" from Dr.
Loring of New York, but the process seems to me
scarcely violent enough to be termed inflammatory, and
it might perhaps be better to speak of a "neuro-choroi-
dal congestion." The appearances just described are
always found in these cases of asthenopia, but others
are occasionally met with, which are not so characteristic.
The development of blood-vessels upon the optic disk
and retina is sometimes enormous, and this depends
more upon the great enlargement of the minute nutrient
vessels of the optic nerve, which in the natural state
are scarcely or not at all visible, than upon the distension of the main vessels of the retina. These numerous
vessels are very tortuous and are interlaced with one
another till a perfect network is formed, and in these
cases the tension of the globe is generally increased.
Of course the natural tendency of such a process is towards inflammation, and there is but a slight transition
to a fully-developed neuro-retinitis.

One remarkable feature in these cases is, that the patient's vision for the distance is perfect. They will tell
ou that they have no trouble in the street or in the
nouse, or in a crowded assembly, but that the moment
they undertake to read or sew, an intense pain comes
on in the eyes and forehead, and everything seems
blurred before their eyes. Of course, if such attempts

are persisted in, the retina becomes hyperæsthetic, the sensitiveness to light increases, and soon the patient takes to green-glasses, shades, veils and a dark room, and becomes practically helpless.

The exciting cause of all these changes in the eye is in the beginning some error of refraction, which is usually hypermetropia. A hypermetrope, the focus of whose dioptric apparatus lies on the negative side of infinity, that is, really behind the eye, must bring a great amount of force to bear upon the ciliary muscle, in order to focus near objects upon his retina. Connected with this extreme and constant tension upon the ciliary muscle, there is an equally constant force acting upon the internal recti muscles to produce the necessary amount of convergence of the optic axes. It has been long recognized that an intimate connection exists between the action of the ciliary muscle and that of the muscles of convergence, that is, in general terms, with every degree of convergence of the optic axes there is · connected a certain amount of accommodation..

It is well known that the action of the ciliary muscle in myopes and hypermetropes is totally different. In a myopic patient, as long as objects are regarded from an infinite distance up to the position of the far-point, the ciliary muscle remains inactive, while in a hypermetropic patient it is constantly in action when the person desires to see distinctly an object at any distance whatever. From all this we are led to suspect a lack of uniformity in the development of the muscle in the two eyes, and this, Iwanoff has proved to be the case. (Archiv für Ophthalmologie, XV. 3. p. 284, et seq.) Our anatomy teaches us that the ciliary body is a direct prolongation of the choroid coat, and looked at from behind, appears as a series of large and small club-shaped projections arranged in a longitudinal direction. These projections or ciliary processes are nothing but folds, in whose anterior concavity lies the ciliary muscle or " tensor choroideæ." This muscle was formerly known as the " ligamentum ciliare," and appears in the form of a tolerably thick, broad ring, which in a vertical section has the form of a three-sided prism. It consists of smooth, unstriated, muscular fibres, which have partly a meridional, partly a circular direction. The longitudinal fibres spring from the most anterior zone of the internal surface of the sclera. The most superficial of these fibres run close against the sclera backward towards the " ora serrata," and are firmly inserted in the choroid. The deeper fibres have a similar origin, and assume generally a similar direction, but curve towards the optic axis and run into the ciliary processes. The circular fibres or " Müller's ring muscle," almost always lie anteriorly close to the margin of the iris.

Iwanoff (loc. cit.) examined microscopically emmetropic, myopic and hypermetropic eyes, and found the following condition of things : In myopic eyes the ciliary muscle was found considerably thicker and longer than in emmetropic eyes, and its thickest part was situated posteriorly. Iwanoff was not able to corroborate Donders' statement, that in such eyes the ciliary muscle showed signs of atrophy. Microscopic examination proved that the increased thickness of the muscle in myopic eyes depended solely upon thickening and lengthening of the muscular fibres, and that the connective tissue had nothing to do with it. Another fact revealed by the microscope was, that the circular muscular fibres were almost entirely wanting in myopic eyes, and the entire ciliary muscle consisted of longitudinal fibres, which, near the sclera, ran parallel to it, while the more internal ones bent forwards and inwards.

In hypermetropic eyes a totally different condition of things was met with. The muscle was found very much lessened in size and pushed forward. The posterior portion was atrophied at the expense of the highly developed anterior portion. A microscopical examination showed that here the thickened part occupied the seat of the circular fibres. These fibres were found enormously developed, while the longitudinal fibres were very much atrophied, and in many places were merely rudimentary.

The resultant of the two lines of action of the circular and longitudinal fibres of the ciliary muscle is directed somewhat from behind forwards, but chiefly from without inwards. By such a combined action the relaxation of the zonula becomes much easier in hypermetropes than in myopes. In the latter the muscle must cause by its contraction a much more extensive stretching of the choroid than in hypermetropes. The muscle in myopes must pull upon both points of fixation, and as the point of origin of the longitudinal fibres is in the firm fibrous tissue around the canal of Schlemm, the greatest effect is produced upon its insertion in the choroid far back towards the optic nerve entrance. Iwanoff thinks it very possible that posterior staphyloma may be the result of this constant tension in myopic eyes. It seems to me quite as likely that the minute changes in the choroid between the macula and optic disk are caused by this same tension, which first sets up a state of congestion followed by a slow atrophic process, and this I believe to be actually the rationale of the whole matter.

In what manner the ciliary muscle acts in producing the same condition of things in hypermetropic eyes, where the circular fibres are enormously hypertrophied at the expense of the longitudinal fibres, I am not yet able to explain. Iwanoff, regarding the ciliary muscle of the emmetrope as the normal muscle, thinks that it is changed into a hypermetropic muscle when the visual axis is accidentally shortened. According to him the completely developed hypermetropic muscle, in consequence of the hypertrophy of its circular fibres, gives to the lens such a form that it throws upon the retina a distinct image, with the least possible stretching of the choroid. Nevertheless, there is produced a certain amount of stretching. With the increase of the necessary accommodation, there may therefore be developed, even in hypermetropes, a posterior staphyloma. This may possibly be the true explanation, though I admit that it is not entirely satisfactory.

The vascular development of the optic nerve, retina and choroid, in these cases of asthenopia, offers a very interesting field for clinical observation. The vascular connection between the central artery and vein of the retina, the small vessels supplying the two sheaths of the nerve, and the branches of the short posterior ciliary vessels has been shown to be very intimate (Leber, Archiv für Ophthalmologie, XI, 1). In a recent article Wolfring (Archiv für Ophthalmologie, XVIII, 2) states that in sections of an injected optic nerve, near the lamina cribrosa, the minute capillaries could be seen always surrounded by connective tissue, and this not only in the lamina cribrosa itself, but more externally;

and not only in transverse, but also in longitudinal sections, and that the vessels present in their course a much more characteristic representation of the cribriform fascia than the connective tissue. This histological structure of the lamina cribrosa, dependent upon the vascular anastomosis, is of great importance from a pathological standpoint. The few small branches of the posterior ciliary vessels do not all pass directly into the optic nerve, in order to anastomose with the central retinal vessels, but some pass backward between the two sheaths of the nerve and here form a rich network of blood-vessels. The scleral vascular circle is formed by an anastomosis between the branches of the short posterior ciliary arteries and minute vessels, which come directly from the brain and run along the surface of the inner sheath of the optic nerve to the sclera. In addition to all these networks, there is still another between the inner sheath of the nerve and the nerve itself, which anastomoses intimately with the vessels supplying the nerve fibrils.

Leber in a recent paper (Archiv für Ophthalmologie, XVIII, 2) calls attention to the following points, viz:

1. The central artery and vein of the retina supply not only the retina and optic papilla, but also in connection with the vaginal vessels, that portion of the nerve-trunk in which they run.

2. The vessels of the optic nerve-trunk always run within the meshes of connective tissue by which the nerve is traversed.

3. The relations of the branches of the vascular circle of the sclera are, with some slight modifications, a repetition of the relations of the vaginal vessels of the optic nerve-trunk.

4. The lamina cribrosa, optic papilla, aud a small portion of the retina are supplied both by the central vessels and ciliary vessels.

All this discussion of the vascular supply of the retina, choroid and optic nerve, is of very great interest, not only when we have to do with a question of true anastomosis, as in the diagnosis of a simple embolus of the central artery of the retina, but also in all cases of inflammatory affections of the deeper tissues of the eye. In this matter of asthenopia with a congested fundus, it seems to me of special importance as a means of explaining the great development or enlargement of vessels seen by the ophthalmoscope. The constant strain upon the choroid, due to the contraction of the longitudinal fibres of the ciliary muscle, must necessarily cause an increased flow of blood to the parts, while the coincident ever-progressive hypertrophy of the fibres themselves, due to continuous action, would of itself tend to the same end.

As regards the treatment of these cases of asthenopia, I think we may safely say that we can do a great deal. In my experience the most obstinate cases to deal with are those in which there is no error of refraction, and in which the exciting cause has been simply long continued abuse of the eyes. The first thing to be done is to look carefully into the acuity of vision, both for the distance and for ordinary near-work. If we find that the vision for the distance is not normal, that is, if the patient cannot read *Snellen XX* at twenty feet, then we should try whether the vision can be improved by spherical glasses. We can thus generally satisfy ourselves of the existence of hypermetropia or myopia, and if the latter, determine its degree. With hypermetropia it is somewhat more difficult, as the patient frequently refuses a weak convex glass, and yet there may be considerable latent hypermetropia present, particularly if he be young. Having determined the vision for the distance, we should try the patient upon *Jæger's* or *Snellen's* test-types for reading, and we shall generally find that there is more or less limitation of the accommodation, and this almost always occurs in a hypermetrope. The near-point will be found to have receded from the eye, and thus to have approached the far-point. We should next examine into the condition of the muscles of the eye, and note whether the excursive movements of the globe are normal. Test the power of convergence, and if the trouble has lasted for any length of time, an insufficiency of one or both internal recti will be discovered, so that when an object is brought to within a certain distance of the eyes, one eye diverges or turns outwards. But sometimes this is not noticeable, and yet the patient tells you that he sometimes sees double. We must then resort to the use of prisms, and by placing one with the base upwards or downwards before one eye, and telling the patient to fix an object like the flame of a candle or a black dot upon white paper, vertical diplopia is immediately produced. The patient will then tell you that the objects do not stand vertically, but that there is also a lateral displacement, and then by placing a series of prisms with the base inwards before the same eye, we at last find one which brings one image directly over the other, and this is the measure of the insufficiency. Finally comes the ophthalmoscopic examination with its revelations.

The first step in the treatment is to ensure the stoppage of all work. The patient must be informed of the danger of continuing work, and to make sure of this, atropine should be instilled thrice daily for from two to four weeks. This paralyzes the ciliary muscle, sets the accommodation completely at rest, and thus aids in stopping the increased congestion. As the pupils are now widely dilated, a pair of blue or smoked glasses should be constantly worn, and a leech should be applied to each temple, and if necessary repeated once every week. If there be much hyperæsthesia of the retina, the lactate of zinc may be given in five grain doses three times a day, and it is better to give it in pill-form combined with iron and quinine. If the intraocular congestion be very marked and venous pulsation present, the heart's action will generally be found to be accelerated, and digitalis is then indicated, in small doses. Attention should be paid to the general health, bathing and exercise should be advised, and the bowels kept regularly open. After three or four weeks the symptoms will generally have disappeared, the congestion of the fundus will have subsided, and the atropine may now be discontinued. If the patient be hypermetropic the proper glasses should then be ordered, and in about two weeks the blue glasses may be laid aside and work be recommenced. And now comes in play what is called the muscular gymnastic exercise of the eyes, or "Dyerizing," to coin a word from the name of Dr. Dyer, of Philadelphia, who recommended the plan to be described. The patient should be told to put on his glasses and read for from two to five minutes in the morning, and the same length of time in the afternoon, and no longer. The next day this time should be increased one minute, and so he should go on for several days, increasing each day by one minute.

After a time the increase may be raised to five minutes each day until finally the patient finds that he can use his eyes for a number of hours continuously. He should carefully avoid working by gas or lamp-light for some time to come, and if possible should change his occupation for another that does not tax the eyes so much, as he is liable to a return of the asthenopia on slight provocation.

1615 Washington Avenue.

ON TETANUS AND TETANOID AFFECTIONS, WITH CASES.

By R. ROEMER, M. D., St. Louis, Mo.

[Continued from page 309]

The internal use of opium is advantageously combined with large doses of camphor, as in the case of Van Bibber. Professor Rochester has reported two successful cases of strychnia poisoning in which he relied upon camphor, and asks the question, "might it not possibly be successfully used in cases of traumatic and idiopathic tetanus?"

XXIV. Cannabis indica.

Authority.	Form of Tetanus.	Remedies and their doses exhibited in the order named.	Result.
Case I.	Acute.	Cannab. ind. gr. 1 every 1 to 1½ hour with quinine, grs. 2. Took in 36 h. 146½ grs. of the extract.	Recov'd.
Case II.	Sub-acute.	Ex. cannab. ind. ½ to 1½ grs. every one to two hours with quinine.	"
Case III.	"	Same treatment.	
Case IV.	"	Same treatment.	
Case V.	"	Opium 3 grs. every two or three hour; ex. cannab. ind. gr. 1 with quinine grs. 2, every hour.	"
Case VII.	Acute.	Morphia endermic., cannab. ind., chloroform and nicotine.	Died.

Authority.	Form of Tetanus.	Remedies and their doses exhibited in the order named.	Result.
Case IX.	"	Tr. aconit. r. gtt 15, quin. grs. 2½ every three, and double quantity every one hour; frictions with aconite lin.; cannab. ind. 1½ to 4 grs. internally, and 1 gr. hypodermic.; took 185 grs. of the ext.	Recov'd.
E. F. Millholland.	"	In the beginning only ex. cannab. ind. gr. 1 every two to one hour.	Died.
W. Farrage.	"	After other remedies, cannab. ind. grs. 6, ex. hyosciam., assafœt āā ʒss in 12 pills, 1 every h., tr. cannab. ind. gtt 30 every two hour, etc.	"
Same.	Sub-acute.	Tr. cannab. ind. gtt 10 to 20 every h.; calomel; counter irritants.	Recov'd.
Jno. Rogers.	" (idiop.)	Opium grs. 5, camphor grs. 12 in 4 pills, one every two h.; ex. cannab. ind. grs. 4, camphor grs. 12 in 4 pills, 1 every ¼ h.; wine, croton oil; enemata.	Died.
Ch. O'Donovan.	Acute.	Cannab. ind. throughout, took 1437 grs. of ex. in 22 days.	Recov'd.
Hague.	Sub-acute.	Tr. cannab. ind. ʒss every h.; croton oil and enemata.	"
E. W. Skues.	" (Chronic.)	Ex. cannab. ind. gr. ¼ to 2 every hours; wine; took daily 4 to 18 grs. (patient 9 years old.)	"
C. R. Greenleaf.	Sub-acute.	For 2 days ex. cannab. ind. gr. ½ to 1 without benefit; other treatment.	"
Jas. Moore.	" (Chronic.)	For 3 days tr. cannab. ind. gr. 1 to 3; lost its influence.—(Why?)—result not given.	
Same.	Trismus.	Narcotics with indian hemp.	Recov'd.
Same.	Idiop.	Opium and indian hemp.	"
H. K. Steele.		Mixed treatment with indian hemp.	Died.
H. H. Toland.	Sub-acute. (chronic.)	Morph. gr. 1 to wound; tr. cannab. ind. gtt 20 every 2 h. for 2 weeks; duration 4 weeks.	Recov'd.
Fayrer.	" (chronic.)	Chlorof., cannab. ind., camphor and opium, duration 7 weeks.	"
Theo. Mack.		Indian hemp; amputation.	Died.
H. Z. Gill.	Acute.	Morphine, chloroform, tr. cannab. ind., for 6 h. narcotized by chloroform, whisky and indian hemp.	"
Same.	"	Chloroform, cannab. ind.; died on second day.	"
S. G. Chuckerbutty.		13 cases; cannab. ind. fairly tried in 8 cases of which one died. Tr. cannab. ind gtt. 30 to 40 every 2 to 3 hours.	} 6 Died } 7 Re'd.
W. B. O'Shaughnessy.		Introduced cannab. ind., was successful in doses of 2 to 3 grs. every 2 h. until its intoxicating effects were produced; gave as much as 1 dr. of the tr. every ½ h; had a wonderful success.	
Poland. (Guy's Hosp.)		Had no success with cannab ind.	
F. Hinkle.	Hysteric. tetanus.	Mixed treatment, ex. cannab. ind. most prominent remedy.	Recov'd.
I. Ashhurst.	Complic. .tetanus.	Ex. cannab. ind. ¼ gr. 4 times daily; mixed treatment.	Died.

Cannabis indica . (the Gunjah of India and the Haschisch of Hindostan and Persia) owes its medicinal properties to the resinous secretion contained in it. The great diversity in its reliability is due to the many and really spurious kinds usually sold, among which the Italian cannabis ranks foremost as the easiest of access. The resin and extract obtained from India possess the therapeutic virtues claimed. In its purity its action is directed first to the motor nerves, whence it is transmitted to the sensorium and nerves of sensation as a hypnotic. Its secondary effect is a paralysis of the voluntary muscles. As a hypnotic it is regarded by Fronmüller to have no dependent excitement of the vascular system, nor does it produce a stoppage of the secretions. He denies a consecutive paralysis. In order to convey a practical appreciation of its reliability of action I quote the following : (Fronmüller in *Am. Jour. M. Sc.* 1861, April, p. 554)—"Out of the 1000 cases (*experimented upon*) it was found that the narcotic property of the hemp was completely developed in 530, partially in 215 and little or not all in 255. With the extract the best effects were produced—

145 times with a dose of 12 grains.			17 times with a dose of 2 grains.		
64 " " 8 "			15 " " 14 "		
63 " " 10 "			14 " " 20 "		
35 16 '			13 " " 6 "		
22 .. 3 "			12 " " 5 "		

He concludes that of all known medicines which cause stupefaction, Indian hemp produces a narcotism most completely supplying the want of natural sleep without great excitement of the vascular system, etc. . . . . that it may be given in all acute inflammatory diseases, that it may be alternated with opium, where it (opium) has failed, and that the lowest dose of

24

the alcoholic extract to produce sleep is 8 grains, given
in pill-form of one grain each." Of course, these 8
pills are to be given successively. Cannabis indica may
be regarded as a cerebral sedative, indicated especially
in that form of tetanus which is complicated with cerebral excitement and is useful therefore in delirium tremens, as I have found in two instances.

The results of Fronmüller, the opinion of Chuckerbutty, a. o.,(that a want of success with cannabis indica
is owing to small and inefficient doses and to the inferior article used, or to its combination with other drugs,
so that neither could be expected to exert its full influence) and a few isolated cases of judicious treatment
place Indian hemp among the best of all known anti-
tetanic remedies. The plan of treatment pursued by
Mr. Skues, and especially the case of Dr. O'Donovan,
though a heroic medication, are analagous to the opium
medication of Prof. Frick, and of Dr. Knight, who
exhibited unintentionally an overdose of laudanum to
an infant with perfect success. The rule in tetanus is
death from want of therapeutic action, and few patients
are killed with medication—a homœopathic course of
treatment is especially in tetanus innocent of shortening life by commission, but the error in omission is pal-
pable and thereby augmented. As high an authority
as Watson endorses the treatment of an Edinburgh
physician, who gave to his own wife, while suffering under
a tetanic affection, over 40,000 drops of laudanum, which
is more than four ounces a day, and in all more than
two imperial quarts. In my cases, now reported, after
determining the remedy to be used, and finding it well
borne, I prescribed the dose and the time of its administration with the effects produced; and I do not hesi-

tate to pronounce such a course as the only one at all promising. A combination of two or more remedial agents is only warranted after a reasonable quantity has been ineffectually given, and then I would prefer either a change in the mode of exhibiting it, from the internal to the endermic use, and *vice versa*, or a complete suspension for a time, until an equivalent has taken its place with a like failure, or has rendered the system susceptible to a renewed action of a moderately increased dose.

XXV. Calabar Bean. (*Physostigma.*)

Th. R. Fraser reports nine recoveries and two deaths, and recommends the extract in pill-form, or 32 grains solved in one ounce of diluted alcohol. He commences treatment by subcutaneous injection to be repeated until a decided effect is obtained; then by the mouth in a dose three times as large. In severe cases he persists with the hypodermic use, for an adult ⅓ gr. being sufficient, repeated in two hours, when the effects of the first injection have generally passed off. As vehicle he uses water.

E. Watson gives the following cases and authorities:

	Recoveries	Deaths.
Alexander, - - -	2	0
Campbell, - - -	1	0
Bourneville, - - -	0	
Ashdown, - - -	1	
Bouchat - - -	0	
Macarthur, - - -	1	◡
Boslin and Curron, -	1	0
His own cases, - - -	4	6

To illustrate his treatment, I give a synopsis of two successful cases:

1. A. W., age 11, acute tetanus; calomel and jalap.;

cannab. ind.; Squire's gelatine paper (1 square) containing ex. calabar bean; in 1½ hours 2 squares; in 4 hours 3, and in 3 hours 2 more squares; 2 squares every hour during night; ex. calab. bean grs. 12 and vinum alb. 1 ounce, 5 drops = ⅛ gr. every half hour: after two grains were taken only momentary twitches; narcotism; continued calabar bean as needed.

2. John, age 13, sub-acute form; tr. calab. bean gtt. 5 every 2 hours, with benefit always for ½ hour; sleeps; gtt. 4 every hour; pupils contract; gtt. 5 every 2 hours and two doses at night; then every 3 hours, again increased to gtt. 6 every 2 hours and during night; lastly gtt. 6, 3 times daily.

A. Boutflower gives a recovery from traumatic tetanus under morphia ½ gr. subcutaneously; calabar bean 1 gr. internally, and ½ to 1⅛ grs. hypodermically; finger amputated; received in 9 days 40⅝ grs. by the skin, and 49½ grs. by the mouth. *C. C. Sherard* gave in a fatal trismus neonat. ex. physostigm. ₁⅟₂ gr. repeated every hour, continued remedy every 30 minutes, and after 3 doses every 20 minutes, then ⅛ gr. every 20 and 10 minutes; remedy had no effect whatever; gave 4 grs. of the extract. *B. Duffy's* successful emprosthotonos received ⅛ gr. of ex. calab. bean endermically every 3 hours for one day; nausea; injection every 2 hours, again nausea, etc., and spasm yielding on the 6th day. *Wm. Haining* had a successful traumatic tetanus with the internal use of calabar bean 1 to 3 grs., and subcutaneously ½ gr. gradually increased to 6 grs.; 41 grs. were injected in one day producing the full physiological effects of the remedy; total amount taken, over 10 drachms and over 140 punctures. *Alexander,* from whose notes the eight cases by Watson are compiled, remarks that one of the fatal cases included was not treated at all, as he only doubtfully swallowed one dose and died. *Andrews* exhibited in a recovery from a sub-acute tetanus, after quinine 8 grs. every hour and anodynes, the tr. calab. bean gtt. 10 every 4 hours, alternately with 10 grs. quinine; after 24 hours gave gtt. 15 every 2 hours, and gtt. 40.; finally in teaspoon doses with quinine 8 grs. every 4 hours. *F. Mason's* fatal case of acute tetanus was treated with the ordeal bean until its physiologic effects were produced, also a like instance treated by *Ridout*, received ⅛ to ⅜ gr. every hour for 13 days without success. *J. T. Newman* gives a recovery from acute tetanus with ex. ealab. bean ⅛ gr. hypodermically. *Ch. R. Greenleaf* had success with this remedy by the mouth and hypodermically for 22 days; *a failure* with the ⅛ gr. every hour; *a second recovery* with the ⅛ to ⅓ gr. every half hour, and ⅓ to 1 gr. every 3 hours hypodermically, using from the 12th day this drug in the form of suppositories; his fourth case *died* under ex. calab. bean ½ gr. every 2 hours, it manifesting its physiologic effects clearly; and his *fifth case* recovered, giving calab. bean and morphine to an equivalent of 54 grs. opium in 4½ hours. *Anderson* reports the fatal case of Dr Jno. Davis with 1/16 to ¼ gr. for 6 days internally, and ⅜ to ½ gr. for another six days hypodermically. *A. M. Brown* gives a fatal issue with ex. calab. bean ¼ gr. every hour, increasing every third dose to ½ gr. than ½ gr. every hour, and hypodermically every 15 minutes until 2½ grs. were used; etc. *Brown* relates the treatment of a sub-acute case then in treatment, in which he gave the ex. calab. bean internally, and 1⅓ gr. (maximum) hypodermically for 10 days, also the tr. in an equivalent of 2½ grs. of the extract every 2 hours. *H. K. Steele* in his fatal case

regards the calab. bean as of the least value. *Holthouse*
gives one recovery and one, death from doses of 3 grs.
every 2 hours, and once 4½ grs.   *P. H. Watson* had 2
fatal cases, in each of which the calabar bean produced
its full effects.

The calabar bean. ordeal nut, or esere of calabar,.
has been fully tested in its physiological effects.   If the
opinion of Dr. Fraser is received, then ⅓ grain subcutaneously must be an equivalent of $3 \times \frac{1}{3}$, or one grain
internally.   This dose effects the system generally up
to two hours, when the exhibition should be repeated—
in tetanus, however, a quicker succession or a larger
dose is to be recommended.   The first case of E. Watson proves how far the tolerance of the body may be
guided in a uniform medication of gradually increasing
doses, but a treatment of ⅛ to ⅓ grain internally and ⅓ gr.
hypodermically, and of $\frac{1}{16}$ to ¼ gr. internally, and ⅛ to ½
gr. hypodermically, as given in a case reported, does
not accord either with itself or with the object to be
gained.

The primary action of the calabar bean consists in
a direct and powerful diminution of the reflex action of
the central nervous system, (Fraser in *Am. J. M. Sc.,*
1868, April p. 502,) and may be detailed as follows :
1. Contraction of the pupils. 2. Paralysis of the motor
nerves without affecting the muscular irritability and
the intellect.   (In other words its action is upon the
spinal cord.)   3. It destroys life by paralyzing the respiratory muscles, and is a respiratory poison.   (*vide*
case I of E. Watson.)   4. It may weaken, but does
not stop the heart's action, and is not a cardiac poison.
(Hence not as antagonistic to atropia as Dr. Harley
affirms.)   Calabar bean excites the lachrymal and sali-

vary secretions and is *collectively* allied to conium and woorara.

XXVI. Curare.

Authority.	Form of Tetanus.	Remedies and their doses exhibited in the order named.	Result.
W. H. Wickham.	Acute.	Aconite in frequent and increasing doses; subcutan. inject. of ex. woorara and repeated; brandy and quinine; cold to spine.	Died.
Lloyd.	"	Woorara hypoderm. every 15 to 20 m. 1-20 to 1 gr.; used 6 grs.	"
T. S. Wells.	Sub-acute. (chronic.)	Woorara hypo. and epiderm.; 6 grs in 6 days.	Recov'd.
Same.	Acute.	Assafœt. injections per an.; woorara inoculated in both arms.	Died.
Same.	Sub-acute.	Opium and ether; woorara; cloroform anæsth.	"
E. T Milholland.		Corroval subcutan. after other rem'dies	"
Busch.		Subcut. inj. of 1-50 to 1-30 gr. of pure curare every 2 hours, in one case the recovery was ascribed to morphia.	} 6 Re'd· } 5 Died
Isambert.		Treatment with curare.	Died.
Same.		Same.	Recov'd.

T. Spencer Wells refers also to two chronic cases on the Continent (Europe) successfully treated by Vella, Maneo and Chassaignac and one additional in England, successfully treated with curare. *Demme* (Austrian army) had 8 recoveries and 14 deaths, but gives neither type of disease, dose, nor mode of exhibition. The cases of Prof. Busch may have been sub-acute. Continental reporters, especially the French, do not discriminate as carefully as they should, and my remark upon Busch's cases is based upon his statement, that in very acute cases curare is unworthy of confidence, and that then he gives generally the preference to other remedies, or to curarine. Profs. Vella and C. Bernard have tested the antagonistic powers of woorara and strychnine, and upon their affirmative report, M. Thiercelin applied the former in the counteraction of artificially produced convulsions and with marked success.

Woorara, curare or urari is represented by two distinct varieties (Harley speaks of five specimens of different strength because made by different tribes): corroval and vao or bao.   The *former* is the most powerful of the curare kind ; acts first upon the heart through the blood and produces paralysis of its muscles ; then upon the voluntary and reflex movements depending upon the heart and upon the sensory and motor functions, destroying muscular irritability and paralyzing especially and primarily the sympathetic nerve.   In this respect it has a similar effect with upas antiar, as we shall hereafter see, which, however, is its inferior in toxic activity, and both are liable to fatal results when exhibited under symptoms of cardiac inaction.   The *second* and milder variety vao induces experimentally paralysis of the extremities, loss of reflex action and of respiration, and may be said to give: 1, Increase of the heart's action; 2, Paralysis of its muscles in rapid, and paralysis of the voluntary muscles in slow poisoning, and 3. Paralysis of respiration and circulation, affecting the sensory nerves first and the motor afterwards.

The action of urari is rapid (according to Prof. Kölliker) when injected into the blood or a wound, and slower through the mucous membranes. He, (Kölliker) believes its action to be first upon the peripheric nerves, then upon the brain, and lastly upon the spinal cord, which retains its reflex activity for some time.   If it is agreed that the paralysis of involuntary muscles proceeds from the pneumogastric nerve (heart) to the sympathetic (iris), thence to the capillary vessels and splanchnic nerve (peristaltic motion), we are forced then to look upon *woorara as little calculated to take its place among anti-tetanic remedies,* especially also if we compare the microscopic investigations of Jacubowich, (who after poisoning with curare discovered ruptured nerve-cells and broken cylinders,) with the post-mortem appearances of the spinal cord after tetanus above detailed. Some writers differ from these views (*vide British Med. Jour.* 1867, June 22, article "Action of Curare") in exempting the cardiac fibres of the pneumogastric and splanchnic nerves from all inhibitory action. To recapitulate, the uncertainty in the action of woorara on account of impurity and variety, its action upon the brain and heart with variable and indefinite violence, and the great difference of opinion from experimental sources (Harley, believing the motory nerves first and the sensory not at all or very late paralyzed, and Hammond and Mitchell teaching that, (*a*) corroval abolishes both the sensory and motor functions, and (*b*) that vao paralyzes the sensory nerves first, and the motor nerves afterwards)—combine to render woorara an unsafe remedy, but one deserving of further attention. It is contra-indicated in all cases manifesting a metastatic tendency upon the lungs and air passages, since it suspends the respiratory act and thus conditions or hastens death by asphyxia. C. Bernard has observed that a nerve tissue is characterized by physical, chemical, and physiological properties, and that the action of woorara and all its kindred poisons is directed upon the physiological. Tetanus is due to the physical combined perhaps with the chemical property of the nerve tissue and a remedy, in counterbalancing one with the other, is said to be curative, when by it a certain degree of positive or negative physiological disturbance is brought in antagonism with an equal degree of a physical or chemical character. In many instances, consequently, the therapeutic virtue of an agent acts either in an obscure and undefined manner, or by a mere numerical strength, by which a certain amount of excitability or irritability is set aside by the greater exponent of a similar cause, which has a tendency to impress itself upon the nerve-center *from a different direction.* Thus, for instance, strychnine may act in its exhibition for the cure of tetanus. The curative value of a remedy, which the experience of most practitioners will admit, is too often restricted in practical application, it being pronounced by one almost a specific, and by another next to worthless. Much of this must be ascribed to a faulty reflection of the physician at the bedside, who remembers the experiments of the physiologist and forgets that the tolerance of a disease for its therapeutic agents is pathologically different from one purely experimental.

It seems to me proper to add here a short notice of a poison, which in many respects is closely allied to the one now considered. *Upas,* an arrow poison among the inhabitants of East India, is supposed to be obtained from arbor toxicaria (Rumph) called by the natives Ipo. Leschenault speaks of a milder poison, *upas antiar,* and of an *upas tiente,* derived from antiaris tox. and strychnos tiente, the former without convulsions until just before death, and the latter with strong tetanic spasm. Upas antiar produces also vomiting, languor and irregularity of and reduction in the heart's action, death being the result of paralysis of the muscles of the heart. Respiration, however, and the cerebral functions remain undisturbed. It is similar in its action with corroval, destroys the properties of the muscular fibre, and arrests the contractions of the heart. The toxic effects are, 1, paralysis of the muscles of the heart, 2, of the voluntary muscles, and 3, of the nerves. The upas tiente produces tetanic convulsions, rigidity of muscles and general exhaustion, its action being expended over the brain. The active principle, according to Pelletier, is strychnia combined perhaps with igasuric acid, while the antiar contains the antiarin, a bitter and in alcohol and water soluble alkaloid. Its action is, 1, upon the spinal cord and brain, paralyzing the voluntary muscles, and 2, upon the muscles of the heart. The usual intermixture, however, of these two poisons has transferred the action of one upon the other, and their antagonism is only established in their purity. The upas tiente resembles, consequently, not only strychnine, but also certain inorganic salts of cyanic acid, for instance the sulphocyanide of potassium, leaving the muscular tissue intact, but resulting in tetanic contractions and paralysis through the brain. Upas antiar and tiente claim an equal attention with corroval, vao and strychnia in the treatment of tetanus.

Before concluding these observations, I would repeat the injunction, that the course of this disease should be taken in consideration as not only modifying the choice, but also the exhibition of the remedy. A routine of treatment is not applicable to tetanus. In progressive tetanus a greater care in the selection of the anti-tetanic remedy should follow a more doubtful and complicated diagnosis, and the employment of the ophthalmoscope may be highly useful in locating cerebral lesions. Its careful and repeated use (and even in tetanus it can be used if proper precautions are observed) is capable of indicating an organic disease of the encephalon, and

acute meningeal affections of the spinal cord and brain
from the morbid changes of the optic nerve and retina,
neuritis and neuro-retinitis.   In tetanus both eyes are
generally alike implicated, and a papillar and retinal
hemorrhage evidence serious disturbances in the cerebral
blood circulation from cerebro-spinal lesions.

My resumé on the treatment of tetanus is as follows :

1.   Division of a nerve can be of benefit only if
practiced very early ; amputation is similarly practicable,
but generally of little avail, because decided symptoms
have already been developed.

2.   Local applications and general attention to the
wound are of the utmost importance to prevent complications, and to insure local quietude and avoid derived
irritation.   Fresh air is for a like reason instrumental
in the successful management of tetanus.

3.   General and unconditional quiet and rest around
the patient are enjoined ; all noises, even to speaking in
an elevated tone, are to be interdicted, remembering
that sudden death has often followed after exciting impressions.

4.   Supporting nourishment in concentrated form,
and stimulants should supply the exhaustion in a disease, which is not characterized by disorganization of
any vital organ.

5.   In cases where the patient is plethoric, the pulse
full but not frequent, and where there exists a disposition to, or symptoms of, isochronic inflammatory action,
venesection, leeching and cupping are indicated in the
outset, and shall be promptly but carefully practiced.
The subsequent action of the therapcutic agent is
thereby rendered more certain.

6. Purgatives of prompt action are necessary in all instances, and should be repeated and interchanged until a desired effect is obtained, aided by enemata if demanded.

7. The selection of the anti-tetanic should be made according to the most promising statistics on tetanus, and with these references :—

(a). As corroval and its kindred remedies act upon the heart by paralyzing its muscular action, the cardiac condition should be carefully diagnosticated, its normal status by commemorative evidence and symptoms, —the tendency of the spasm, flushed face, etc., with the general phenomena of functional or organic disease—and the effect of the remedy, especially in cases in which no morbid action of the heart was found, but in which medication tends towards interfering with the cardiac action, should be considered.

(b). When the remedy in a quick but cautious exhibition sustains itself by the systemic tolerance, then the same should be continued in adequate doses until its full therapeutic virtues are elicited.

(c). The remedy should be given in a form easiest taken up in the system, to insure its action as soon as possible, to avoid accumulative effects, and with due regard to the difficulties of deglutition.

(d). It should be continued in its full effects upon the system until the abnormal condition of the spinal cord and nerves has been exhausted or annihilated.

8. As standard remedies, opium, cannabis indica and the calabar bean are entitled to the greatest confidence (in their purity of preparation), and their mode of exhibition is exemplified in the cases reported by

Frick, Knight, Greenleaf and V, VI, and VIII, reported by me (opium), O'Donovan, Chuckerbutty, O'Shaughnessy and my cases, I, III, IV and IX (cannabis indica), and Fraser, Watson, Boutflower and Haining (calabar bean).

704 Chouteau Avenue·

ASIATIC CHOLERA; ITS HISTORY, CAUSES AND PREVENTION.

By H. A. BUCK, M. D., St. Louis.

We have very good authority for believing that epidemic cholera had its origin in the *Black Death,* or *Oriental plague* of the 14th century. And cholera, unquestionably, in all of its various forms, has destroyed more lives then all of the other epidemics taken together.

We are informed by historians that it swept off one-fourth of the inhabitants of the Old World, in the short period of four years.

England lost one-half of its population—London lost 100,000 in four months, and other cities in proportion.

It was preceded by great revolutions in the earth. From China to the shores of the Atlantic, the foundations of the earth were shaken, the atmosphere was in continual commotion; and endangered by its poisonous influences, both vegetable and animal life. These terrible convulsions are said to have began in 1333, fifteen years before the *plague* broke out in China.

According to the traditions of the Chinese, the pestilence was followed by torrents of rain, and great floods, and more then 400,000 people perished in consequence of the floods. A few months afterwards an earthquake caused an extensive range of mountains to sink and disappear, and in its place a lake was formed, more than 100 leagues in circumference—where thousands found a watery grave.

It is estimated that 4,000,000 people perished in China in the year 1337.

Europe was also visited with earthquakes and other atmospheric phenomena. These convulsions continued till 1347, when the plague or cholera, in its primitive form, broke out in the East.

This epidemic entered the Western countries of Asia from China, in the year 1347, and here the historian obtains the first certain knowledge of the character of the disease. From China the route of commerce ran to the North of the Caspian Sea through Central Asia —from thence to Constantinople, the medium of communication between Asia, Europe and Africa. Thus in all directions contagion made its way, and doubtless Constantinople and the harbors of Asia Minor were the great centers of infection, whence it spread all over the world. People were struck down by " *Black Death*" as if by lightning, and the young and the strong were more frequently its victims than the aged and infirm. The descriptions of the disease given by historians, are rather indifferent. They inform us that sometimes it commenced with bleeding at the nose, which was a sure sign of death. Both in men and women, tumors in the groin, and inside of the thigh appeared at the beginning. These varied in size, but were frequently as large as an egg.   Similar tumors appeared afterward all over the body, and black and blue spots came out on the arms and thighs.

These spots were indications of the fatal termination of the disease.   No power of medicine brought relief; almost all died in from one to three days, and generally without fever or other symptoms—such was the form that the "*Black Death*" assumed in 1347, and three years following.   In 1360 and 1373, it assumed a milder form, and then it was called the "*Oriental plague.*"   The tumors no longer appeared, and bleeding at the nose was seldom known to occur.

It has been supposed by excellent medical authority, that the form thus assumed by the "*Oriental plague,*" is identical with the cholera of the present age, and that the term of *Black Death* applied to it, was derived from the livid, and frequently spotted appearance of patients in cases of malignant cholera.   The most reliable estimates given, state that China lost 13,000,000 by *Black Death* or *Oriental Plague.*

India was almost depopulated, and Tartary and Syria, and all the adjoining countries were literally covered with dead bodies.

Cyprus, it is said, lost all of its inhabitants ; and ships without crews were seen, long after, floating about in the Mediterranean.   It was reported that in the East, excepting China, 23,000,000 fell victims to this pestilence.

No climate was a barrier to its devastating and death dealing power, it penetrated the icy regions of Greenland, Iceland, Norway and Denmark.

It reached the British Isles in 1349, and Russia in 1351, and according to all accounts it was not as fatal in the cold climates as it was in the hot climates. Thus we have the form and character of what is supposed to have been epidemic cholera in its primitive state.

Quite a period of time elapses before we have any description of this epidemic again, although it is supposed by some to have prevailed in a milder form in these countries where it first made its appearance.

It visited London again in the year 1666, and the mortality averaged one-fourth part of the population. During the cholera of 1832, the worst plague that has visited London since 1666, the deaths were only one out of two hundred and fifty inhabitants. This decrease of mortality was owing to the sanitary improvements in regard to cleanliness.

The next description that we have of it, is by a physician attached to the Dutch East India Company. His book was published in Batavia, in 1629. In describing what he calls epidemic cholera morbus, he says: "It is a disease of the most acute kind, and therefore, requires immediate application.

"The animal spirits are speedily exhausted, and the heart, the foundation of life, is overwhelmed with putrid effluvia.

"Those who are seized with this disease generally die, and that so quickly as in the space of twenty-four hours at most.

"This disease is attended with a weak pulse, difficult respiration, and coldness of the extremities to which are joined great internal heat, insatiable thirst, perpetual watching, and restlessness and incessant tossing of the body.

"If, together with these symptoms, a cold and fetid sweat should break forth, it is certain death." This I

consider a very good description of the epidemic cholera of the present age.

During the latter part of the 17th century, and until
the year 1774, the cholera appeared to have confined
its ravages almost exclusively to the Hindoos.

Hindoo practitioners appear to have been familiar
with its symptoms, or at least a disease closely resembling it, which they called *vishuchi*, a term in their language signifying vomiting and purging. In the first
campaigns of the British troops in India, in the year
1774, cholera presenting all the symptoms known
to characterize the epidemic, made its appearance at
Madras, and proved very fatal to both, the European
and native soldiers, carrying them off very quickly after
they were attacked. It is asserted that over 60,000
people perished between the years 1774 and 1781. The
disease prevailed at various times between the years
1783 and 1790, and always with the same symptoms
and with the same fatal results.

In the year 1783, the cholera broke out at the sacred
bathing place on the Ganges. This was the year of the
great pilgrimage, it is said 2,000,000 were assembled at
this time. In eight days 20,000 fell victims. It did
not extend beyond the place of bathing, and ceased on
the dispersion of the multitude. In 1817, it broke
out again on the banks of the Ganges, causing a greater
destruction of life then at any other time.

By the end of 1818 its ravages embraced nearly all
of Hindostan, and in 1819 it appeared in Java,
in the Isles of France and Bourbon, and over India
and China. In 1821, in Bagdad, Arabia, and in
1822, in Persia and Syria. In 1823 it broke out in
Antioch, Tripoli, and all along the Mediterranean

coast. In 1823 and 1827, the disease continued its ravages in China and India—in 1828 the Russian Empire was again invaded. The cold of the preceding winter stayed its progress, but the summer of 1829 found it committing terrible havoc in the same localities.

In 1830 it appeared in the Georgian cities, and in Poland. In 1831 in Warsaw, St. Petersburg and all the principal cities of Russsia, Prussia, Austria and Italy; and the same year made its appearance in England, Scotland and Ireland. In 1832, in the month of March, it appeared in Dublin, and in May, in Paris.

Its first appearance in the New World, was in June, 1832, at Montreal and Quebec, and during its prevalence the mortality was great.

Since its appearance on our shores it has been almost periodical, visiting a place in its epidemic form once in sixteen or seventeen years, and remaining from one to three years during the hot months of the year, if it found a soil congenial for its germs, to propagate in.

Epidemic cholera has appeared in St. Louis twice* at an interval of about sixteen years. On its appearance in 1849, there were some 65,000 inhabitants in St. Louis. It is thought some 15,000 left the city; the statistics give the mortality at 6,000.

Let us compare the mortality of St. Louis with Boston and Baltimore, where strict sanitary laws were enforced in the same years. Boston appropriated a sum of money sufficient to clease and purify the streets and

---

*[*Three times.*—First in 1833 and 1834. We have little more faith in the sixteen or seventeen year periodicity of cholera than we have of the "forty-year flood of the Mississippi."]

alleys and yards. The work was done thoroughly and effectively.

In St. Louis no attempt was made to remove the filth, or any way to improve the sanitary condition of the city, except what may have been done by a few individuals on their own premises.

Now compare the results, Boston, out of a population of 140,000, lost but 327 by cholera, from all causes, 5,000—while in St. Louis, with less than 65,000 inhabitants, 6,000 persons died of cholera alone.

In Baltimore $40,000 was appropriated by the city council, for the work of purification in anticipation of the coming epidemic. The result was, that out of a population of 160,000, but 853 died of cholera. Showing, I think, conclusively, that cholera can be prevented from appearing in an epidemic form.

I was in New York when epidemic cholera prevailed in 1850, 1851 and 1852. It was the last of September when the cholera boke out in an orphan asylum. The Superintendent took the orphans out on a picnic, and immediately on their return the cholera attacked them in a very malignant form. The Superintendent and some thirty out of ninety cases died. I think the great mortality in the asylum was in consequence of worthless nurses, (as they had to depend on the alms-house for nurses on that occasion,) badly ventilated rooms, and not separating the sick from the well. I was a student of medicine, and helped to take care of them, and formed a very unfavorable opinion of the curative properties of medicine in epidemic cholera at that time. In 1866, when the cholera attacked the inmates in any of the public institutions and hospitals in New York, they removed them to wards by themselves, and they disinfected the wards, and the consequence was, there were very few cases compared with former epidemics. I was one of the Ward physicians of the Sixth Ward, in St. Louis, in 1866. Our Ward extended from the levee to the city limits west

The cholera that year was confined mostly to the crowded tenement buildings on the principal streets and alleys. There were a few cases in the Western portion of the city where the buildings stood isolated, and it was thought by some it was in consequence of drinking the well water in those localities that were subject to surface drainage.

Its second appearance in an epidemic form in St. Louis (as you all know) was in 1866. I have not the statistics of the number of cases and deaths at its last visitation in St. Louis, but there were not as many according to the number of inhabitants as in 1849. But I believe we had more cases than there were in New York in the same years, 1866 and 1867.

According to the statistics of the Board of Health for New York and Brooklyn, they only had 1,909 cases of cholera in the year 1866, they do not give the number of deaths for that year. In 1867 they only had twenty-seven deaths from cholera. And I think it can be attributed to the great vigilance of the Board of Health of New York, that it was prevented from making such ravages as in its former visitations in that city. Now, unless there is a new departure in the perodicity of epidemic cholera, we need not fear another visitation of it again until 1882 or 1883, and not then if there is a strict observance of sanitary laws and hygiene.

We stated in the fore part of this paper that there were great floods, converting immense tracts of land

into swamps.   And as the water subsided, the flooded
districts were drained, foul vapors arose everywhere,
from decomposing vegetable and animal matter, made
more horrible and poisonous by the odor of putrified
corpses, the victims of floods, famines and earthquakes.

It is probable that the atmosphere thus contaminated
gave origin to the Black Death, whenever the organs of
respiration came in contact with it.   At a later period it
was stated that its origin in several instances was traced
to the pilgrims, who visited the banks of the Ganges,
in the observance of their religious rites.

And still later, the havoc committed by the epidemic
at Alexandria, suggested official inquiries, and the President of the Board of Health addressed a communication on the subject to the Minister of Foreign Affairs.
In this paper it is stated as the opinion not only of the
President himself, but of all the scientific and professional authorities in Egypt, that the poison is generated
by crowds of pilgrims periodically visiting the holy
places of Arabia.   The pilgrims congregate at certain
periods of the year, from all parts of the Mohamedan
World, to the number of seven or eight hundred thousand.

It is ever a point of religion with them that no pilgrim should change his clothes during the whole time of
his pilgrimage.   Under these conditions they are hud-
dled together in enormous crowds beneath the fiery sky
of the desert.   It is an indispensable incident of the
ritual that each pilgrim should sacrifice at least one
sheep, and the skin and offal of these countless victims
are left to decompose under an Arabian sun.   The
result of all this is that thousands of pilgrims perish on

the spot, leaving their bodies to be shuffled hastily under a coating of sand which the first sirocco will disperse; and their clothes to be packed up and carrried off as relics to be distributed among their relations and countrymen. The Egyptian minister thinks that here is the seed-plot and hot-bed of cholera.

It will scarcely be questioned that epidemic cholera is a disease originating in a specific principle pervading the atmosphere; this acting in combination with miasmata rising from the earth creates a positive poison, and this is productive of the same results wherever it comes in contact with the vital organs.

But while it produces but one disease there are distinct stages of the same, the different stages, in some cases, being more or less merged into one; but in nearly every instance the peculiarities of each are plainly observable. How this atmospheric poison originates, or in what manner it attacks the system, we can only venture to express our opinion. It may act indirectly through the nervous system, thence affecting the organs of sympathy and sensation. Some distinguished medical gentlemen contend that it enters through the medium of the lungs. The discussion of the subject must be after all a mere matter of speculation, as it is not known how it enters the system. Neither is the nature of the cholera-poison known. The fact, however, is well-known that a malarious poison does exist ; that, combined with local causes, it operates with deadly power. By imprudence in living, fatigue, want of sleep, gorging the stomach with food, stimulating the brain with alcoholic drinks, giving way to fear, or in fact, any irregularity having a tendency to derange the course of nature, the magazine is prepared with explosive material, only waiting the epidemic match to hurl its victims to destruction.

How to prevent epidemic cholera?' In reference to this subject the first thing to be considered is the fact that cholera is dependent primarily on atmospheric conditions, and proximately on local conditions, impure air, being the most conspicuous. The mysterious principle, whatever it may be, generated in the great crucible of nature—whether in the jungles of India, the simoons of Arabia, or the craters of Vesuvius—may be carried on the wings of the wind over the surface of the earth, without producing more than a slight disturbance of the functions of animal life, manifested in a tendency to disease of the bowels, and general depression of the vital powers. Another poisonous principle is generated in the laboratories of terrestrial filth. Every city and town sends up its deleterious gases, its disease-laden malaria which combines with the poisonous principle with which the atmosphere is already impregnated, and thus a compound is generated, which may be the fatal cholera-poison.

Predisposition and susceptibility favor the operation of the prevailing cause, therefore sanitary measures should be promptly instituted for the thorough purification of these gas-generating foci all around us in full blast; from the offal in vacant lots; from the alleys reeking with pollution; from the gutters and back yards of tenement houses.

This is where sanitary labors should begin. Competent sanitarians in every community, great or small, should inspect this work.

Timely and thorough *cleansing,* and *disinfecting* is what "stamp out" Asiatic or sporadic cholera, better than any other means yet known to civilization.

Hospital Reports.

ST. LOUIS (SISTERS') HOSPITAL.

Clinic of Prof. E H. GREGORY, reported by Dr. CHARLES GARCIA.

CASE I. *Jan. 9th, 1873.* A young man, farmer by occupation, has varicose veins. I advised obliteration. You see this large vein, both dilated and elongated; as it increases in length it must become tortuous, indicating growth. A cluster of similar vessels would make a tumor, and a corresponding involvement of the small vessels would constitute a nævus. Aneurisms are probably growths. Thus you perceive the probable close alliance of varices to aneurism, and the probable connection of both with inflammatory over-growths. We may palliate this condition, or attempt a radical cure. Some surgeons doubt the propriety of obliteration, insisting that nature thus equalizes abnormal pressure of the vessels and to obliterate at one place is to induce this formation in another site. Operation: Patient stands on the table; veins are pinched up and pins inserted under them every one, two, or three inches as required, and then tied by the figure 8, (silk thread) and allowed to remain eight or ten days till the vessels ulcerate through.

We may palliate in these cases by using a roller bandage; a starch bandage might be useful, a laced bandage, an elastic bandage; a starch bandage might be worn for several weeks and then be renewed. Patients suffer most when standing, least when walking. Thrombi sometimes form, inflammation and abscess follow, with spontaneous cure. Rupture may occur ; but bleeding ceases when the patient is recumbent. You constantly see ulcers in connection with varices of the lower extremities. Not unfrequently an eruptive trouble, " exema," occurs with intolerable itching requiring, some special application.

CASE II. Observe the symptoms in this case. Here is a small opening ; I press in the vicinity, and pus wells up. I introduce a probe and it passes, as you observe, along a sinus. I suspect diseased bone, and as it is near the extremity of the bone—tibia, it is probably caries. The history of this case is : some weeks ago there was an abcess, acute in its character; there was fever and this little opening is where the abcess opened, and this track along which this probe passes is the contracted cavity of the former abcess. At the bottom of the cavity is the diseased bone into which the probe sinks. Observe the site of the disease is the cancellated structure. The cause is not so clear ; probably it originated in some constitutional predisposition, Certainly the slight violence to which the part was subjected was insufficient to produce the large result which we see. This is a case of caries, which implies decay of the bone. Abcess is almost always present in these cases, yet decay and absorption may go so exactly together, that a bone may lose materially in weight and strength, become rarified, exhibiting the condition of " interstitial absorption " without the formation of pus.

We have already shown you a macerated specimen of bone illustrating this condition. Inflammation is probably always present in caries, and whilst the inflammatory process seems in its main features to be essentially the same in all circumstances, its products vary much, sometimes solid, sometimes fluid, sometimes high in organization, sometimes most degraded, sometimes simple, sometimes specific, sometimes contagious, sometimes infectious, sometimes acrid and offensive, again bland and creamlike, then like cheese, and again like wash or starch. Thus you perceive how strangely varied are the results of this most mysterious process. As you advance you will come to take much interest in this subject.

CASE III. Necrosis of the superior maxilla. You see a depression in this patient's cheek. Move the skin and the dimple adheres to the bone. This is positive proof of the former involvement of the bone. The patient was here several months ago, and a particle of bone was removed from the site of this depression. She yet complains of pain, but the part has healed and the scab is depressed, one of the best signs we have that the morbid action has ceased. Her suffering is at night. The surgeon soon becomes familiar with nocturnal exacerbations of pain after injuries of all kinds, in many local affections, especially in diseases of bone and periosteum it is the rule to suffer most at night. It is said to be a physiological habit to repair the body at night, which has been wasted during the day. If the idea is true, congestions, or active fluxions occur at night as the condition of repair. There is nothing unreasonable in this supposition. We have heretofore ordered five grains of iodide of potass. for this patient, three times a day, and with seeming benefit. The prescription will be repeated to-day.

CASE IV. *Jan. 11th.* This man says he has a piece of cat fish bone in the palm of his hand, but we are not sure of it; I press with the back of my knife to limit the site of the pricking sensation, which probably fixes the precise locality of the foreign body. As the patient seems so sure of its presence, I will incise this part, puncturing as you observe with this narrow, sharp pointed instrument, and cutting from within. Were I to cut from without, I might drive the body deeper into the part. I now search with the forceps which I use as a probe. I discover nothing. I will insert this lint, and wait for suppuration. After a few days we will explore the part.

In seeking for needles, or other slender bodies, press with the back of the knife over the suspected surface, and not with the finger, using a narrow edge, we can find the pricking sensation and cut down on the point, and if you do not find the foreign body, suppuration will uncover it in a few days.

The man returned in three days, and the bone was removed.

Reviews and Bibliographical Notices.

A HANDBOOK OF MEDICAL ELECTRICITY. By Herbert Tibbels, M. D., L. R. C. P., London. Philadelphia: Lindsay & Blakiston, 1878. pp. 164.

[For Sale by the St. Louis Book & News Co.]

This book is well illustrated, and is intended for beginners in the employment of electricity for medical purposes, franklinism, voltaism aud faradism, are the terms adopted for static or frictional electricity, for dynamic or current electricity, and for induced electricity. Why voltaism is chosen instead of galvanism, generally adopted, is not explained.

The first half of the book is taken up with a description of apparatus; the latter half with their application.

" The scientific electro-therapeutic, application of electricity, is the growth of the last thirty years. Prior to this date, the difficulty of obtaining apparatus adapted for the purpose, and the consequent inconvenience of the whole proceeding seems to have stopped all inquiries at the very threshhold.

" To Duchenne, who was aptly called the father of electro-therapeutics, may fairly be ascribed the birth of medical electricity as a branch of therapeutics, and his writings undoubtedly impelled to its study some of the most painstaking physicians, especially in Germany.

" Before Duchenne no one had attempted any local application of electricity that could be properly so called. The only effort towards this end had been that of Sarlandiere in 1825, who conceived the ingenious idea of using acupuncture in order to direct and limit the power of electricity within certain nerves and muscles. The pain of this application, especially when a large number of muscles were inserted, and many other disadvantages precluded it from being adopted in practice. But it appears to have suggested to Duchenne that in some way it might be possible to arrest electricity in the skin without stimulating the subjacent organs, or, on the contrary, to cause it to penetrate the skin without influencing it, and concentrate its power on the deep-seated muscles or nerves. The result of his experiments was entirely successful, and we owe to him the fundamental principle of all methods of localized electrization.

"He applied to the dry skin the dry metallic conductors of an induction instrument in action. Sparks and crackling were produced, but no physiological phenomena. The electricity did not penetrate the skin. He replaced the dry conductors by well moistened sponges. The current produced nether sparks nor crackling, but very variable phenomena of contractility, or sensibility, according as it acted upon a muscle, a nerve, or upon an osseous surface."

The paragraphs quoted afford a specimen of the rhetoric, which is bad while the meaning is still very clear. Though careless in expression, the subjects discussed are rendered clearly comprehensible. After a brief account of the application of the thin forms of electricity, the diagnostic value is briefly described.

We have not room to follow the author through his treatise. He does not prescribe the agent for all manner of diseases, and he mentions as special contra-indications, "actual softening of the brain or spinal cord. Active or severe inflammations, or congestions, whether central or peripheral, great exaltation of reflex action after recent paralytic seizures, and those conditions generally in which active medication is contra-indicated."

"The mild continuous voltaic current only should be employed."

There is throughout a want of definiteness as to what kind of electric current is best adapted to particular forms of disease, probably because the science of the application of electricity is not yet sufficiently matured to enable one to know—more definite knowledge may be expected in a few years.   P.

THE SCIENCE AND ART OF SURGERY : being a treatise on Surgical Injuries, Diseases and Operations. By John Eric Ericksen, Senior Surgeon to University College Hospital, and Holme Professor of Clenical Surgery in University College, London. A new edition, enlarged and carefully revised by the author. Illustrated by upwards of seven hundred engravings on wood. Philadelphia: Henry C. Lea. Two vols. pp. 1699.

Ericksen's Science and Art of Surgery is now presented to us in a "New American Edition," in two volumes. In the preface to this edition, we are told by the author: "In consequence of delays that have unavoidably occurred in the publication of the Sixth British Edition, time has been afforded me to add to this one several paragraphs, which I trust will be found to increase the practical value of the work."

Several changes have been made in the work, in order to keep abreast of the general advance of surgical science. That which was regarded as obsolete has been omitted. "Several chapters have been recast, and some almost rewritten." "Many wood cuts have been redrawn, and nearly a hundred new illustrations have been added." The author is a strong advocate of the *starched bandage* in the treatment of fractures. Ericksen's Surgery has been so frequently reviewed and noticed in the journals, and is so well known as a reliable authority that it needs little recommendation at this time. It is a most excellent work, very popular, as the numerous editions prove. Its publication in two volumes is an advantage. The typography is well done, and reflects credit on the publishing house of Mr. Lea.

FUNCTIONAL DISEASES OF THE RENAL, URINARY, AND REPRODUCTIVE ORGANS, with a general review of Urinary Pathology. By D. Campbell Black, M. D., L. R. C. S., Edin. Member of the General Council of the University of Glasgow, etc. Philadelphia: Lindsay & Blakiston, 1872. pp. 300, 8 vo.

[For Sale by the St. Louis Book & News Co]

This work on Functional Diseases of the Urinary Organs, etc., is divided into seven chapters, the most important of which is the sixth, "on the pathology and treatment of nocturnal enuresis, and spermatic incontinence." The profession it seems have come to look upon spermatorrhœa as a name without a corresponding disease, or if a disease exist it is of trifling importance. "Absolutely *there is,* or *there is not,* such a disease," says our author. "If there is, it is ours *to treat it*; if not, it is ours *to expose the fallacy.*" On this subject the remarks are judicious; and numerous cases are selected from both recent and from older writers.

On Suppression of Urine in Cholera, the writer remarks: "It is possible that by these copious evacuations (from the bowels), the *vis medicatrix naturæ* is in operation, but in thus attempting to rid the system of the noxious material, the constitution of the

blood is compromised, and the interchange of elements generating heat in the depths of the tissues, and constituting life by the
proper performance of this function, is impaired. In a chemical point of view, the alkaline salts constitute the most important principle of the blood, as their presence greatly promotes
oxidation; even vegetable acids are converted in the system
into carbonates for this purpose. If, then, the alkaline and
saline matters are in cholera removed therefrom to any considerable extent, the practice of recruiting the blood through the
veins, with such material as that removed by the disease, the
absorptive function of the stomach and bowels being suspended,
cannot be impeached; and taken in conjunction with the invariable improvement in the patient's condition, in all the cases
described by Dr. Little, such as the marked increase of the
temperature, the sudden change of color from deep lividity to
diffuse redness. The fact cannot be gainsaid, that salines act
by oxygenation, and that the practice of saline injections as
used by Dr. Little, is founded on the soundest physiological
basis. In confirmation of our opinion that the salines do so
act, we may refer to the analysis of Dr. Lithely [London Hospital Reports, see *Glasg. Med. Journal,* 1867.] "As the patient
improved, the quantity of urine voided was augmented, its
color improved and the percentage of solid residue increased
most markedly. An impetus, as it were, had been imparted
to the process of secondary assimilation, and the system became
thus enabled to resume its proper function."

"Choleraic suppression may therefore be taken as typical of
the *variety, of suppression due* to *altered chemical composition of the
blood."* page 83.

"The treatment choleraic suppression involves that of cholera
itself, viz: what we believe to be the rational treatment, al-
coholic-saline injections into the veins, keeping up the warmth
of the body, and maintaining in every possible manner the
strength of the patient, until the poison is dissipated from the
system." page 87.

In speaking of the surgical means for relieving retention of
urine, no mention is made of the use of the *aspirating needle*
now frequently made use of.

Our author is by no means a novice with the pen, but in some
respects, his style is not such as we would recommend. It is

stiff; many unusual words are applied where others would have
been better, and too much Greek, Latin and French for the
ordinary reader. The ablest writers are the plainest. The
work has merit, and the writer has displayed ability as well
as learning.

Proceedings of the St. Louis Medical Society.

June 7th, 1873.—Asiatic Cholera being under consideration
it was said to be a subject so vast and so full of undecided
points, that only a cursory glance over the subject can be attempted in the few moments allowed us here. It may be defined to be a specific disease, indigenious to certain areas and
parts of India, but capable of being disseminated over the surface of the earth, through the atmosphere and by the intercourse of the healthy with the sick.

For reasons yet unexplained, it has proved more virulent or
fatal on its first outbreak than at the close of an epidemic.
Hence the diagnosis is usually easy at the outbreak of the disease.

The most common premonitory symptom is diarrhœa, (but we
have witnessed many cases in which this warning was not given,
but the disease was announced by debility, vertigo, tremors, a
sense of "goneness" at the pit of the stomach, vomiting and
purging of a serous "rice water" fluid (alkaline), coldness and
lividness of the lips and tongue, feeble, rapid pulse, restlessness, suppressed urine, blueness of the surface of the body, and
sunken, deathly, countenance. The amount of pain and cramp-
ing of the muscles varies greatly; one of the first malignant
cases we saw in this city at the outbreak of the disease in 1849,
was so free from unpleasant sensations of any kind, that the
patient (an intelligent gentleman) said, " he felt to be dissolving
into water, that his sensations were never more pleasant," and
thus he passed away without a pain. In view of the fact that
the disease spreads over countries where the moral and physical habits of the people, also the climate, soil and geological
formations differ as widely as possible, is conclusive evidence,

we think that the remote cause of cholera is a specific poison. Whether this poison acts primarily through and upon the fluids of the body, or nervous centers, or upon the mucous membrane of the alimentary canal, is not fully demonstrated; and the questions: Is the poison produced in the human organism and propagated through the excreted matter? May it be produced in dead animal or vegetable matter, or in these matters mixed with the excretions of cholera subjects? May it be propagated through water, air, or contact; either, or all, of these channels? The London College of Physicians have expressed the opinion, "That human intercourse has a share in the propagation of the disease: that the poison may attach itself to the surface of bodies, walls of rooms, and furniture, clothing, etc., in infected dwellings; but that it may spread independently of communication of the sick with the healthy, *i. e.*, be carried by currents of air.

A committee of eminent scientists appointed by the Board of Health of London in 1858, when cholera prevailed in that city, found or concluded, that, the meteorological changes which renew the purity of the air are defective, where cholera prevails; and eminently so in low, wet situations, which show high barometric pressure, absence of ozone and of electricity, in which localities the epidemic was most marked. They also concluded that the poison acted as a *ferment,* and therefore takes effect only under congenial circumstances. That organic impurity is the material out of which the ferment bears or begets the poison. Hence the susceptibility of a given locality for a cholera epidemic is somewhat in proportion to the above soil relations and atmospheric conditions. No theory so far includes and harmonizes all the facts observed, as to the origin and spread of cholera. But that it is due to a specific poison, which originates among the vapors of the wet, uncultivated deltas of the large rivers of Central India, that these are the "breeding grounds" of the disease all agree. A good degree of concurrence also exists as to the fact, that the poison is cast off from the cholera patient in the discharges, and may be transmitted to other persons in the following ways, viz: by soiled hands from attendance on the sick, by means of bed-clothes and other tainted articles, or through atmospheric dispersion. The poison may be dried and preserved for a period not yet determined, also the poison may exist in the premonitory diarrhœal discharges.

26

As quarantine cannot be made absolute, it cannot exclude the disease, particularly in these days of railroad travel; but it may lessen the rapidity of infection; it is becoming obsolete. Dr. Lionel S. Beale says of the cholera-poison : " That the infecting material consists neither of insects, of animalcula, nor any kind of vegetable organism; but of living matter, formed in the organism of man, the particles being exceedingly minute and capable of maintaining their vitality a long time, and under various conditions, although separated from the body; that the living contagious particle is not of the species of the parasite, nor species at all, nor has it originated in the external world and grafted itself on man; but has originated in his organism, and that it is degraded living matter. As to the support of the organic theory, direct observation or positive proof is yet wanting. Future microscopic investigations after the manner of Pastuer, may possibly settle the question." Many other observers of less reputation as microscopists differ with Beale, and describe organisms, fungi, etc. Aitkin remarks in concluding the evidence; that "so far, therefore as fungi are concerned in the spread of cholera, I am satisfied that we have no grounds for such a belief."

Dr. Thudicum, who made careful chemical examinations, says, " there is no chemical evidence of any special cholera-poison in the blood." Niemeyer speaks of the period of incubation, and limits it from thirty-six hours to three days; others make the time longer. The temperature of the body in cholera falls from five to seven degrees below the normal standard. Dr. Fair's investigations show that males suffer more than females, at all ages *under 25 years;* from 25 to 45 the females suffer most. As a rule in all countries, the lower classes have suffered more than the upper. The anæmic are predisposed. To prevent the extension or spread of cholera, according to the theories held at present, we cannot do better than to thoroughly disinfect or neutralize all dejections from cholera patients immediately. For this purpose carbolic acid, sulphate of zinc, and sulphate of iron, are particularly recommended. Dr. Kühne prefers strong acids or alkalies, permanganate of potassium and sodium. He recommends two parts of permanganate of sodium (solution), 45 parts acid sulphate of iron, and 53 parts of water in 100 parts. This solution to be used freely to disinfect all dejections from the sick, water closets, etc. Aerial disinfection is best effected by burning sulphur; for washing clothes a solution of zinc salts is preferable. If thorough and intelligent use could be made of these agents early, on the first approach of cholera, it is possible it might be confined to sporadic cases.

We have heretofore alluded to the establishment, by the city authorities, of a *sanitarium,* on the high ground in the suburbs of the city, convenient to street car travel; particularly to avoid the loss of children by *cholera infantum.* We believe tents could be procured from the Army Quartermaster, in sufficient number for the experiment; a pine floor, and shed back of each tent to cook under, is all the lumber needed. The expense of fitting up a thousand tents would be trifling; allow any poor family with an infant to have the use of a tent *free of cost,* during the hot weather, and they would soon be occupied. If we are threatened with cholera, the more important: as it would doubt-less prove the best sanitary measure, in case of that epidemic.

We will conclude this report with a brief allusion to what was said on the *treatment* of cholera. Dr. Fergus, of Glasgow, recommends the following rules:

Avoid all depressing passions and exhaustion of nerve-force, avoid brandy, or other stimulants, as they are not preventives; make no change in the usual diet, if that is simple, digestible and nutritious. Avoid excessive fatigue; if over-heated, beware of chill, but see that the skin is kept comfortably warm; should the slightest diarrhœa occur, the patient should *lie down immediately,* and if chilly, have bottles of hot water placed to the feet and legs, also take thirty drops of laudanum, and if a physician is not at hand, the following recipe may be used:

> R Oil Anise, ol. cajuput, āā ʒss.
>
> Ether, Sulph., ʒss.
>
> Liquor Acid Halleri, (which consists of
> one part of concentrated sulphuric acid
> to three parts of rectified spirits.) ʒss.
>
> Tinct. Cinnamon, ʒii.

M. Give 10 drops every 15 minutes in a tablespoonful of water. The opiate may be given with this *once or twice,* but not more. The patient should remain in bed two or three days after the diarrhœa has ceased: ice to dissolve in the mouth to relieve the thirst; no food for a few hours, then the lightest kinds. This is strictly for the first stage; should the case go into the second stage, the particular treatment must be dictated by the physician at the bed-side. We have no specific for the disease, neither can the poison be eliminated from the blood, more than small-pox or measles; to sustain the vital power while the poison is expended is the most successful plan. Remidies which are acid rather than alkaline, or neutral reaction, have been most beneficial, says Aitkin.

The Indian Army Sanitary Commission states in the *London Lancet*: That in fully developed cholera verging towards collapse medicines were simply of no use. That when recovery took place, it was due to good nursing, rest, in a strictly recumbent position, etc.

It would seem that cholera does not add so much to the average death-rate as is supposed; for instance, in England the rate being 22.3 to the 1,000 of population. In 1847, the death-rate was 25.4 for male and 23.8 for females ; in 1848 and 1849— cholera years—24.8 males and 23.8 females. The cholera year 1854, 24.4 males and 22.7 females. From which it would appear that about the same number die of some disease; if not of this epidemic.

Dr. Hodder of Toronto, gives details of three instances in which transfusion of milk was practiced in cholera, latter stage; the first case was in collapse, pulseless, blue and shrivelled. The man rallied almost immediately, and made a rapid recovery; the second case, an intemperate woman, also recovered ; the third case, proved fatal, but was said to be in articulo mortis, when the transfusion was practiced. (For method of operation see March number of this JOURNAL.)

Dr. Hodgen mentioned a plan of treatment pursued by him in a few cases at the close of the epidemic of 1866, with results considered sufficiently encouraging to merit further trial. In the *stage of collapse*, the doctor injected subcutaneously from a sixtieth to a thirtieth of a grain of sulphate of atropia, and injected freely into the bowels warm water with a little salt in it, reaction and convalescence followed in over half the cases without fever, the doctor also referred to the importance of promoting the action of the kidneys as early as possible, by diuretics and warm poultice or fomentation over the kidneys not to eliminate the cholera-poison, but to obviate uremia.

Dr. S. C. Townshend, Sanitary Commissioner at Nagpore, holds that for the production of cholera two conditions are necessary—the presence of the specific contagion, and a susceptibility to its influence on the part of the person to whom it is applied.

That a high temperature and extreme dryness are no obstacles to the diffusion of the contagion, which, having secured lodgment is farther diffused by human intercourse.

Dr. Robert Martin, of Manchester, England, in a report before the British Medical Association, holds that alcoholic liquors directly favor the development of zymotic agents.

Also Dr. French, the medical officer of health for Liverpool, supports the same views. That the drunkard is a source of the greatest danger to himself and the community. That incentives to intemperance should as far as possible be suppressed. Reference was made to Dr. ᴜaniel W. Parsons, who read before the Liverpool Medical Institution a paper in which he set forth the advantage of the self-registering thermometer as the surest guide to *prognosis*. In the first stage, temperature about normal, 98° in the axilla, and from 97° to 98° on the tongue. Second stage, axilla from 95° to 97°, tongue, 87° to 89°. Third stage, axilla 93° to 95°, tongue 85° to 87°. In all cases he had examined, a difference existed between the axilla and tongue of some 8°. One case only recovered with the axilla 93° and the tongue 85°. A sudden rise of temperature often preceeds death.

The disease, or something very like to it, being reported at various points on the lower Mississippi river, a lively interest was manifested in the discussion which was resumed at the following meeting, when an interesting paper on the history of epidemic cholera, by Dr. Buck, was read, and the benign effect of thorough sanitary measures was urged, but nothing particularly new on the origin, nature, mode of action of the poison, or its treatment was presented.

Editorial.

In the medical profession are men of every type. Solid men of learning; brilliant men of genius; strong men of logic; true men, ever loyal to make known their discoveries and advances in every department of science. Free men, to investigate fully, faithfully, and fearlessly, any and all questions of fact or theory, pertaining to medical science and practice.

The profession imposes no creed—no "thirty-nine articles," to be confessed. Truth, the search for facts in nature, the love of truth; and to practice according to our convictions of truth, is all that is required. How could the profession be more liberal, more free, more promotive of progress? In view of these facts, how can we respect the men who leave our ranks to establish or join either of the *sects* or so-called schools of medicine? What motive except personal ambition, or hope of pecuniary gain can the broadest charity accord them? A commendable motive to found or join a sect, under such circumstances, is highly improbable, yes, too absurd to be entertained for a moment; and this is the reason why the true members of the regular profession do not, and cannot respect the men who thus seek to advance their personal fortunes, at the expense of truth and honor, as the former understand it.

The weakness of a cause could not be better confessed than by submitting it of choice to the *uninformed*, and incompetent, for a verdict in its behalf: and however learned or highly cultivated persons may be in other matters, if they know nothing of anatomy, physiology, chemistry or therapeutics, how is it possible for such persons to judge of the comparative merits or demerits of the various theories of practice in medicine. It matters little how learned they may be as divines, how profound as lawyers, or shrewd as merchants; their judgment in matters of which they are uninformed cannot be of much value.

Again, for a young man, casting about to determine what his life work shall be, to elect, to become a disciple, an advocate, a practitioner, of one of the *sects in medicine,* while he is without knowledge of the facts needful to judge of the comparative merits of the various theories of medical practice, seems to us the consummation of error. Or that parents or guardians should influence or advise their sons or wards, to discard the regular schools of medicine, where the foundation may be laid deep and broad for a medical education, which shall *include a fair and impartial consideration and examination of each of the sects or schools, as to their real comparative merits,* is a fearful abuse of their sacred trust. It is no less than to consent that their ward's young mind shall be *cast in the mould* of the sect of their choice, or grow into their shell, which may limit and dwarf their opportunities or faculties, instead of enjoying the freedom of nature, to extend their growth and culture in any direction, and thereby finally attain that diversity and extent of knowledge which the physician should ever possess.

Meteorological Observations.

METEOROLOGICAL OBSERVATIONS AT ST. LOUIS, MO.

By A. WISLIZENUS, M. D.

The following observations of daily temperature in St Louis are made with a MAXIMUM and MINIMUM thermometer (of Green, N. Y.) The daily minimum occurs generally in the night, the maximum about 3 P M The monthly mean of the daily minimum and maxima, added and divided by 2, gives a quite reliable mean of the monthly temperature.

THERMOMETER FAHRENHEIT.

MAY, 1873.

Day of Month	Minimum.	Maximum.	Day of Month.	Minimum.	Maximum.
1	52.5	78.5	18	54.0	68.0
2	49.5	55.0	19	60.5	87.4
3	46.	53.0	20	57.0	75.0
4	41.0	68.0	21	61.0	86.5
5	53.0	73.0	22	65.5	89.5
6	56.0	75.0	23	61.0	88.0
7	58.0	68.0	24	67.5	90.5
8	56.0	74.0	25	67.5	82.5
9	57.5	65.0	26	66.5	88.5
10	50.0	67.5	27	62.0	80.5
11	48.0	71.0	28	60.0	83.5
12	54.0	87.5	29	64.0	86.5
13	60.0	75.5	30	59.0	74.5
14	55.5	74.5	31	54.0	77.5
15	50.5	69.5			
16	49.0	71.0	Means	56.5	75.9
17	55.0	67.0	Monthly Mean 66.2		

Quantity of rain : 3.91 inches.

Mortality Report.

FROM MAY 31st, 1873, TO JUNE 21st, 1873, INCLUS.

Date	White Males	White Females	Col'd Males	Col'd Females	Under 5 yrs.	5 to 10	10 to 20	20 to 30	30 to 40	40 to 50	50 to 60	60 to 70	70 to 80	80 to 90	90 to 100	Total.
Saturday 31	63	43	6	2	48	9	6	12	9	15	9	6	2	...	...	114
" 7	58	46	5	4	54	3	12	15	7	9	9	3		2	...	113
" 14	60	40	5	2	54	5	4	8	15	10	6	3	3		...	109
" 21	83	70	2	4	96	5	8	10	15	16	4	3	1		...	159
Total,	264	199	18	12	252	22	30	45	46	50	28	15	6	2		493

Atelectasis 1	Cerebritis 2	Fever, typhoid 8	Ovarian Tumor 1
Alcoholism 2	Consumption 48	Gastritis 5	Paralysis 5
Abscess 3	Convulsions 35	Hemorrhage 3	Peritonitis 4
Abscess of Liver 2	Croup 1	Hepatitis 2	Pertussis 4
Albumenuria 5	Cyanosis 1	Hemoptisis 1	Pneumonia 25
Apoplexy 1	Disease of Bladder 1	Hydrocephalus 4	Premature Birth 2
Ascites 2	Debility 11	Icterus Gravis 1	Rubeola 3
Asthma 2	Delirium Tremens 1	Inanition 3	Scald 6
Atrophia 9	Diarrhœa 9	Inflammat'n Bowels 2	Small Pox 20
Bright's Disease 1	Disease of the Heart 1	" of Liver 1	Strict of Esophagus 1
Bronchitis 3	Diphtheria 2	Injuries 4	Septicæmia 2
Burns 2	Dropsy 4	Intemperance 2	Suffocation 1
Cancer 4	Drowned 5	Laryngitis 2	Suicide 3
Carditis 2	Dysentery 1	Lockjaw 9	Summer Complaint 2
Cerebro-coletis 1	Eclampsia 5	Marasmus 8	Tabes Mesenterica 3
Cholera, Infantum 33	Encephalitis 1	Measles 7	Teething 1
Cholera Morbus 35	Enteritis 1	Meningitis 18	Unknown 2
Concussion Brain 3	Erysipelas 4	" cereb-spin 38	
Conges. of Brain 11	Fever, Cong 5	Metro Peritonitis 1	Total...... 493
Conges. of Lungs 2	" puerperalis 3	Œdema 1	
Conges. of Abdomen 1	" remittent 2	Old Age 4	Stillborn 29

THE SAINT LOUIS

Medical and Surgical Journal.

AUGUST, 1873.

Original Communications.

REPORT ON THE PROGRESS OF MEDICAL SCIENCE.

To the Missouri State Medical Association, May, 1873, Moberly, Missouri.

To note accurately the progress in any department of human knowledge, made in the brief space of a year or two, if possible, would certainly be difficult: for facts in nature when fairly brought to view are often found to have been partially uncovered by former explorers; hence, it is difficult to say just how much is to be credited to any one man, or particular period of time.

Again, theoretical changes in practice, growing out of the discovery of facts in etiology, pathology, or therapeutics, may as surely define true and valuable progress, as absolute discoveries with the microscope, micro-spectroscope, or other delicate contrivance to wrest from nature her most retired secrets.

Opinions thus gradually modified to better accord with facts of recent discovery help to fill the chain which connects all scientific truth in one harmonious and symmetrical whole; and as certainly, if not as sharply, define progress as the direct results of work with the microscope, or test tube.

Of course, nothing is finished. No man or generation *achieves*; instead of reaching the end of the chain of knowledge as we advance, the end recedes: and thus the pleasure of investigators is perpetuated.

We think it a good custom, for our profession to assemble from time to time from various and distant fields of observation, to compare notes and generalize; that *all* may share the benefit of the observations of *each*, and attain to a more certain and perfect knowledge of any progress made, than would be possible otherwise. Who could describe accurately a mountain or other object with many sides or surfaces, without changing his point of observation from time to time, or trusting to others (which might be better) for facts bearing upon the same object, that his conception of the whole may be more complete and accurate?

It has often been observed that carefully taken observations of the same object from opposite standpoints were so diverse, as to be unreconciliable, until notes were compared, when it was found that both were right, and yet consistent with each other.

As the term " Progress of Medical Science " includes so vast a field, we hope to be indulged to wander about, with little or no system, seeing it is quite impossible that our report should be exhaustive. First of

DIAGNOSIS.

What continues to characterize advance in this important department, is *accuracy, certainty*. The ophthalmoscope and thermometer, microscope, and test tube, with many other appliances continue their contributions to accuracy in diagnosis, and certainty in prognosis. The former indispensable to scientific clinical practice, and the latter promotive of a sound reputation at least; differentiating *various* diseases where a short time ago *one* only was believed to exist.

By the ophthalmoscope not simply the organ of vision is now explored, but the condition of distant organs, through their influence upon *cerebral circulation*, is more than hinted: thus it is highly prized as an aid to diagnosis, before the more obvious or outward symptoms have been declared.

In dermatology, the microscope continues to give new light upon the nature and mode of development of many diseases; also to acquaint us with the delicate structures of the tissues and circulating fluids, noting the changes indicating disease of a *progressive* or *retrogressive* character.

In a recent paper, by Prof. G. Simon, (translated from the German for the *New York Medical Journal*, by Alfred E. Walker, M. D.,) *on Dilatation of the Anus and Rectum*, he recommends carrying the process to an extent, which is at least not common; that is, not only for surgical operations, but also for examinations of the abdominal viscera; he gradually and carefully forces the whole hand into the rectum. By this means he claims "one is able to get behind and above the uterus and detect tumors the size of cherry stones, to examine the ovaries, and in man, to determine accurately the condition of the bladder, and ascertain the existence of calculi, their volume and number, indeed, all the viscera in the lower two-thirds of the abdomen. The operation favors the cure of ulcers in the lower bowel by allowing a free escape of the morbid products, and, in case of fistulæ, may be followed by the use of Sim's speculum, making surgical procedures much easier than when performed through any of the common anal specula.

Claiming all these advantages for the process of visible dilatation, he declares it produces no injury to the structures acted on. In some cases he incises the sphincter ani, in other cases merely distends it. Under the influence of chloroform the rectum of an adult, if there is no contraction of the pelvis, he claims, may be so enlarged, as to gradually admit the hand and part of the forearm, permitting the fingers to be introduced into the sigmoid flexure; and this but rarely causes a slight tearing of the anus. Where the anus is particularly unyielding, or when it is necessary for surgical operations, lateral incisions may be made near the raphe or at the sides of the coccyx."

Concerning that most important and interesting field of inquiry, the *etiology* of disease, nature has proved most reticent as formerly, unwilling, it would seem, that we should have this help to "preventive medicine" which might rescue so many from premature graves. No department of science so successively challenges human sagacity and industry to discover its secrets as the *causes* of disease. The pestilence, the presence of which is doubly assured by its effects on every side, still challenges us to say from what, or how it originated, or how it is conveyed; whether the poison must have contact or fomites? and what of malaria? what is the nature of the ultimate disease germ? Does it propagate itself as a vegetable ferment, emitting spores to be conveyed by the atmosphere? Or is it a "contagium animatum," a parasite, which may so occupy the atmosphere as to be swept over a continent in a few days? Or is it true, according to another theory, that epidemics are not due to specific poisons, but to predisposing influences everywhere present, waiting to become effective through incidental exciting causes?—a promising field this, for much thorough work, which must ultimately yield results of vital importance to practical medicine.

In a recent monograph by A. Wolff, F. R. C. S., on the causation of *Zymotic Diseases*, the theory that all zymotic disease is a process of *inflammatory disintegration* is ably defended. The means of extending this class of diseases, in the author's opinion, is the contact of decaying organic matter from various sources; and the difference is determined by the diversity of the organs or tissues upon which the poison takes effect, to-wit: in typhus, the *blood* is primarily affected; in enteric fever, the *bowels;* in cholera, the *alimentary canal;* in variola, the *skin;* and in measles, the respiratory tract, etc.

Dr. James Ross, in a book of near three hundred pages, advocates the *graft theory* of disease. That it is living particles which give origin to this class of affections. "Anatomical units modified and individualized by a diseased process, and impressed on the healthy organism with which they come in collision, a succession of changes similar to that which precedes their own modification in the body from which they were detached." According to Wolf it is the extention of death from one body to another. According to Ross it is the extention of an anomalous *life* from one organism to another.

The following is a contribution to our report on

THERAPEUTICS.

By David Coggin, M. D., of St. Louis.

This *resumé*, containing some of the latest views respecting the employment and action of both old and new remedies in disease, is written with the hope that its perusal may induce medical men in this vicinity to place at the disposal of their professional *confrères* the results of their experience.

The reporter is aware that his paper is far from being exhaustive, but he trusts the limited time allowed for its preparation, and the inconsiderable amount of material available for reference, will be accepted as sufficient excuse for all short comings.

Chloral Hydrate.—Since its introduction into this country, now a little over three years, has been extensively used as an anodyne and hypnotic.

From the experiments of Dr. Richardson, and other physiologists, it seems probable that on coming into contact with the blood (an alkali) it is converted into chloroform.

Dr. C. H. Clark, of Boston, thinks chloral acts with greater rapidity and power in fevers of a typhoid type, in which the blood is highly charged with ammonia than when it is less alkaline.

From fifteen to thirty grains is sufficient for a dose for an adult. That manufactured in England and Germany seems to occasion less nausea than does that made in the United States. If administered largely diluted in the proportion of eight grains to the ounce of water, it is less liable to produce nausea and is more quickly absorbed than if it is given more concentrated. To give an adult over sixty grains within twelve hours may be attended with danger.

One case is recorded in which sixty grains was given and it terminated fatally. It should be stated however, that at the autopsy the tricuspid valves were found to be diseased, while the walls of the right heart were thin.

Jolly reports the death of two insane patients. They had been taking 75 grain doses one for four, and the other for twelve days. In both patients the respiration and the action of the heart suddenly stopped. The autopsy showed œdema of the lungs while the blood in the several organs was fluid and dark.

Dr. N. R. Smith, of Baltimore, lately reported three cases from the use of chloral. He has also noticed the occurrence of erythema and ulceration of the skin around the finger nails, in persons who had taken the salt in moderate doses but long continued.

Chloroform and Morphia.—The discovery by M. Barnard that the anasthesia produced by chloroform can be prolonged by subcutaneous injection of morphia has been made use of by MM. Labbé and Guyon. Twenty minutes before the amputation of the foot, about ⅛ of a grain of morphia was subcutaneously injected. Chloroform was then given; the anasthesia was complete after the lapse of seven minutes and lasted long after the operation was terminated, and the patient was awakened and answered questions; about an ounce of chloroform was used in this case.

Lactic Acid.—Dr. G. W. Balfour, of Edinboro, reports the successful employment of lactic acid, in diabetes, as first proposed by Dr. Cantani, of Naples. He gave from 77 to 154 grains in 8 or 10 ounces of water daily in connection with an exclusively meat diet, all vegetables as well as milk and eggs, being forbidden, and only salt, oil, or a little vinegar, allowed for seasoning. Dr. B. W. Foster treated a case of diabetes with lactic acid, which gave rise to symptoms of rheumatism in the joints, but they subsided on withholding the acid only to return when it was resumed. This circumstance deserves notice as it gives weight to the lactic acid theory of rheumatism.

Digitalis.—Recent physiological experiments have confirmed the clinical experience of many practitioners, as regards the action of small doses of digitalis in cases of insufficient cardiac power. Dr. Fothergill, of Edinboro, thinks that in all cases in which the heart-muscle is inadequate to do its work well, either from valvular or other disease, *digitalis* can be given regularly for months or even years with great benefit.

Atropia.—Dr. R. A. Vance, of New York, has employed the sulphate of atropia, with marked success, in the treatment of Writer's cramp, or Scriomer's palsy. He injected subcutaneously an aqueous solution containing one-sixtieth of a grain three times a week. The injections were continued for a time varying from one to six months.

Xylol.—This remedy was introduced in the treatment of small-pox over a year ago, but its use has failed to realize the great expectations its discovery promised. It was claimed to lessen the secondary fever and to arrest the disease by acting in the blood as a disinfectant. The latest observers (in Germany) consider that xylol diminishes the pustular eruption in the throat and therefore the angina, and it also acts as a deodorizer, but no other effect can be ascribed to it.

Carbolic Acid.—Dr. J. H. Bell, U. S. Army, reports cases in which he used carbolic acid locally as an anæsthetic. He applied for a quarter or a half hour a compress wet with a saturated solution of the acid to the abscess, felon or bubo that was to be opened, and then made the incisions without causing pain. In some in- stances, after dividing the integument, he brushed out the wound with acid, if any pain was felt, before cutting deeper. This experiment has been reported by other surgeons with the same experience : but it seems there is some danger lest the acid acts as a necrotic, instead of a simple anæsthetic. Dr. Ollier, of Lyons, gives an ac- count of two cases of gangrene from the application of this strong solution. Dr. Wilde found traumatic erysipe- las disappeared in three or four days after the subcutane- ous injection in the borders of the wound of a solution of one part of the amorphous acid to twelve of water. Mr. Ashmead has employed carbolic acid in combina- tion with tannin and glycerine as an injection in gonor- rhœa after this formula :

Carbolic Acid,	gr. viii.
Tannic Acid,	gr. viii.
Glycerine,	℥ss.
Water,	℥i.

It appeared to act as an antiseptic, arresting the dis- charge and cutting short the disease.

*Quinia and Cinchonia.**—M. Briquet recommends the use of the sulphate of cinchonia in the place of the sulphate of quinine, in intermittent fever, as being less costly and equally efficacious, and its taste being far less bitter, while he considers the dose as the same, and gives from nine to fifteen grains in divided doses be- fore the expected chill.

Ergot.—Von Langenbeck successfully treated two

---

*[Cincho-Quinine has recently appeared in the drug market as a substitute for quinine, at half the cost of the latter ; it is worthy of a trial.]

aneurisms, one in the right supraclavicular fossa and the other of the right radial artery, by the subcutaneous injection of ergotin. This method has been repeated by others, and it lead Dr. Ritchie, of Manchester, to employ it in hæmoptysis. Finding five grains of ergotin in ten minims of distilled water to occasion too much irritation, he pursued Von Langenbeck's plan and injected three grains in equal parts of glycerine and rectified spirits. One injection was generally all that was required,—an immediate lowering of the pulse, by five or six beats following its use, and there is generally a slight increase of temperature. Hildebrandt has treated nine cases of intra-uterine tumors with ergotin. The most annoying symptoms soon disappeared, and after a while the tumors themselves diminished. He supposes this to be due to the interference with the nutrition of the tumor by the contraction of the blood-vessels supplying it, and also by the compression it undergoes from the walls of the uterus. Pain and hardening of the place of injection somewhat interfered with this plan of treatment. Ergot has been used considerably of late in this country, in the treatment of cerebro-spinal fever, either alone or in combination with physostigma (calabar bean), belladonna, or the bromide of potassium, but the results attending its use appear to be conflicting and uncertain.

Dr. Beatty "has concluded that most of the fatal cases in children in ergotic labor are induced by an exposure of more than two hours to the poisonous effects of ergot through the blood of the mother." Dr. F. W. Draper, of Boston, considers its effects on the child as deleterious in three ways:—first, by compressing the brain and limbs, and interfering with the circulation ; secondly, the constant tonic contraction acting on the muscular tissue and on the vessels of the womb tends to impede the uterine and the fœtal circulation and to prevent fresh blood from entering the partially emptied vessels ; while the secondary sedative action on the heart of the mother also modifies the normal circulation ; thirdly, while the child is attached by the umbilical cord to the uterus and derives its nourishment from that source, it is exposed to the toxic influence of the ergot through the maternal circulation, and it may be born with symptoms of acute ergotism. A prominent American ovariotomist was once heard to say : "nearly every young physician kills one or more patients with morphia in the first years of his practice!" Whether this is true or not, how can we call to mind the common and oftentimes injudicious use of ergot in labor without thinking of the "slaughter of the innocents?" The French government has recently interdicted the sale of ergot to midwives.

Peruvian Bark.—Dr. Montverdi prefers the action of peruvian bark and its salts to that of ergot of rye in obstetrical practice either in cases of deficient pains or in hæmorrhage during gestation or labor. Many eminent physicians in this country and abroad recommend opium in the highest terms, in cases in which the os uteri is rigid and the pains are flagging. Morphia in doses of one-fourth to one-third of a grain seems to exert a marked oxytoxic effect.

Ice Bags.—The recently introduced plan of lowering the body temperature in typhoid and other fevers by subjecting the patient to a bath of 66° F. at frequent intervals has been attended with flattering results. This course can be readily followed in hospitals, but in private practice, for obvious reasons, it is not always practicable. In the place of cold baths ice bags applied to the spine and abdomen have been found to be more agreeable to the patient and quite as efficacious in the abstraction of heat. Ice bags placed on the spine often give immediate relief in the obstinate vomiting of pregnancy, dysentery, etc., when other remedies have been tried without success. Their use has been suggested in the treatment of cerebro-spinal fever.

A New Rule for Doses.—Dr. E. H. Clark proposes a new and simple rule for the administration of medicines. That such a one is needed, must be allowed by all physicians, and more especially by those just commencing to practice who, oftentimes refer to works on materia medica in vain for information as to the proper doses particularly for children. The dose must naturally vary according to the disease and temperament of the patient, of which the physician can judge the best, but the principle remains unchanged. Dr. Clark supposes the average weight of an adult to be one hundred and fifty pounds, for whom an appropriate dose is 1 or 1½ drachm, the dose of most medicines must be increased or diminished in the proportion of the weight of the patient to the number of pounds. This proportion is represented by a fraction, whose numerator is the patient's weight and whose denominator is 150. If a child at birth weighs six pounds the dose would he $\frac{6}{150}$ or $\frac{1}{25}$; a child two years old weighing twenty pounds would require $\frac{20}{150}$ or about $\frac{1}{7}$ of an adult dose. A person weighing two hundred pounds should have $\frac{200}{150}$ or 1⅓ of an average adult dose.

CHANGE IN PHARMACOPŒIA.

A practical pharmaceutist of St. Louis, Mr. Hubert

Primm, 14th and Washington Ave., writes us of changes in the pharmaceutic art, as follows: " I beg leave to state in reply to your favor of recent date that the committee to whom was referred the duty of revising the U. S. Pharmacopœia have concluded their labors, and issued the work, which contains many new articles and preparations, as follows, changes in the mode of preparation of well known articles resulting in altering their sensible properties, taste and appearance. Some few articles have been discarded altogether.

" Thus in the primary list of the materia medica, there have been added twenty-four articles, and to the secondary list three; one article from the primary list and four from the secondary have been dropped. Among the new preparations admitted to the list with working formula are, carbolic acid water, hydrate of chloral, charta cantharides, prepared mustard leaves, flexible collodion, aconite plaster, extract of American hemp, extract of calabar bean, extract of stramonium seeds, fluid extract of belladonna root, glycerates of carbolic acid, gallic acid, tannic acid, tar, and borate of soda, yellow oxide of mercury, liquor of the arsenite of soda, citrate of lithia, preserved juices of conium and taraxicum, suppositories of carbolic acid, tannic acid, aloes, assafœtida, belladonna, morphia, opium, and acetate of lead and opium. Among the articles dropped are acetate of colchicum, fluid extract of conium, and tincture of aconite leaves.

The following changes modify the finished preparations either in result, appearance, flavor or activity. Thus the saffron is dropped in acetate of opium, Tr of aloes and myrrh, pills of aloes and myrrh, Tr cinchona comp. which is made without the cochineal; unguentum (formerly ung. adipis) is now made with yellow wax instead of white, which is an improvement as it obviates the tendency to become rancid; ointment of nitrate of mercury is now made with lard instead of neat's foot oil, savin cerate, with fluid extract of savin.

"All the fluid extracts which heretofore were made with sugar now contain glycerine, and the process of manufacture is substantially the same as is known as the "Campbell Process." The strength of the fluid extract of cinchona and wild cherry being doubled. The foregoing are considered the most important changes, not comprising all; as regards local pharmaceuticals, mention may be made of the following: *fluid extract of palma christi* used with apparent benefit in lactation.

"*Pancreatic Emulsion.*—Particularly that of English make has been extensively used the past winter in the treatment of consumption, especially in connection with cod liver oil.

"*Pepsin* of some particular makers is still held in favor by many practitioners for digestive troubles.

"The bromide of quinine, iron and calcium are much used, the latter being preferred where *prompt* action as a hypnotic or calmative is desired.

"*Codein.*—One of the opium alkaloids is used more than formerly.

"*Carbozotate, or Picrate of Ammonia,* has lately come into use as a cheap substitute for quinine in the treatment of intermittent fevers, with what result it is not for us to say, objection has been made that it *yellows the skin* temporarily.

"*Dioscorein.*—The active principle of dioscorea villosa, or wild yam, in bilious colic is gaining favor.

"*Citrate of Lithia.*—In its effervescent granular form, and the *benzoate of ammonia*, are now much prescribed in renal disorders.

"*Lacto-Phosphate of Lime.*—Not in much favor, (the fate of many drugs from more being expected from them than they could accomplish.)

"*Peroxide of Hydrogen.*—Prescribed in the treatment of diabetes, but owing to the high price perhaps, is but sparingly used.

"Among the pharmaceutical specialities which have met with deserved favor should be mentioned the *gelatine coated pills* of the house of *McKesson and Robbins*, New York, which are superior to the ordinary sugar-coated pills with which the stores are stocked; they are inviting and readily dissolved in the stomach, hence are likely to come into general use. The vital importance of *purity of drugs*, as well as *accuracy* in dispensing the same, is being appreciated in the better and special education of the manufacturing and dispensing pharmaceutist of this city and State."

Electricity.—Dr. Prince, in the St. Louis Medical and Surgical Journal, for February, 1873, remarks of electricity that faradization, or the interrupted electrical current, is preferred to stimulate organs in a sluggish condition or paralyzed muscles, if not continued too long, for the exhaustion of *irritability already enfeebled*, must do harm.

For electrolysis, *i. e.*, decomposition of the tissues so as to set their elements free—hydrogen and the alkalies going to the negative pole, and oxygen and the acids going to the positive pole—for the purpose of electrolysis the negative pole in the form of a needle, or a number of them, is employed to develop hydrogen in the tissues; if the action is only continued a very short time, the vitality of the tissues is not destroyed, but a new action is set up which in many instances is sufficient to stop the morbid growth. If the action is continued long, the tissue is torn apart by the development of hydrogen, and a slough is the consequence. Electricity from its perfect manageability is to become the king of *caustics,* and is destined to rescue from the monopoly of quacks those morbid growths which are not treated by the knife.

Electro-therapeutics, opens up a wide field of usefulness in skin diseases, and in a short time will doubtless rank with the salts of mercury and arsenic as a curative agent. Dr. Beard prefers the galvanic to the faradic current, and thinks he has had better results from applying the negative pole to the affected part. Subsequently he speaks of brilliant results from his method of *central* galvanization.

ABSTRACT OF A PAPER ON DERMATOLOGY.

By W. A. Hardaway, M. D., St. Louis.

Progress in this department of medicine is more demonstrable than in some others where neither the pathology nor the results of treatment are so readily appreciated.

Recently two representative books of English and German dermatologists have appeared, one by Neuman, of Vienna, the other by Fox, of London.

Neuman follows the example of the distinguished Hebra, that we place by far the greatest value upon external treatment, while Fox wisely urges attention to appropriate constitutional measures and lays great stress upon the proper performance of the kidney function.

Hebra has described a peculiar new formation about the nose which he has called rhinoscleroma, the disease seems to consist in ivory-like tubercular indurations upon the nose and upper lip ; and is most intractable in its nature, resisting both constitutional and local treatment.

The existence of the parasite element in eczema marginatum, tinea kerion, and various other diseases, as demonstrated by various observers, is constantly being confirmed ; a notable thing is the enlargement of the group of parasitic affections, until a large proportion of skin diseases are believed to be due to this or other external agencies, to the exclusion of their constitutional origin.

Dr. Izard, at l'Hôpital du Midi, testifies that *iodoform* is a therapeutic agent of more certainty, and which acts more promptly than the remedies ordinarily employed for promoting the cicatrization of ulcerative syphiloids in general, under whatever form they present themselves ; and that in the treatment of soft chancres iodoform is in some sort a specific by the promptness with which it promotes cicatrization without pain. He has also used it in the form of ointment to bubos with excellent results : in fact its range of application seems to be wide, and Dr. Damon, the translator of Izard's book, advises its internal administration in certain syphilitic conditions.

TREATMENT OF THE PHARYNGO-NASAL CAVITIES.

To the Chairman of the Committee on Medical Progress.

The following is respectfully submitted in answer to your favor of the 10th, concerning any progress in the *treatment* of inflammation, acute or chronic, of the mucous membrane of the nasal and pharyngo-nasal cavities, the pharynx and larynx.

Carbolic acid stands with me at the head of the list of remedies for *local application.*   My method is—

> ℞ Carbolic Acid cryst.   ℥ss.
> Glycerine,   ℥i.
> Water,   ℥vii.

M. Use one or two drachms in each inflamed cavity with the spray daily.

For the posterior nares the syringe or catheter douche is the instrument with which the remedy is to be applied, and three times this quantity of glycerine and water should be added.   The strength should be such as to produce only a *slight* smarting sensation, lasting from five to ten seconds.   The relief from each application should be evident to the patient.   On your (Dr. Edgar's) recommendation, (August 1872,) I was induced to try the extract of pinus canadensis; and have since been combining one drachm of it with the above carbolic acid solution. It has proved to be a decided improvement in the treatment of those cases which require an astringent and local tonic;   that is, where the secretions are abundant, and the mucous membrane flabby. Unlike any other astringent I have used it with benefit from the first treatment to the last, in almost every case.   I have found no remedy to be so good a cleanser of the cavities under consideration as *common salt* and warm water (one drachm to one ounce).   But it will not deodorize an ozæna; for this purpose the bromochloralum is preferable.   The most offensive cases yield to it;   being at the same time a good remedy from two drachms to an ounce may be dissolved in a pint of warm water.

The fluid extract of geranium maculatum, when added to the carbolic acid solution, is also a valuable astringent, but must be discontinued as soon as the excess of secretion has been checked. After this its application will occasion pain and harm.

The tincture of calendula officinalis is to be preferred in some cases of flabby condition of the mucous membrane, but it is of no particular benefit after this condition is overcome; one fluid ounce may be added to the glycerine and water solution.

The tincture of aconite root, half drachm to the carbolic acid solution, is a valuable remedy in pharyngitis with pain, without much swelling or secretion; but so soon as the pain is relieved it is well to discontinue it.

Muriate of ammonia (ʒi to water ℥viii) is beneficial in cases in which there is a varicose condition of the blood-vessels, and either have a great excess of secretion or where the membrane is in a dry and glazed condition, but as soon as the secretion of the membrane is regulated, the remedy should be discontinued, as it frequently aggravates the symptoms if longer continued.

Chlorate of potash is a remedy which does not sustain its former reputation in the treatment of these surfaces. It may be beneficially employed in acute conditions when there is not much swelling but great excess of mucous. It is of no benefit in the chronic form, while in the acute or chronic state where there is *ulceration*, it is very injurious; in every case of this kind which has come to my knowledge the last nine years it has resulted in injury to the diseased parts.

In cases of phagedenic ulceration, the sulphate of copper in solution of from xx to cxx grs. to the ounce of water has proved useful in promoting healthy granulations, but previous to its application with the brush or sponge, the ulcer and surrounding parts should be well cleansed by the spray of muriate of ammonia solution.

The foregoing is respectfully submitted from my personal observation and experience, which, if not as extensive as some others, is quite sufficient to demonstrate good results from the agents and methods advised.

THOS. F. RUMBOLD, M. D.

No. 1205 Washington Avenue.

VARIOLA.

We will refer to another disease and to that briefly. Variola you are aware has been epidemic at various places in the State, particularly at St. Louis during the past winter. The superior abilities and extended opportunities of the contributor of the following communication for personal observation, and trial of new remedies, have been such as to entitle his opinions to much weight.

Dr. Robert Burges, physician in charge of the Grand Avenue Small Pox Hospital, writes April 7th, 1873, as follows, in reply to my invitation for him to contribute his experience to this report: "Your letter of the 5th instant, inquiring as to what knowledge I have of progress being made in the treatment of small pox the past year or two has been received. In reply I can only say that the treatment of small pox is still symptomatic, not specific. While the greater part of my patients have been treated according to the symptoms presented, and according to the methods most approved among the profession, I have not failed when occasion presented to try the various so-called specifics, and have not yet found one that is deserving that title.

"The 'sulphate of zinc and digitalis' remedy is an unmitigated humbug both as a preventative and cure. Xylol does not accomplish what is claimed for it. The antiseptics, carbolic acid, sulphurous acid, and their various salts have all been tested and have betrayed the confidence which has been placed in them; though apparently acting well in some cases in others they have most miserably failed.

"My assistants have been enthusiastic in praise of the *hyposulphite of soda,* in forty grain doses every four hours, and not without cause, but I would desire to put it to further test before giving a positive opinion.

" There is, however one positive step which has been made in the treatment of small pox, and that is the application of a solution of the *silicate of soda* to the face, to prevent suppuration and pitting, when the application is thoroughly made for the first day or two of the eruption the pustules are aborted, and no pits remain. I have · seen a number of cases where the pustules on the face were aborted by this treatment, while those on the rest of the body went on to suppuration. We make the application with a camel's hair brush from one to six times a day, the object being to make and maintain a thick, glassy, impenetrable covering."

SANITARY REFORM.

All who have noticed the mortality reports in our large cities during the summer months must have observed how large the proportion of deaths were *children under five years,* and principally from *cholera infantum* ; heat, moisture and impure air being chief factors in the production of this infant mortality. It has been proposed by Dr. J. M. Toner, of Washington City, to establish camping grounds, or sanitariums, near our large cities as a resort during the summer months for the poor who have young children.

If one-fourth of the public attention bestowed upon criminal abortion and infanticide could be given to devising sanitary measures for the better preservation of infant life among the poor of our cities, many thousands of those who now perish annually might be reared to the credit and advantage of the nation and world. I would not say too much attention had been given to the *inhuman* practices referred to, but that too little attention has been bestowed upon the preservation of the lives of infants of *legitimate birth.* How fruitless all attempts to invigorate and maintain infant vitality in our large cities during the hot season our mortality reports demonstrate. It is not better doctoring or feeding that will save them, although these are bad enough the Lord knows. To *remove them* from the heat and foul air of our "tenant houses" is what is required, with the temperature outside night and day near 100° F. (for the reflected heat from walls and pavements keep up the heat at night) intensified by the heat within from a cooking stove in almost every room, with the impurities of the exhalations from the bodies of half a dozen persons, more or less, sleeping in the same room, leave but slight margin for struggling infancy. To expect infants under such circumstances to be "tided over the heated term" by doctoring and dieting, is the extreme of absurdity. What shall we do then—continue to swell this tide of infant mortality with the general increase of population? or adopt some plan of removing these people from their unhealthy city abodes during the summer months? The appreciation of human life throughout the civilized nations of the globe makes the latter a necessity. We only wait a practical feasible plan to accomplish the much desired and vitally important end. Dr. Toner has proposed the establishment of camping-grounds for temporary use near and accessible to our large cities. The details may be difficult, but by no means impossible. With regard to our city of St. Louis, we would suggest that if cheap temporary abodes·could be erected by the city or benevolent associations, on leased property now vacant at the outskirts of the city, high and airy, but within the corporate limits, to be subject to proper police regulation, and near enough to be reached by street car travel, so that the male supports of families could remain at home nights, we believe it would result in the saving of thousands of lives yearly who must otherwise perish as heretofore

In conclusion, we ask your indulgent attention to a few thoughts on the contagious disease ordinance now on trial in St. Louis, strictly as a measure of sanitary reform.

Every municipal, state, national and international association of physicians, or sanitary boards, agree in recommending quarantine as the safest and surest way to limit the spread of, and finally to eliminate, any contagious disease from any city or community.

Is there any good reason for making an exception of the contagious diseases pertaining to the social evil?

Is it a just and veritable objection that because *all*

prostitutes, men as well as women, are not alike subjected to examination ?

From a sanitary standpoint, is it possible for any one
in his senses to believe that the number of cases will be
increased or intensified by promptly removing one half
(if you please) of the sources or centres of contagion
from the community ?

If you could not quarantine every case of small-pox,
would that be a reason for doing nothing ?   Everybody
knows fresh cases are constantly coming into the city
from all quarters.   Is that any reason for abandoning
the Small-pox hospital and Quarantine?

And what of the inequality and injustice of the operation of this law we hear so much of, that it discrim-
inates to the prejudice of women, etc. ?   The variations of sex and circumstances are such that where one
case of disease is propagated by a diseased man, one
hundred are by a diseased woman ;   and in view of the
variation referred to, there is better reason to believe
these diseases originated primarily with women than
that sin did.   We have said it was exceptional where
disease was propagated by a *man* (being himself diseased) ; he *may* be the instrument, and doubtless sometimes is, of conveying the poison from a diseased woman to one in health, while he has not the disease himself.   Cases of this kind are on record, and have fallen
under the observation of many practitioners.   Again,
men suffering from primary disease are not prompted
as a rule to acts which are necessary to extend the
direase.   Also men more promptly and certainly seek
medical advice and treatment when first attacked, total
separation from females being imperatively enjoined by
the medical adviser at once and in all cases; least of all
are men incited thereto by pecuniary considerations as

women are; hence the fallacy of all this wordy objection of unjust discrimination against women.

But we are told the friends of quarantine (for that is all the present law amounts to) have failed to furnish the figures to demonstrate the sanitary benefit of the law; that, so far as appears, there are as many cases of disease as formerly.

Without record or enumeration of the cases in the city prior to the enactment of the law, how is it possible at this early day to institute a comparison in *figures*, particularly as St. Louis is a city in the midst of this continent, with population flowing in upon it from all parts of the globe. The only testimony possible in the circumstances is that of the physicians who see and treat this class of diseases, and that is decidedly to the effect that there are less cases of disease, that they see less of it by one-half, notwithstanding the influx of population and the numerous cases which come from the surrounding country for treatment. Many good people seem to be under an apprehension that, notwithstanding the law may be a good thing as a sanitary measure, in the same ratio moral degradation is increased. They cannot disabuse their minds of the superstition that the disease is a curse upon the evil practice, and not a consequence simply. Yet they must admit a grosser insult cannot be offered to a good citizen than to intimate that his virtue is due to his fear of the penalty of violated law.

We have thus attempted to embody a *few* of the recent advances in the science of medicine, and our thanks are especially due and hereby gracefully tendered to the gentlemen who have (on so short notice), contributed so largely to this report.

WM. S. EDGAR, M. D., *Chairman.*

STATISTICAL REPORT OF TWO HUNDRED AND FIFTY FIVE CASES OF DISEASES OF THE EAR.

By H. N. Spencer, M. D., St. Louis.

It has been urged against the prosecution by individuals of special departments of medicine to the exclusion in practice of everything else that the tendency is to indifference to advances which are made in other special departments than one's own, and the consequent fruits of that—the failure to appreciate oftentimes organic connections at the base of which may lie the origin of a disease.

When this observation has been confirmed, when the test has been made in the crucible of years and the final decision is against us, it will be time to consider if this even affords a sufficient argument for the abolition of such practices at the sacrifice of what is likely to accrue from the assiduous and persistent efforts, and the accumulative experience of one man engaged day after day, and year after year, upon one subject of investigation and thought. But it does not occur to us how it is possible that such a result of such labors should obtain; co-laborers in the same great vineyard of science, co-workers for the good of humanity, we are moved to regard with interest the progress others are making. But on a more important, if not on a morally higher, than a *philanthropic* ground the work of every one is *essential* to every other. The specialist if he be a true man of science, cannot in the very nature of things neglect to use every collateral aid to an understanding of his subject. He is more apt than another to discover whatever lays desecrating hand upon the object of his love, and it will be within his reach more readily to discover fallacious references.

Our science is of such nature that to understand one part involves a knowledge of the whole. The gynæcologist cannot say to the psychologist " I have no need of thee." This intimate relation of one part to the whole, and the influence which is exerted by one part in a disordered state upon every other, makes it incumbent upon every specialist striving for a good understanding of the truth to be a *whole physician.*

A plain sequence of the foregoing statements: it is the duty of every one so engaged to let the result of such special labors be known from time to time. This is but discharging indeed an obligation which every physician owes to the profession at large. And a second deduction to be urged is this—that hereafter the general ·practitioner or the physician engaged in some other special department of medicine (by selecting a case I shall make a practical illustration of my meaning), in the broad light of these results and the facts which have been elicited in the developement of them, becomes culpable, inexcusably culpable, who, shrinking from the responsibility of treatment in a case where he is confessedly ignorant, and ignorant, *it is to be hoped,* of the consequences that may ensue, tells an alarmed and anxious parent making solicitous inquiry that his child suffers only from an *otorrhœa* (which word he pronounces with due gravity) and that he will *outgrow it.* Mr. President and gentlemen, that physician can *never* outgrow the terrible reprehension which that case stamps as a blot and a reproach upon his professional escutcheon, and his accountability is measured in every instance by the degree of inconvenience or absolute loss

his advice has occasioned; he has violated a trust he
had assumed in the presence of men and before God.
It is his duty to know or to confess his ignorance. He
should be so far informed at least as to be able to read
the probable results of a diseased process. It has been
but a short time since I sat by the death bed side of a
patient who had been lulled into a feeling of security
by a such character of advice. Her otitis media purulenta culminated in an intercranial inflammation, and
this the result. I cannot envy her adviser his feelings.

Actuated purely by such motives as these preliminary remarks imply, I give the subjoined report, laying
stress as occasion allows on the connection of the ear
in its varying pathological conditions to other structures adjacent or remote.

I have had occurring to me in my private practice,
from the time of a last similar report to this one, (from
1st December, 1871, to 1st December, 1872,) embracing
a period of twelve months, two hundred and fifty-five
cases of diseases of the ear. They have been distributed as
follows—of the external ear fifty, of the middle ear
one hundred and ninety-eight, of the internal ear seven.
It will be remarked how large a proportion are classed
under the head of middle ear diseases, and how very
few are designated as affections of the internal ear or
labyrinth. This is not the proportion as diseases of
the ear absolutely exist, but does not vary essentially
from the usual proportion in practice, excluding from
statistics those belonging to institutions for the deaf
and dumb. Under any and all circumstances the
affections of the middle ear are greatly in excess of
either the external or internal ear, or both combined,
and we shall see the reason, if it is not already patent
to every one.

I shall pass over the first division of our subject—the diseases of the external meatus—under which head are classed furuncular inflammation, eczematous eruptions, inspissated cerumen, and foreign bodies, to consider the more important division of the middle ear. The diseases to which the tympanic cavern is liable are of inflammatory nature, whether of traumatic or idiopathic. origin. It is convenient to designate them as acute and chronic, and for the present we shall say they are inflammations of catarrhal or purulent nature.

I shall take it for granted that it is known how readily acute affections of the middle ear are recovered from where the proper means are instituted to that end, and it is my purpose to call attention more especially to those affections which, having for a long time existed, have involved beyond the superficial structure and have wrought changes upon which the impaired hearing is more dependent even than upon the diseased condition itself in whatever stage, and frequently the loss of function is more than seems to be warranted by the measure of extension of the disease.

The *otitis media purulenta chronica,* the chronic supurative inflammation of the middle ear, exists in a variety of forms in its objective appearances, and in its subjective manifestations, attended quite universally with greater or less destruction of the membrana tympani, and from being localized to including the whole tympanic cavern. *These* are the cases of *otorrhæa* which *some* would let alone. Patients are not usually left to outgrow a corneal ulcer or a necrosis of the inferior maxilla; there is no indication for granting greater privilege here, or taking advantage of your license: it is an insidious enemy that in an unsuspected

moment may lay violent hand upon the subject of your
confidence and crush it. I believe it would be a safe
assertion to make, that more inter-cranial complications
result from a neglected ulcerative process in the cavity
of the tympanum than there are ear complications arising
from meningeal inflammation, which it is known, in this
section are of frequent occurrence, to the sad experiences of many of you. It may not be known how frequently deaths have occurred in these cases where a
correct diagnosis has been made out, but the physician
has been innocent of any knowledge whatever as regards the exciting cause. But the outlook for the
future is more hopeful than the retrospect is pleasing to
contemplate, and from the advanced state of our
knowledge, and the now general diffusion of it, we can
confidently asseverate that there will be hereafter fewer
untoward results from chronic purulent processes affecting the middle ear. They are not any longer being
called *simple otorrhœæ*, for an otorrhœa of any character is recognized as indicating a complicated state of
things and of grave import.

Referring to the table we find out of fifty-four cases
of otitis media purulenta chronica these results were
obtained : Six were cured (*i. e.*, there was restoration of
the deficient membrane and the hearing was restored to
a normal condition); thirty-six were improved (in
these cases the ulceration was entirely healed and the
hearing power much and permanently amended) ; six
unimproved; four unknown, and two died.

In the treatment of these cases we have obtained a
great advantage when a good patency of the Eustachian
tube has been established, fluids are made to pass readily through into the naso-pharynx, insuring greater

cleanliness and frequently removing a lurking obstacle in the way of improvement.

In the cases which indicate its use at all, I have received better results than from other means heretofore employed from using strong solutions of nitrate of silver, 240-480 grains to one ounce, in alternation with the milder astringent solutions, at the head of which, I feel disposed to place the sulphate of zinc. The sulpho-carbolate of zinc may be used where there is a fetid discharge. A natural consequence of the long continuance of this suppurative process is a depleted blood, and a judiciously chosen general treatment is of efficient aid.

We come to consider next in order a more interesting class of inflammations of the tympanic cavity, the *non-suppurative*—the *otitis media catarrhalis chronica* according to the German nomenclature. Dr. D. B. St. John Roosa, who has probably done more than any other in this country to inspire an interest in this department of medicine, and has done much for its advancement, gives a better definition in my mind and a better nomenclature for this class of diseases than we have had heretofore. Roosa says, " I have never been fully satisfied with the nomenclature of Von Tröltsch—vast improvement as it was on those classifications which had preceded it. Some of them were crude, others fanciful and altogether too refined. Von Tröltsch classified all non-suppurative diseases as catarrhal, and then separated those in which the catarrhal symptoms, excess of secretion, was not very marked, by placing them under the head of sclerosis, or hardening or rigidity of the mucous membrane. After looking at many ears in which there was no trace either in the pharnyx, Eustachian tube, or cavity of the tympanum, of an excess of secretion from the mucous membrane, but in which there were marked changes in the way of increase, hypertrophy or proliferation of tissue, I felt that aural catarrh was a meagre and incorrect name with which to describe such a state of things.   The very name of catarrh as applied to a sunken drum-head, immovable chain of bones, dry phanryx, easily permeable Eustachian tube, is repugnant to all our notions of scientific nomenclature." *   Roosa then divides the chronic non-suppurative inflammations of the middle ear into two great classes :—"catarrhal and proliferous." Upon this subject I cannot refrain from giving you these further observations of Dr. Roosa, because they are so eminently practical and satisfactory.   " Some authors and practitioners would admit another classification, based upon the parts involved, and speak of chronic myringitis, or chronic inflammation of the membrana tympani, and of chronic catarrh of the Eustachian tube. Whatever we may believe of *acute* inflammation of these parts, I can scarcely accept the idea of one that has existed for any considerable space of time without involving either the cavity of the tympanum or the mastoid cells, or both.   The nomenclature tubal catarrh leads, as I believe, to incorrect notions as to the therapeutic value ᐟof the Eustachian catheter and of Politzer's method of inflating the drum cavity.   These methods of ᐟtreatment are useful not so much for what they do to the tube, but for their effect upon the cavities into which it opens when air-bubbles are crackling in the cavity of the tympanum, as in catarrhal inflammation,

* From a paper read before the New York State Medical Society, 1872.

or when the tube is greatly narrowed by the hypertrophy of its lining membrane, but at the same time we
have as we always do in the latter case, a sunken drum-
head, altered light spot, signs of proliferous inflammation of many of the structures making up the
middle ear. I do not see how we can with propriety
speak of a tubal affection even if its symptoms are predominant, and even if treatment of and through the
lining membrane of the tube does place things in such
a condition that nature will complete the cure. No
time need be spent upon this question, which may perhaps seem to some a comparatively unimportant one,
had not incorrect notions in the past led to an incorrect
treatment. In former times the membrana tympani, under the assumption that such an affection as an independent chronic myringitis existed, was vigorously treated
by instillation of various fluids and by perforation,
and of late under the idea that we have a great deal of
tubal catarrh without further progress in the morbid
action, undue stress is sometimes laid upon application
to the mouth of the tube. Politzer's method is substituted for the catheter when its true place, valuable
and indispensable as it is, except in the case of very
young children, is an adjuvant to that instrument."*
It is not our purpose to enter into details of symptoms—
either to describe the appearances or subjective phenomena—they are obtainable from any of the late
works on aural surgery.

I would preface a consideration of results of treatment with saying that we have here, *ex concesso*, the
ground of scepticism for those who libel the practice of
aural surgery.

*Idem.　　　29

At the first blush the results obtained may seem as
very inadequate, and the more especially if called to
consider the weeks and months of patient treatment
employed in almost every instance where treatment was
pursued at all, and they may be considered excusable
who despair laboring in such a field.   But when we consider the relentless nature of the enemy disease we have
here to meet and cope with—and reflect that as has
been said "a person with this variety of aural disease
may have the best general treatment the world affords,
and be under the most appropriate hygienic conditions ;
he may live in a climate like that of Nice, Mentone,
Naples, or St. Augustine, and then he will not recover
from his aural disease.   *Nay, more,* he will continue to
grow *slowly but gradually worse* if his pharynx, Eustachian tubes, and middle ear are not treated by the appropriate appliances and remedies."*   It is this statement
of the case which encourages us, and we are *comforted*
by our *improved* cases which we have been able to save
from this impending fate, for our improved cases are
cured except in the restoration of ability to the parts to
perform their natural function.

To be considered among the influences modifying
treatment in this variety of affection, are prominently
naso-pharyngeal complications, which exist as a rule,
specific infection and affections of the labyrinth and of
the auditory nerve.   The naso-pharyngeal complication is placed chief, for the uniformity of its presence
and the plague of its persistence, and when success in
treatment depends much upon the removal of this em-
barrassment, in this climate, in a manufacturing city
using the character of coal peculiar to this region, and

* Dr. Roosa.

where in addition limestone dust is as free as air, it cannot be surprising that better results have not been attained. The ear affection involved with one of the other conditions requires a local treatment at the same time that the complicating circumstances must have most earnest attention. (For results of treatment see Table.)

Under the third head of internal ear diseases and affections of the auditory nerve, (which I have chosen to put in one class in order to simplifying the subject,) I desire to refer but briefly to those cases of deafness where the impairment of hearing is traceable as a consequence upon cerebro-spinal meningitis. Within the time covered by this report, I had six of these cases coming under my observation. In every instance the diagnosis was clearly made out, though in one case the mother of the child was satisfied upon the authority of her family physician (a homœopath) that typhoid fever had been the ravager. I elicited from her such symptoms as these: There was in the beginning a headache, followed by vomiting and convulsions, *predominant opisthotonos*, unconsciousness and delirium, and when the child came to my office, three weeks after her recovery, there was an unsteadiness to be observed in her gait, with a tendency to fall sideways. I felt warranted in adding this, when I had also taken into account the nature of her ear disease as I found it, to the number of cases of deafness consequent upon a meningeal inflammation. In these cases the deafness was of the highest degree and bi-lateral. The ear affection in cerebro-spinal meningitis is not always of this extreme character. One side may be more seriously affected than the other, and the degree of hearing lost is variable. The complete loss of hearing is the rule to which these diverse conditions are the exceptions. It is the rule again for the ear complication to occur when the disease is at its acme, but to this also there is exception. Knapp says in a paper given to the *Medical Record* (August 15, 1872)," I find in my notes some cases in which hearing was still present some weeks after the disappearance of the severe symptoms, and was lost during the recovery."

Knapp, who claims to have had opportunities for observation, describes the appearance and manifestations of disease as referring to the ear, thus: "In the early stages, hyperæmia of the middle ear is commonly present, the drumhead being dull yellowish, the region of the handle and upper portion red, and the light spot faint, smaller or absent. The pharynx is generally red. The tympanum is inflatable with a rough blowing sound, after which the appearance of the membrana tympani is not essentially changed. In very rare cases only the affection rises beyond this condition of a mild acute otitis media, developing in purulent inflammation of the drum with perforation of the drumhead and otorrhœa, which ceases in one or several weeks." I give these observations of Dr. Knapp for the opportunity has not been afforded me as yet of seeing the cases in this stage, and I find nothing on the subject searching the authorities which are available to me. An objective examination later reveals nothing. In four of the six cases that have come under my observation there was little or nothing in the appearance of the membrana tympani, or in the condition of the tube, or the middle ear, as we ordinarily interpret its condition, that was abnormal. In the two remaining cases there was nothing to be discovered to which could be referred this high degree of deafness. There was opacity of the membrane with slight retraction of the handle, and a consequent change from the normal appearance of the light spot, but the tubes were pervious to Valsalva's method, a condition referable beyond doubt to a disease preceding this present affliction.

I am asked, what is the nature of this ear disease and where its seat? It should be as readily diagnosticated from the ear affection which follows upon typhoid fever, as the diseases which have originated them are distinguisable from one another. Indeed more so. If there are symptoms in common between these affections that in one stage of the disease might lead to confusion, here there is nothing in common. The ear complication growing out of the exanthematous diseases is one of the middle ear, which, however seriously affected, never gives rise to so extreme impairment of hearing as this. In one case we have a disease of the middle ear with pharyngeal complication; in the other we find a deeper seated and graver affection. In one case the conducting apparatus is involved; in the other the sensory nerve upon which hearing depends.

Dr. Knapp states that the disease is a purulent inflammation of the labyrinth, and in confirmation of this, refers to post-mortem examinations which have been made by Lucae and others. I regret that he did not make more definite reference by which his authorities could be consulted. He also fails to state upon what data his own opinion has been based. I have been unable to find any sufficient evidence for sustaining me in the belief that this affection arising from cerebro-spinal meningitis is of this nature at all. The membranes at the base of the brain come in contact with the nerve going to supply the ear and may become involved at this seat with the disease of whatever nature it is: or an effusion taking place and afterwards contracting would occasion such a constriction upon the nerve as would paralyze its functions. This might be the explanation in Knapp's cases where the deafness came on after recovery, and there might be a possibility of restoration of the lost function, recovery occurring with absorption. From purulent inflammation of the labyrinth there could be no recovery, no more than from the purulent choroiditis, having originated under like circumstances, there would be, of course, in each case a destruction of the membranes.

255 CASES OF DISEASES OF THE EAR SEEN IN PRIVATE PRACTICE.

	Cured.	Improved.	Unimproved.	Unknown.	Died.	Total.
EXTERNAL EAR.						
Furuncular Inflammation...........................	9	...	...	...	...	9
Eczema..........	6	...	...	...	...	6
Inspissated Cerumen....................../........	30	...	...	...	...	30
Foreign bodies..........	5	...	...	...	...	5
MIDDLE EAR.						
Otitis Media Purulenta, Acute......................	29	...	...	...	...	29
" " " Chronic................	6	36	6	4	2	54
" " Catarrhalis, Acute................	12	...	...	...	...	12
" " " Chronic............	8	38	33	6	...	85
" " " "Proliferous".......................		2	7	9	...	18
INTERNAL EAR.						
Primary Disease of Labyrinth......................	...	...	...	1	...	1
Total deafness from Cerebro-Spinal Meningitis..	...	...	...	6	...	6
	105	76	46	26	2	255

1615 Washington Avenue.

LARYNGEAL SURGERY.

By W. C. GLASGOW, M.'D., St. Louis.

Prior to the invention of the laryngoscope laryngeal operations held an obscure place in the annals of surgery. They may well be said to have had no existence, if we except those performed by external incision or division of the thyroid cartilage, the thyro-hyoid, and thyro-cricoid membranes. The extraction of foreign bodies has been successfully accomplished both before and since that time without the aid of the laryngeal mirror ; but as the position of the body is unknown, a great deal of suffering and often danger results from the blind introduction of the forceps or the probang.

Cases have been reported of growths removed from the epiglottis and interior of the larynx, but they are with few exceptions very problematical. In those well authenticated cases reported by Rignoli, Horace Green, and Sir Ashley Cooper, the tumors were of large size, and plainly visible from the mouth.

The variety of tumors on the epiglottis must be the reason why so few cases have been recorded, for the number of persons is quite large in whom, with a properly shaped tongue depressor, not only the top of the epiglottis, but the greater portion of it may be brought in view.

The honor of having invented the laryngoscope has been warmly contested by different men : Babington in the year 1829, Warden in 1844, Garcini in 1855, and Türck in 1857, all claim to be its originators, but it is undoubtedly to the inventive genius of Türck and the practical adaptation of his ideas by Czermak that a revolution in this branch of surgery has been rendered possible, and laryngoscopic operations taken their place amongst the most delicate and satisfactory efforts in surgery. Since that time, the number of operators skilled in the use of the laryngoscope has steadily increased, until at the present time, with the improved instruments now in use, a foreign body or a growth may be removed with the same facility from the larynx, as a body impacted in the eye, or a polypus from the middle ear.

The essential requirements for a laryngoscopic examination are a concave mirror attached to the forehead, and a small round plane mirror to be introduced into the posterior pharyngeal space—which must be previously warmed to prevent condensation of the breath and a cloudiness of the mirror. For the purposes of illumination any kind of light can be used—from the simple tallow candle to the light of the sun,—the most convenient and most available at all times is the common illuminating gas used with an original burner, a large sized burner using coal oil also answers all requirements. The magnesium light has been used, but aside from its cost and the complexity of apparatus necessary for its production, it offers no advantage over sunlight, indeed, it presents some disadvantages, for the brilliancy of the light often dazzles the eye of the operator in a critical moment.

Many contrivances for illuminating have been lately introduced, but they are entirely useless and unnessary ; they serve at most the purposes of ignorance and charlatanism, serving to inspire awe in the minds of patients and concealing to a degree the lack of knowledge under the mask of a multiplicity of mechanical contrivances. The same may be said of the innumerable modifications of the laryngeal mirror, for to-day, the simple round mirror as used by Türck answers every requirement of a laryngoscopic examination or operation.

Although the laryngoscope has given us the power of bringing the offending body directly into view, still there are many difficulties peculiar to this special branch of surgery. The peculiar function and position of the parts affected, the important relations they bear to the function of respiration, each renders operations difficult and at times impossible.

An essential feature is the absolute necessity of proper co-operation of the patient with the operator, hence, extreme youth and feebleness, or want of self-control renders them impracticable. Excessive sensibility of the pharyngeal or laryngeal mucous membrane, a large thick tongue, great hypertrophy of the tonsils, and a pendant epiglottis, each presents its peculiar difficulties.

The sensibility of the pharynx may be diminished by local applications, a strong solution of bromide of ammonium used as a gargle often serving to reduce it. The same end is accomplished by the oft repeated introduction of the mirror, the mucous membrane soon becoming, as it were, accustomed to its presence; very often a slight congestion or catarrh of the pharynx produces a degree of hyperæsthesia of the parts, and it is only after this morbid condition has been allayed that an examination is practicable. The obstacle to success however lies oftener with the operator than the patient, and is due to an unskillful handling of the mirror, for it is only in very rare cases that an examination may not be made at first sitting. Should the tonsils be so much enlarged as seriously to interfere, they must previously be removed. A pendant epiglottis can be raised by making the patient intone vowels *a* and *e*—should this not suffice, proper instruments must be used to elevate it. To reduce the sensitiveness of the larynx the laryngeal sound should be repeatedly introduced, and when this is too tedious or ineffectual, local anæsthesia may be applied. This consists in the introduction into the interior of the larynx of a strong solution of morphia, a somewhat dangerous procedure as the constitutional effects of the drug take place long before the local anæsthesia becomes evident. On account of the difficulties and tediousness of inter-laryngeal operations, it has been proposed by some to replace them by the extra-laryngeal, especially the operation of thyrotomy or division of the thyroid cartilage. This is almost always unwarrantable and in the majority of cases totally unjustifiable. Of all the cases reported, which have come to my knowledge, in which an effort at extirpation was demanded, but very few could not have been operated upon through the fauces, either alone or after having been preceded by tracheotomy, neither operation, nor both combined being as dangerous as thyrotomy.

Inter-laryngeal operations are as a rule devoid of danger, as far as this can be said of any surgical operation, given of course, a proper experience, a dexterity in the handling of instruments—such experience is absolutely essential, for we have not here as in other branches of surgery, a free view of the parts to be excised, but the cutting must be done and the hand guided solely by the reflected view we obtain in the laryngeal mirror, and it requires considerable practice to discriminate justly and accurately the distances to be traversed by the instrument. The first touch of the instrument causes spasmodic contraction of the parts, so that the least mistake, especially with cutting instruments, may cause serious and perhaps irremediable danger. Tracheotomy is performed now daily with the happiest results. The same cannot be said of thyrotomy, for even in the most favorable cases aphonia, or a permanent hoarseness, often perichondritis and trachitis come. In condemning thyrotomy, I am sustained by the most eminent laryngoscopists of the present and past time. Morell Mc-Kensie, of London, uses very forcible language when he says in his work "Growths in the Larynx," page 86: "It may be stated as a cardinal law that an extra-laryngeal method ought never to be adopted, even when laryngoscopic treatment can not be pursued, unless there be danger to life from suffocation or dysphagia. Direct incision into any part of the air-passage is always attended with both immediate and remote danger to life, the amount of risk being dependent on the situation of the opening, and the mode in which the treatment is carried out. The existence of dysphonia does not justify operations, which though easy to perform, may be regarded as 'capital.' Hence an extra-laryngeal operation is not justifiable for the removal of a *small* growth in the larynx unless that growth give rise to dangerous dyspnea and cannot be removed by a less serious method—an external operation, when laryngoscopic treatment could be ultimately successful, is not less reprehensible than to perform lithotomy in a case of calculus in which lithotrity could be effected, or to amputate a limb where resection could be accomplished." The two great conditions requiring the use of instruments in the larynx are, the removal of foreign bodies and the extirpation of growths, although we might well include under this head the opening of abcesses, the scarification of œdematous swellings, and the local application of medicaments to the parts in all cases of laryngeal disease, for in the present state of laryngeal therapeutics, the direct contact of the medicament to the effected part constitutes the greater part of the treatment. In a large number of cases in which a foreign body has been swallowed, it is forced by the deep inspiration which the person takes in his anxiety and fright at the moment of swallowing into the interior of the larynx—rarely, however, does it pass at once below the vocal cords—for the moment it impinges upon any portion of the larynx or even the epiglottis, then follows a spasmodic contraction of the thyro-arytenoid muscles or false cords, and the entrance to the trachea is closed, it is only subsequently, when the glottis is distended through some cause, that it falls below it. Experience shows that there are certain portions of the larynx in which bodies are most commonly found lodged. Small, light bodies, like pins and small fish-bones, are often caught on the anterior surface top of the epiglottis, and becoming entangled in the mucus remain fixed in this position, causing little distress. They are often found in the hyoid fossa, or space external to the ary-epiglottidean fold; if they are of hard consistence they may remain here an indefinite time without danger, except it may be from subsequent swelling of the parts. Should the body succeed in passing into the larynx, the fossa innominata, or space between the false cords and the ary-epiglottidean fold, often receives it. These are the class of cases in which the result depends a great deal upon the judgment of the practitioner. Should he, as is too often done, introduce his probang and force it down the œsophagus, he takes the best possible means to dislodge the body, but to dislodge it only to have it fall into the trachea, for in the effort of introducing the probang the patient gaps, and taking a full inspiration, throws open the glottis to its fullest extent, and the body falls below it; the introduction of the forceps or the action of an emetic may cause the same disastrous result.

The result of this class of cases proves conclusively the necessity of a laryngoscopic examination in all cases of foreign bodies supposed to have entered the air-passages, as there is no impediment to respiration in this class of cases, and the impossibility of determining from the sensations of the patient whether the body is lodged in the superior portion of the œsophagus, or one of the fossæ of the larynx; an examination should be made in all cases of foreign bodies lodged in the throat, if he would certainly preclude an unfavorable result. Should the body become lodged in the ventricle or pocket between the true and false cords, the diagnosis may be made at once, for with the sudden and great dyspnea and cough, the patient becomes at once aphonic. It is remarkable how large a body may be embedded here and still a considerable amount of respiration continued. The cough is not excessive as a rule, but of a croupal character and the pain is slight. I call to mind a case in the practice of Dr. Gregory, seen last fall in which a large sized cockle-burr found lodgment in the ventricle, and after tracheotomy had been performed, was extracted through the fauces. Bodies having entered the trachea, unless they are large enough to become fixed between its walls, generally fall into the right bronchus, which is explained by the statement of Goodnell that the septum of the bronchial tubes lies somewhat to the left of the median line.   Sudden and violent attacks of dyspnea and cough occurring in paroxysms give the greatest cause for uneasiness, and the great danger lies in the possibility of the body becoming fixed in the glottis during the violent efforts of expiration.

In a certain number of cases they may be recognized and extracted by means of the laryngeal mirror, but there is always more or less danger of spasm of the glottis.   As in many persons a clear view may be obtained to the bifurcation of the trachea, a questionable diagnosis could thus be rendered certain.

If the laryngoscope has proved an invaluable instrument for the extraction of foreign bodies, it has shown its greatest triumph in the power given us for the removal of growths blocking up the air-passages and impeding respiration.

Tumors of the larynx are of frequent occurrence, their diagnosis, however, is quite rare, owing to the fact that comparatively few physicians are acquainted with the use of the laryngeal mirror.   The subjective symptoms to which they give rise are, except in marked cases, of such a nature as not to enable us to make a diagnosis, and it is only through inspection by the laryngeal mirror that they are discovered.   Some give rise to no symptoms except a slight and persistent hoarseness. In others there is a complete aphonia with more or less dyspnea and cough, the symptoms varying according to the size of the growth and its position in the larnyx, a tumor situated on or between the true cords always produces more or less loss of voice, it serving to interfere with the vibrations necessary for the production of the tone of the voice. If it is situated on the epiglottis or lateral portions of the larynx, the sensation of a foreign body is produced or it may interfere with deglutition. Cough, when present, is of the dry, hacking character similar to the cough of incipient phthisis, although if the growth is large it becomes croupal.

Laryngeal tumors may be conveniently divided according to their character into benign, malignant and specific—under benign we understand those which having been thoroughly removed show no tendency to return, the great majority, not only of this class but of all other growths, are the papillomatæ, or warty growths, consisting essentially of a hypertrophy of the normal papillæ. These are generally multiple and their usual site is the true vocal cords, although they also occur in the other portions of the larynx—they present a villous, velvety appearance, and vary in size from a pin's head to a hickory nut. The fibrous or fibrocellular growths occur next more frequently, and more rarely we find the cysts, the myxomata and the glandular tumors.

The papillomatæ are readily removed, being quite soft and friable, and tearing away readily in the grasp of the forceps, sometimes they contain more or less fibrous tissue, and the use of cutting instruments is required. In a certain number of cases they show a disposition to return, especially when their bases have not been thoroughly eradicated. A case which I operated upon, one year ago last August, (reported in the August number (1872) of the St. Louis Medical and Surgical Journal) in which several tumors the size of a hazelnut were removed from the true cords, returned, and a second operation was necessary in the following March. The second operation proved decisive, and there is at the present time not the slightest trace of the neoplasm—previous to the operation the patient suffered with great dyspnea and was completly aphonic, at the present time the only thing perceptible is a slight deepening in the tone of the voice.

Fibrous tumors are generally small and situated in the true vocal cords, they are of slow growth and often present no symptom except aphonia. There is always a question of the propriety of an operation in these cases where there is no interference with respiration, and when the loss of voice does not seriously interfere with the business and well-doing of the patient. Cutting instruments and powerful escharotics are the means employed for their removal.

The malignant growths include the carcinomata, they invade all portions of the larynx, varying in size, from the small epithelial growth to the medullary cancer covering the greater portion of the larynx, and extending into the trachea, the œsophagus and up into the pharynx. The characteristic symptom is great pain, often radiating up into the ears, and the difficulty of swallowing ; they finally ulcerate causing vast destruction of the tissues. The only treatment justifiable is the local application of morphine, or a mild astringent which serves to deaden the pain, and to render the taking of nourishment more practicable. Excrescences or condylomata occur in the early stages of syphilis as well as the gummy tumors in the later stages. They can be recognized by their general appearance and the readiness with which they disappear under constitutional treatment. The rugged ulcerations of phthisis often present the form of excrescences and have the appearance of tumors, they generally appear late in the disease, when the diagnosis may be readily made. The aphonia of the latter stages of phthisis is often the result of this condition, although this must not be mistaken for the paralysis of the cords arising from a loss of force in the nerves of the larynx, or ulceration and destruction of the arytenoid cartilages.

My object in presenting this paper to the Association is to make evident to you how absolutely essential the knowledge of the use of the laryngoscope is to every practitionei. It is not to be expected that every one can become a skillful laryngoscopist, but a certain amount of knowledge can be readily acquired such as will help all to recognize morbid conditions of the larynx, and in many cases to give the patient the benefit of appropriate treatment.

Let us hope that with the present advancement being made in medical education, that the time is past when every disease of the throat shall be ascribed to some mysterious disease of the tonsils, which organ seems in general estimation to bear the same relation to throat disease, as formerly the liver held in obscure diseases of the general system ; and then we shall not hear of so many persons being condemned to death through the oracularly spoken word " consumption " who are simply suffering from chronic laryngitis ; or of persons being compelled to remain year after year in a state of aphonia, cut off from one of the greatest of God's gifts, when the removal of a growth or the stimulation of the nervous apparatus of the parts would at once restore them to health and happiness. (*Trans.M.S.M.A.*)

Reviews and Bibliographical Notices.

HALF-HOUR RECREATIONS IN POPULAR SCIENCE. Dana Estes, Editor. Part 6. *Unconscious Action of the Brain and Epidemic Delusions.* By Dr. W. B. Carpenter, F. R. S. Boston: Estes & Lauriat.

This lecture is one of a series, by eminent men in science, published in Boston by Estes & Lauriat. The name of the writer, Dr. Carpenter, author of "Human Physiology," is sufficient to bespeak for the lecture a careful reading. We are of the opinion that there is too much of the solidity of fact and of truth in the lecture for it to be very popular at this time; but the advice is so judicious, and there is so much set forth which people do know, from which conclusions are drawn, that the attentive reader must be at once entertained and instructed. We are told that the *unconscious action of the brain*—"unconscious cerebration"—is largely dependent in its productions or results upon the previous discipline and action of the mind, not merely in acquiring a knowledge of facts, but in considering those facts for the purpose of arriving at a correct conclusion as to the *true* and the *good*. He speaks much of *common sense*, of which he says, page 217 : "We fall back upon this, that common sense is, so to speak, the general resultant of the whole previous action of our minds." Again, after hearing evidence on both sides of a question, a mind which has been properly trained will, if left to itself, be most likely to arrive at a correct conclusion. "And this conclusion will be the resultant of the whole previous training and discipline of our minds."

This lecture, which was delivered in Manchester, England, December 1, 1871, is full of correct principles.

The second lecture, delivered by Dr. Carpenter, one week later, at the same place, is on *Epidemic Delusions.*

The terms may be accepted as meaning simply "a delusion which affects the popular minds." He speaks first of states of mind in the individual, and then of those which affect a number of persons or almost a community. Cases are referred to of the *flagellants* of the thirteenth century who, under the idea that the world was coming to an end, went about with banners and music, with scourges and at given signals partly stripped and beat themselves or one another; also, the dancing mania, fortune telling, witchcraft, as in New England in its early settlement, mesmerism, spiritualism, table-turners and table-rappers. The author accounts for the existence of such strange belief in such strange things, by the previous possession of the mind in some cases, and our earnest desire for communications supernatural in their nature. It is generally the ignorant who readily embrace such nonsense, because of the abnegation of their common sense, or because "the resultant of the whole previous training and discipline" is so weak as to be overborn by a morbid curiosity.

These lectures should be distributed among, and read by all classes.

HANDBOOK FOR THE PHYSIOLOGICAL LABORATORY. By E. Klein, M.D., Assistant Professor in the Pathological Laboratory of the Brown Institution, London, etc.; J. Burdon-Sanderson, M. D., F. R. S , Prof. of Practical Physiology in University College, London; Michael Foster, M. A. M. D., F. R. S., Prælector of Physiology in Trinity College, Cambridge; and T. Lauder Brunton, M. D., D. Sc., Lecturer on Materia Medica, in the Medical College of St. Bartholomew's Hospital, London. Edited by J. Burdon-Sanderson. In two volumes, with one hundred and thirty-three plates, containing three hundred and fifty-three illustrations. Vol. I,—text, pp 585, 8vo.; vol. II—plates.
[For Sale by the St Louis Book & News Co.]

In considering and estimating the work before us we must not loose sight of the object of the work, viz: a guide for the *Laboratory.* We could have wished the work had been more after the plan of "Hassall's Microscopic Anatomy;" but that could not have been accomplished, and the present object fulfilled, without greatly increasing the size of the volumes.

The *text* is divided into suitable chapters and sections, but the references to the plates are infrequent, indeed the deficiency in this regard is, for the student, very unfortunate. As an example in the text, page 38, figure 7 a and 7 b are referred to while the number of the plate is not mentioned. They are found, however, in a plate with Fig. 25. So with Fig. 15, found with Fig. 64, no reference in the text to the number of the plate, which is xxvi.

Histology, by Dr. Klein, is divided into *two parts* : Blood corpuscles, and tissues ; and compound tissues and organs.

Physiology into three parts : I. *Blood circulation, respiration, and animal heat*, by Dr. Burdon-Sanderson; II. *Functions of muscle and nerve*, by Dr. Foster, *digestion* and *secretion* by Dr. Brunton.

It is intended to give the method of demonstrating in each of the propositions set forth.

Concerning the "varieties of colorless corpuscles," Dr. Klein speaks, page 18, of three forms of colorless corpuscles which "differ from one another both in size and aspect, and in their property of spontaneous movement."

1. *Common large colorless corpuscles.*

2. *Granular corpuscles.*

3. *Colorless corpuscles of the third form :* (a) small well defined bodies, resembling nuclei, which retain only a very short time the spheroidal form which they had at first ; (b) large corpuscles, consisting of finely granular protoplasm, with jagged outline, containing three or four distinct nuclei, which may be either roundish, or flattened against each other, exhibit a double contour, and contain a few fine nucleoli which are relatively of a large size, so much so, that they often appear to be surrounded by a narrow zone of protoplasm ; (c) large masses of finely granular protoplasm, which commonly are of irregular form, and inclose bodies similar to the nuclei above described, varying in number from five to twenty in each mass.*

Zooids and Œcoids : In speaking, page 30, of the action of *boracic acid* on a salt solution of blood, especialy that of the newt, as serving to illustrate the intimate structure of the colored blood disk, he says, a two per cent solution of this acid does not differ, in its action on the colorless corpuscles, in general from other weak acids. "If however, a salt preparation of newt's blood, in which the colored corpuscles have already sunk, is irrigated with the solution in question, we observe that those bodies swell and acquire a circular contour, showing at the same time a pale oval nucleus. It is now seen that, as the disk

---

* Free nuclei of colored corpuscles, which may be seen if the preparation has been subjected to pressure, must not be confused with these structures.

gradually pales, the nucleus becomes more and more spheroidal
and yellow, while, at the same time it increases in size. At first
it is smooth, subsequently uneven. Here and there corpuscles
are met with in which the yellow central body (*zooid* of Brücke)
is not round, but beset with processes which stretch like rays
towards the periphery. Occasionally it can be made out that
the processes are withdrawn, so that the yellow centre acquires
a roundish form. The zooids eventually lose their central
position, and if the preparation is protected from evaporation
for a sufficient length of time, the observer is sure to see many
corpuscles in which they lie, some partly, some entirely, outside
of the outline of the pale disk. The latter (again following
Brücke) we designate *œcoid*. Brücke teaches that the zooid consists of the nucleus and the hæmoglobin; that it withdraws
from the œcoid which it previously, as it were, inhabited, and
collects itself around the nucleus, so as to form an independent
individual, capable of a separate existence." The author (Dr.
Klein), however, says, on page 32, in speaking of the appearance, disappearance, and reappearance of the zooids : "It is
not difficult to explain all these appearances by coagulation."

Action of Carbonic Acid and of Oxygen on Ciliated Cells:—The
alkalies are not the only stimulants of ciliary action; distilled
water, half per cent. solution of common salt, dilute acetic
acid, carbonic acid, or the induced current act similarly. "The
investigation of the respective actions of *carbonic acid gas* and
oxygen upon ciliary movement is a very important experiment." After a specimen has been prepared, we now allow a
stream of carbonic acid to pass, we perceive * * * that
for a few moments the ciliary motion becomes quicker, but, by-
and-by, slower, until it finally ceases. On now substituting
atmospheric air (oxygen) we find that the movement slowly
recommences, and before long is quite as active as before the
passage of the carbonic acid. * * * Oxygen is therefore as
essential for the continuance of motion in the individual ciliated cell as for the maintenance of animal life in general."
(page 36.)

     *   *   *   *   *   *   *

We regret want of space to extend this notice to include more
of the author's methods of manipulation, to secure accuracy in

experimentation, on which the demonstration of facts in physiology so much depends. We trust enough has been said, however, to indicate the admirable adaptation of the work to aid
the physiological student in the laboratory, to become skillful
and accurate in the delicate manipulations for which he is responsible. The publisher's work is well done.

BOOKS AND PAMPHLETS RECEIVED.

THE PASSIONS IN RELATION TO HEALTH AND DISEASE. By Dr.
X. Bourgeois, of Paris, France. Translated by Howard T.
Damon, A. M., M. D.
[For Sale by the St. Louis Book and News Co.]

NORMAL OVARIOTOMY. By Robert Battey, M. D., Rome, Ga.

REPORT OF COLUMBIA HOSPITAL FOR WOMEN AND LYING-IN
ASYLUM. Department of the Interior, Washington, D. C.
By J. Harry Thompson, A. M., M. D., Surgeon-in-charge.
With appendix. Government printing office : Washington.

STRICTURE OF THE URETHRA, Results of operation with the
dilating urethrotome, with cases. By F. N. Otis, M. D. New
York : D. Appleton & Co.

MINERAL SPRINGS OF THE UNITED STATES AND CANADA, with
analysis and notes. By Geo. E. Walton, M. D. New York :
D. Appleton & Co.
[For Sale by the St. Louis Book & News Co.

PRINCIPLES AND PRACTICE OF MEDICINE. A treatise designed for
the use of practitioners and students. By Austin Flint M. D.
Fourth edition. pp. 1090—8vo. Philadelphia : Henry C. Lea.
[For Sale by the St. Louis Book & News Co]

INSANITY IN ITS RELATIONS TO CRIME. By W. A. Hammond,
M. D. New York : D. Appleton & Co.
[For Sale by the St. Louis Book & News Co.]

ANDERSON ON DISEASES OF THE SKIN, with an analysis of eleven
thousand consecutive cases. By McCall Anderson, M. D.
Philadelphia : Henry C. Lea.
[For Sale by the St Louis Book & News Co.]

CHEMISTRY, General, Medical, and Pharmaceutical. By John
Attfield, Ph. D., F. C. S. Fifth edition. Philadelphia :
Henry C. Lea.
[For Sale by the St. Louis Book & News Co.]

CLINICAL MEDICINE, Study of. Being a guide to the investigation
of disease. By Octavius Sturges, Cantab. Philadelphia :
Henry C. Lea.
[For Sale by the St. Louis Book & News Co]

Meteorological Observations.

METEOROLOGICAL OBSERVATIONS AT ST. LOUIS, MO.

BY A. WISLIZENUS, M. D.

The following observations of daily temperature in St. Louis are made with a MAXIMUM and MINIMUM thermometer (of Green, N. Y.). The daily minimum occurs generally in the night, the maximum about 3 P M The monthly mean of the daily minimum and maxima, added and divided by 2, gives a quite reliable mean of the monthly temperature.

THERMOMETER FAHRENHEIT.

JUNE, 1873.

Day of Month.	Minimum.	Maximum.	Day of Month.	Minimum.	Maximum.
1	58.0	85.5	18	68.5	89.5
2	68.0	91.5	19	73.0	94.5
3	67.0	91.5	20	64.5	80.5
4	70.5	91.0	21	68.5	91.0
5	66.5	84.0	22	72.0	93 5
6	67.0	87.5	23	77.0	96.5
7	67.5	92.0	24	75.0	94.0
8	71.5	84.0	25	76.5	97.0
9	68.0	91.0	26	72.5	94.0
10	67.5	73.0	27	70.0	98.0
11	61.5	80.0	28	69.0	88.5
12	62.0	85.5	29	65.0	93.0
13	67.5	86.0	30	65.0	85.5
14	65.5	88.0			
15	67.5	93.0			
16	71.5	92.5	Means	68.5	89.5
17	71.0	92.5	Monthly Mean 79.0		

Quantity of rain : 5.24 inches.

NOTICE.

INFORMATION WANTED.—Circulars calling for information for the MEDICAL REGISTER AND DIRECTORY OF THE UNITED STATES are being rapidly sent out, and this portion of the labor will soon be completed. It is earnestly desired that the responses be as prompt and as full as possible. *It is important to physicians, who have any education or standing, that they appear properly on this record,* as the work will be one of permanent value, and will be constantly referred to. The forms containing the Directory of the first set of eleven States and Territories (Alabama to Georgia, alphabetically, inclusive), are now in the hands of the printer, and there are but a few days in which informat on can be inserted in those pages.

Officers of public medical institutions of *all kinds,* hospitals, asylums, dispensaries, colleges, medical societies, etc., are particularly requested to furnish us with lists, catalogues, announcements, etc., in order to give brief histories of these institutions, and for use in perfecting the REGISTER AND DIRECTORY in all its parts.

It is intended that the work shall be exhaustive, and as nearly *correct* as may be, and it will be issued as speedily as possible; but the labor is immense, and the work is delayed by the want of promptitude in receiving replies to circulars and letters.   S. W. BUTLER, M. D.,

115 S Seventh Street, Philadelphia, Pa.

Mortality Report.

FROM JUNE 21st, 1873, TO JULY 19th, 1873, INCLUS.

Date	White. Males.	White. Females.	Col'd. Males.	Col'd. Females.	Under 5 yrs.	5 to 10	10 to 20	20 to 30	30 to 40	40 to 50	50 to 60	60 to 70	70 to 80	80 to 90	90 to 100	Total.
Saturday 28	152	99	4		173	4	6	17	23	12	11	4	3	1	...	255
" 5	125	111	4	1	150	8	10	18	18	11	10	10	4	2	...	241
" 12	141	95	4	1	139	15	12	18	22	13	8	6	8		...	241
" 19	163	120	1	2	133	15	13	28	30	28	26	5	9	4	...	292
Total.	586	425	13	4	595	32	41	81	93	64	55	25	24	7		1029

Alcoholism 6	Conges. of Lungs. . 2	Gangrene.......... 2	Œdema............ 1
Asthenia 1	Consumption........ 41	Gastritis 7	Old Age............ 8
Abscess 1	Convulsions........ 48	Hemorrhage . 3	Pertussis..... . .. 4
Abscess of Liver.... 1	Croup 2	Hemoptysis 1	Pleuritis......... 1
Albumenuria........ 2	Cyanosis 2	Hepatitis 5	Pneumonia... 12
Anemia............ 1	Collapse 1	Hydrocephalus..... 14	Poison, Morphia... 1
Apoplexy.......... 7	Debility 25	Hyperemia . 1	Scarlatina 1
Arachnitis ... 2	Delirium Tremens 5	Inanition 7	Sarcoma........... 1
Ascites 1	Diabetes Militus 1	Inflammat'n Brain 4	Scrofula 2
Asthma 1	Diarrhœa 25	" Bowels. 4	Small Pox . 12
Atrophia 5	Disease of the Heart 6	" Lungs 1	Suffocation .. 2
Bright's Disease ... 2	Dropsy. 1	Injuries 5	Softening of Brain 2
Bronchitis.......... 7	Drowned 4	Intussusception. 1	Summer Complaint 170
Burns 2	Dysentery. 8	Lockjaw........... 14	Sunstroke. . . 13
Cancer.............. 7	Eclampsia 5	Marasmus ... 39	Tabes Mesenterica 3
Catarrh 2	Enteritis 8	Measles 8	Thrombosis ... 1
Cerebritis 5	Exhaustion 1	Meningitis ... 41	Ulcer of Stomach . 1
Cholera 14	Fever, Cong 5	" cereb-spin 19	" Intestines . 1
" Infantum 40	" puerperalis.. 2	Nephritis 2	Vomitus........ . 1
*Cholera Morbus 210	" remittent.... 2	Morbus Maculosis 1	
Conges. of Bowels 3	Fever, typhoid 7	Necrosis .. 1	Total......956
Conges. of Brain .. 20	Fracture 1	Nervous Shock . 1	Stillborn.......... 45

*[Misnomer]

R. H. O'BRIEN, M. D.
Clerk of Board of Health.

PAMPHLETS RECEIVED.

A TREATISE ON THE DISEASES OF REFRACTION AND ACCOMMODATION. By C. S. Fenner, M. D., Louisville, Ky.

REPORT OF THE MUNICIPAL HOSPITAL, Containing statistics of 2,377 cases of small-pox. By Wm. M. Welch, M. D., Physician-in-charge.

A REPLY TO DR. H. C. WOODS' REVIEW OF THE MEDICAL TESTIMONY IN THE TRIAL OF MRS. WHARTON. By Philip C. Williams, Baltimore, Md.

OBSERVATIONS UPON THE TREATMENT OF YELLOW FEVER. By Joseph Jones, M. D., New Orleans, La. Published by John P. Morton, & Co., Louisville, Ky.

THE SAINT LOUIS

Medical and Surgical Journal.

SEPTEMBER, 1873.

Original Communications.

EXCESSIVE VOMITING DURING PREGNANCY.

By M. M. PALLEN, M D., formerly Professor of Obstetrics in the St. Louis.
Medical College.

I was requested by Dr. J. B. S. Alleyne to see Mrs. P——, who, according to his statement, was in the 6th month of pregnancy and would not retain anything on her stomach—no food, no drink. He stated that unless she was relieved, she would die for want of nourishment, and that the induction of abortion was the remedy.

He had consulted two well-known medical gentlemen in this city, one of whom had advised purgation with mercurials, which was tried, as were also the various remedies recommended in such cases. But all of these had been of no avail. The other physician, who was subsequently called in, concurred in the opinion that she was in great danger, advised a certain course, but would not consent to the procuring of abortion, as he rightly contended, that the fœtus was not viable, and as he was a zealous adherent of the Roman Catholic church, he plead the well-known doctrine, that it was not right to destroy the child, even to save the mother.

On the 16th of July prepared to do whatever was necessary to save the mother, or both fœtus and mother, if it could be done. I found Mrs P—— as described by Dr. Alleyne.   Pulse 96 ;   incessant nausea ;   vomiting whenever anything was taken into the stomach ; sleeplessness at night or during the day ;   no delirium, no tinnitus aurium ; no dimness of vision. I claimed a delay of twenty-four hours to try two remedies heretofore untried.   One was the hypodermic injection of morphia over the region of the stomach, and the other was the injection of beef essence and brandy into the rectum.   On the next day we again visited our patient. The remedies had done no good.   She vomited, as ever, the little ice-water she took, and the injections could not be retained at all.

My mind was now made up as to the course to be pursued.   I examined the' neck of the womb with my finger.   I could readily introduce the index finger into the os tincæ and carry it up to the internal os, and the examination convinced me there was granular erosion of the cervix.

Nothing effective could now be done, short of abortion ; the method of procedure was the only question. To dilatation by means of tents, there were these objections : it is slow in its operation ; and in this particular case, the pathological condition would lead to a metroperitonitis, or to a pelvic cellulitis.   I have seen these arise after dilatation, even when there was no granular erosion of the cervix, nor any other lesion of that part of the womb, and when dilatation was practiced for other objects.

The detachment of the membranes according to the method of Kiwisch is also objectionable on account of its slowness and uncertainty.

I determined to puncture the membranes and for the following reasons: The child was not viable and could not be saved. I have known cases, when the child was viable, as in the eighth or ninth month of pregnancy, and when I brought on premature labor to allay excessive and uncontrollable vomiting, that the vomiting did cease, almost immediately after the rupture of the membranes and before the emptying of the uterus.

With a small-sized uterine sound, I punctured the membranes. On the evening Dr. Alleyne called for me and told me that in an hour after the operation, she took, with decided appetite, some beefsteak and retained it; at night she did the same, and when we saw her in the morning, she and her mother informed us that she had slept well, and that she had a good appetite, having eaten various things for breakfast. About forty-eight hours after the operation, fœtus and secundines came away, and she made a rapid recovery.

I am aware that there is high authority against the emptying of the uterus in cases of excessive vomiting during pregnancy. I am aware, too, of the sudden and favorable changes which sometimes take place in such cases The experienced physician can often foresee that such will be the result, and he will persevere with his remedies. I will admit, that it does happen, even when he despairs. But it also happens, that although our patients occasionally get well, when we expect them to die, on the other hand, they sometimes die when we expect them to get well.   We must reason from a general rule, and not from an exception.

In regard to authority, I can oppose it with authority.   I intend to quote one; but previously to so doing, let me cite the remarkable words of Prof. Huxley. Referring to science, he says: "I believe that the greatest intellectual revolution mankind has yet seen, is now slowly taking place by her agency.   She is teaching the world that its ultimate court of appeal is observation and experiment, and not authority." *

The only authority I will quote, is that of Dr. Tyler Smith, who writes as follows: "When all other means fail, and when the exhaustion of the patient cannot be arrested, the remedy is the emptying of the uterus, and this should never be delayed so long as to put the patient in a state of imminent peril.   Nature herself, often terminates the distress by spontaneous abortion.   It has happened to me to have been twice consulted, within a recent period, in cases in which the induction of premature labor artificially was so long delayed, that the patient died before abortion could be induced.   Paul Dubois has stated that he met with twenty fatal cases in thirteen years.   It is a reproach to our art that such cases should occur."

Dr. McClintock, in a communication on this subject before the Dublin Obstetrical Society, March 12, 1873, gives some very interesting statistics.   A table of 36 cases was presented where abortion had been produced to rescue the patients from the fatal effects of excessive vomiting.   In 27 of these cases the vomiting was arrested, and the patients perfectly recovered; whilst in

---

* Culture Demanded by Modern Life, p. 144.

nine instances, although the vomiting was arrested, still, ultimate recovery did not take place, partly in consequence of the operation being too long delayed, and partly from the effect of some intercurrent complication (*e. g.* diarrhœa, hemorrhage, puerperal fever, etc.) not fairly attributable to the operation itself. He cited fifty cases, (from various authentic sources) where death had actually taken place in consequence of the persistence and uncontrollable severity of the sickness. (See the *American Journal of the Medical Sciences* for July, 1873, p. 275).

The rules of action in these cases and other matters appertaining to them, I propose to continue in the next number of the St. Louis Medical and Surgical Journal.

A CASE OF PUERPERAL CONVULSIONS, CRANIOT-
OMY, PNEUMONIA, AND FINAL RECOVERY.

By Dr. J. W. Charles, Maryville, Mo.,

I was called on Saturday night, July the 26th, 1873, to consult with Dr. Mulholland in the case of Mrs. R., *æt.* 20, primapara, who had been in labor since the Thursday evening before. Upon my arrival at 11 o'clock, I found her in violent puerperal convulsions, the face turned towards the left shoulder and horribly distorted, frothing at the mouth, jerking the limbs, found she had had five convulsions ere my arrival. The doctor seemed completely paralyzed, at the mishap (as such I term it), and had not done anything to ward off the impending danger, except to apply cold wet clothes to her head.

Dr. Ramsbotham says that "An attack of puerperal convulsions is one of the most frightful accidents that can happen to the patient under labor." We immediately drew some twenty ounces of dark venous blood, with favorable result (temporarily) ; also gave 30 grains of bromide of potassium. Upon examination of the womb and pelvis, found the fœtal head greatly disproportioned to the pelvis, and that the child could neither be expelled by natural powers, nor extracted by the forceps, which the doctor had tried to do time and again, before my arrival ; and I immediately tried, but to no avail ; and in consultation with the doctor, decided upon craniotomy. Some hours had elapsed in effort to deliver by the forceps, and in the mean time she had several convulsions, but not so hard as before. We administered chloroform, and by hard labor were successful in bringing the child down, when the woman had one of the most terrific epileptiform convulsions, which delivered the child. This convulsion was terrible to witness, her lips and face were livid, her eyes expressive of agony, she breathed as if the air passages were in rigid spasm. We administered chloroform until the convulsion ceased, and then gave the bromide of potassium in 30 grain doses every hour, until relief was obtained. After delivery there was very little hemorrhage, but fearing inertia of the womb and its attendant flooding, we gave a dose or two of ergot combined with opium. The patient remained stupid with stertorous breathing for two days, and was nearly a week in more or less unconscious state. She voided her urine two or three times a day, which was of a smoky character, and loaded with albumen. On the third day there were unmistakable signs of pneumonia, crepitation over left lung, troublesome cough, pathognomic expectoration, pulse 130. Treatment was now directed to the pneumonia.

July 31st.—Considerable fever, pulse 130, cough still troublesome, bowels moved several times, but slight lochial discharge.

August 2nd.—Fever, pulse 130, coughs but little, mind more rational; lochial discharge disappeared altogether; ordered injection of warm water with five to ten grs. carbolic acid to the pint of water, every three or four hours ; warm poultice of flaxseed to the vulva and hot fomentations over the uterus.

Aug. 4th.—Still some fever, pulse 90, bowels regular, mind improving, the lochial discharge not returned, coughs seldom, keep up the injections three or four times daily.

The subsequent history of this case presents no points of interest except that the patient had one or two sinking spells overcome by stimulating treatment. The albumen disappeared from the urine, the mind became clearer by degrees, and she is convalescing quite rapidly this the eighteenth day after confinement. The pneumonia, I think was possibly caused by the poisoned state of the blood from great torpidity of the liver; and that hyperæmia of the brain in pregnant women is the probable cause of convulsions. This patient had twelve convulsions during this confinement, none after the delivery of the fœtus. The remedies we give credit in this case are copious venesection, inhalation of anæsthetics, cold applications, and bromide of potassium. In the pneumonia, gave sustaining treatment all together,—opium, quinia, nutritive diet, etc.

INVERSION OF THE UTERUS.

Reported by O H. BLACK, M. D., Mirabile, Mo.

Practicing in a country village where I cannot have the benefit of counsel or interchange of thoughts and views with other physicians, I send you an account of a case under my care, believing it of rare occurrence and of general interest to the profession.

On the morning of April 5th, 1873, I was called to wait on Mrs. G—, in labor (second child). She is about twenty-six years of age, slender make, and during pregnancy was in poor health, but was "able to be around all the time," complaining of nothing but debility. The labor was an easy one, lasted about four hours, child when born weighed 5¼ lbs.; the last pain was rather a light one, expelling the child without any assistance further than supporting the perineum, no traction whatever was used. The child when born appeared lifeless, and as the last pain passed off the woman looked easy and natural as any case of labor could—whilst busy endeavoring to restore life to the child I happened to look towards the mother, she was pallid, eyes turned back in the head, pulseless at the wrist, and to all appearances moribund—instantly leaving the child, I tried to pass the finger into the vagina, the first thought being hemorrhage, but was surprised to find a large smooth body lying outside the vulva,. which on examination proved to be the *uterus* completely invested with the placenta wrapped around it; it was as smooth and even as a plate of French glass, the rough or rugous feeling of the placenta being altogether wanting. Here was a case—Dr. Meigs doubted if such a case could happen ; here I had proof that it could.* What could I do ?—should I send for counsel ? It was five miles to Dr. Scott the nearest physician that I could depend on, the woman might be dead a long time before he could be present. These thoughts and many others ran through my mind in an instant. I determined to thrust my fingers through the placenta and strip it from the uterus, then carefully drawing the uterus through the hand so as to remove all adherent remnants of placenta or other matter, I pressed my fingers into the fundus as you might into the bottom of a rubber bottle, and, by steady and continued upward pressure, succeeded in restoring it to its place.

The woman did well for ten days, when she was attacked with phlegmasia dolens, which readily yielded to ordinary treatment, and she is now (August 15th) doing well.

CREASOTE IN THE TREATMENT OF GONORRHŒA.

By Ulysses L. Huyette, M. D., Relfe, Phelps Co., Mo.

The tendency to routine practice in our profession has long been its bane, and is ever to be reprobated by its friends. In no instance is this proneness so manifest as in the treatment of venereal diseases. Well nigh

---

*Dr. Black has mistaken the views of Dr. Meigs. The latter says: "the accident is a rare one."—[Obst. 5th edition, page 610.]

every practitioner has a specific method—walks in a
beaten path—and can give you a concise answer when
interrogated concerning his treatment of syphilis or gonorrhœa.   To this prëeminence of the *specific plan* is
doubtless due the slow progress in this direction in
comparison with that of the other branches of our profession.   We do not in this paper propose to attempt
to set right the profession upon this subject—nor
yet to add much to what is already known—but wish
humbly to present the results of an experience which
if it but stimulate to further research will amply repay the writer.   Having long been in doubt as to the
efficacy of the ordinary plans of treating gonorrhœa,
and having frequently suffered disappointment and
chagrin at the tardy convalescence of my patients, I
naturally was led to inquire into the *rationale* of my
treatment, and to consider what indeed was the true
course to pursue.   The following considerations presented themselves: 1st, this is not an ordinary inflamation, but a specific disease—the result of a cause *sui generis*—a peculiar poison whose toxic properties are manifest in the pathological condition of the part affected;
2d, not only is the origin of the disease due to this
cause, but its duration also is dependent upon the same
element present in the pus secreted from the mucous surface of the urethra.

For, if gonorrhœal pus will give rise to the disease
when brought in contact with healthy mucous surfaces,
we cannot but think it capable of renewing it constantly
as it comes in contact with the lining of the urethra from
which it emanates.   Hence, if the origin and duration
of the affection be due to a specific virus, what is the
indication?   Certainly not an antiphlogistic course,

which does not destroy the materies morbi present. We naturally look for some means by which we may rob the pus of its septic properties, and render it harmless. And almost intuitively we look to the class of antiseptic agents for the means to accomplish the work. Creasote, whose powers are well known, is the remedy we selected, and after an ample trial in numerous cases in all stages, we are safe in asserting its claims upon the attention of the profession. Another question arises: Shall we use it locally or internally? We deem the former insufficient, from the fact that in many instances we are unable to teach the whole diseased surface by an injection, however well executed; so we should trust to its internal use—by which it is eliminated by the kidneys and passes over the entire mucous tract.

That creasote is the only remedy of this class which will destroy the toxic power of the pus we do not claim, but deem it highly probable that carbolic acid, and other agents of the kind will effect the same end. We are aware that we render ourselves liable to the charge of "*specifist*," which we reprobated in the beginning of our paper, but of this charge we plead not guilty, from the fact that we are not proposing a specific for a disease, but a means of removing a constant specific cause, of the extension and maintenance of the disease; a poison upon which the malady depends, which must be neutralized ere we can hope for a cure. Hence the propriety and the necessity of some agent or class of agents by which to combat it. The mode of administration which I have adopted is in the form of an emulsion from 1 to 3 gtt., *ter die*, and at late bed-time. I find this applicable to all cases, save, perhaps, in some advanced stages of gleet, in which the poisonous element is not present.   The astringent properties of creasote have been recognized, and some may be disposed to attribute any good effects which flow from its use to that property ; but we cannot admit this argument, for there are many more highly astringent remedies which would be preferable if that effect alone were desired. We claim for it a higher virtue, and trust those interested will give it a trial.

Thus, in short, we claim that gonorrhœa is a disease *sui generis*, due to a specific virus or toxic agent, and that the only rational method of cutting short its operations is to rob the disease of its chief characteristic ; to deprive the pus, which is constanly bathing the mucous surface, of its virulent power, when the case will be virtually closed.

By an antiphlogistic course we may reduce the inflammatory action, but only to be excited again by the effects of the pus ; and the disease if treated so, will only end when the toxic element will have been exhausted and the pus ceases to be virulent.

CHOLERA MORBUS.

By H. A. Buck, M. D., St. Louis.

It is a disease, the pathology of which, old writers knew but very little about.   It is derived from the Greek word χολή, bile, and the Latin word *morbus*, disease, rendered *bile disease.*

Late pathologists have decided that there is no disease of the liver or any of its functions in this disease, therefore the name is inappropriate, and should not be used. A better name, and one describing the organs affected in this disease, I believe, would be gastroenterorrhœa, taken from the Greek, γαςτήρ, stomach, ἐντερον, intestine, ἠἐω, to flow, rendered flowing from the stomach and intestines, or vomiting and purging.

Sydenham, who wrote two hundred years ago, called it cholera morbus. He called the epidemic that prevailed in London in the years 1665 and 1666, pestilential fever or plague; this disease by recent writers has been called Asiatic cholera. In the chapter on cholera morbus, he says, "this disease prevailed in 1669, three years after the plague; and in the character of its symptoms it is not altogether unlike the common cholera of intemperance and drunkenness which may occur at any season. Neither is its treatment very dissimilar. Still it is a disease of another family. Its presence is understood at once. There is vomiting to a great degree, and there are also foul, difficult, and strange motions from the bowels. There is intense pain in the belly, there is wind, there are distensions, heart-burn, and thirst. The pulse is quick and frequent, at times small and unequal. The feeling of sickness is accompanied with heat and disquiet, the perspiration sometimes amounts to absolute sweating. The legs and arms are cramped, and the extremities are cold. To these symptoms and others of a like stamp, we may add fainting. The disease terrifies the looker-on, and sometimes proves fatal within twenty-four hours. This disease, however much it may be epidemic, very rarely occurs beyond the month of August—the month in which it begins. This makes me admire the beautiful and subtle mechanism of Nature in the determination of the origin and decline of epidemics; since even although the same causes—viz: the abundance of fruit— are common to the months of August and September, the effect is different."

Now whoever carefully studies the phenomena of the true and legitimate cholera morbus, the only form with which we now have to deal, will certainly own that although produced by the same causes, and accompanied by the same symptoms, it differs from that sort of common cholera which may occur at any time of the year. The two diseases are as far as the poles asunder. It seems as if in the air of the particular month of August there was some hidden and peculiar property which impresses on the blood, or on the bowels, some specific alteration, adapted to this disease and to none other. Sydenham's hystory of cholera morbus in the middle of the seventeenth century compares very favorably with the same disease, or the cholera morbus of our day, that is prevailing at the present time in the cities and towns of the Southwest, and is quite prevalent in St. Louis at the present time. The only disease that cholera morbus assimilates is Asiatic or true cholera, also some forms of poisoning, as by tartar emetic, and the different antimonials—sulphate of zinc and copper.

How are we to differentiate the two diseases? First, we must inquire into the history of the cases, and ascertain if any vessels have arrived in our ports with Asiatic cholera on board, and whether it existed in the foreign ports at the time of the sailing of such vessels. A very little of the Asiatic cholera leaven would soon leaven a whole city, unless energetic or active measures were adopted to prevent its spread. Some of the prominent causes of cholera morbus are, extreme heat following a wet spring, causing infected well-water; intemperate and irregular habits; improper food; unripe fruit, and stale vegetables. It can generally be traced to something the patient has been eating or drinking, or irregularity in living. I believe that it will originate in our climate in any of the hot months of the year, under the above influences, without any combination of the Asiatic cholera poison.

In cholera morbus, in its emeso catharsis, there is bile and fecal matter without suppression of urine. In Asiatic cholera there is seldom any bile in the emeso catharsis, but the characteristic rice-water discharges with suppression of urine. The termination of both diseases when they end in death are similar—a state of collapse. The medical profession differ in opinion relative to the character or nature of these two diseases. Some think that they are one and the same disease, but assuming milder forms in some seasons and in some individuals. I believe them to be two distinct diseases, and that they arise from altogether different causes, and seldom prevail at the same time or place. We had cholera morbus in our country before Asiatic cholera ever left the shores of the old world. Cholera morbus is a disease that is more or less prevalent every summer or autumn. It is not so with Asiatic cholera, it has made its appearance periodically.

The treatment, as given by writers in these two diseases is similar. I have found hypodermic injections of morphia to relieve the nausea and vomiting, and the epigastric pains, and I seldom have had to repeat it if called in season.　Follow twelve hours after with a mild laxative if the bowels do not move before that time.　Such has been my treatment this season in cholera morbus.　I have not seen a death from the disease this season.

[Still it is so exceptional for cholera morbus to kill, that it would seem a little of the foreign *killing poison* had crept in this year.]

THE MEANS OF CLEANSING AND APPLYING REMEDIES TO THE NASAL AND PHARYNGO-NASAL CAVITIES.

By Thos. F. Rumbold, M. D., St. Louis, Mo.

There are no cavities of the body not open to inspection of the unaided eye, that are more easily examined than the nasal and pharyngo-nasal ; at the same time I think there are none so difficult to clean without injuring the already inflamed mucous membrane.　The importance of thoroughly freeing the surfaces of these cavities of the extraneous products of inflammation, is not superceded by the therapeutical effects of the remedial agents employed.　Repeated observations, during the last few years, have shown that if the inflamed surfaces are maintained *clean*, a large majority of the patients will *grow* well without other treatment.　This is especially true of the young.

Experience has shown that whatever method is chosen, it should, while thoroughly cleansing the cavities and applying the remedies to them, cause *no* irritation. For this purpose a Spray Producer is the mildest and the most complete, blowing the muco-purulent secretions away from their lodging place, while forcing the medicated solution into every irregularity ; into places that cannot be reached by the brush or sponge, or even viewed during life. It will be necessary for the Spray Producers to be of different forms, that is, to throw the stream in different directions, to completely treat every portion of the inflamed surface.

Fig. 1.

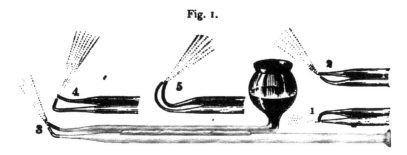

Fig. 1.—Nos. 1 to 5, inclusive, are the forms that may be found necessary to thoroughly cleanse and treat these cases. If the entire diseased surfaces are not medicated, the treatment will be greatly protracted, or may prove a failure.

When the muco-purulent secretions have become hardened, adhering closely to the mucous membrane, the Spray Producer has not sufficient force to remove it, then the posterior-nares syringe may be employed, but this instrument, although very efficient, causes such an unpleasant sensation when applied behind the soft palate, that patients frequently refuse to submit to its use. The Weber Nasal Douche (improperly called Thudicum's) is almost universally called into requisi-

:32

tion in such cases, but from the lack of the adaptation of it to accomplish the end aimed at, it must very frequently fail.   Here is an instance in which the novelty of the appearance of the liquid escaping from the opposite nostril has captivated the judgment of many of the profession, and only because they allowed themselves to forget that in a large majority of the cases, the location of the disease and that of the fluid employed to treat it cannot be the same.   That this mode of treatment is beneficial when the disease is situated low enough for the medicated stream to wash it, or when the secretions are so abundant as to flow down to the inferior portion of the cavity, is not doubted, but it is needless to say that it is of no benefit when these conditions are not present.   Let us examine the adaptibility of this nasal douche (Weber's) as a means of cleansing this cavity,

Fig. 2.

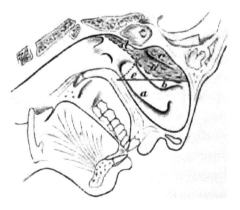

Fig. 2 represents an antero-posterior section of the face and head—in the *proper inclination* for using the nasal douche—exhibiting the turbinated processes, *a, b* and *c,* and the location of the inspissated secretions in the superior portion of the cavity to be washed out, *d d*. The line *e*, starting at the place where the posterior border of the septum nasi joins the hard palate, indicates the surface of the fluid employed ; the soft palate being closed up against the posterior wall of the pharynx, or not, will not alter this turning place for the liquid. After this showing, is it not manifest that this procedure will end in a failure? If that portion of the nostrils that is so washed be examined previous to the use of the douche, it would be found that nine times in ten it is entirely free from any noxious secretions, therefore requiring no such irrigation. Yet it is well known that large masses of fetid secretions do frequently come out of the nostrils after such treatment, but this is an evidence that secretions were so abundant as to fall down to within the reach of the irrigating fluid, or it may be that the irritation of the liquid excited a greater flow of mucus in the whole cavity, thus loosening the scab, having a similar effect to that of an irritating powder if snuffed into the nostrils. Even in those cases, if the practitioner will carefully examine them after this apparent thorough cleansing, he will find in the superior portion of the cavity, as much of the purulent secretions remaining, or more, than has come out ; also, that any amount of washing by this means, that the patient *can* submit to, will not remove this remaining product of inflammation.

The Cathether Douche, about to be described, cannot fail to reach this diseased portion of the cavity. I have employed it daily during the last three and a half years, and find it to be efficacious and mild in its effects. The only sensation it produces, when warm salt-water is used, is that of tickling.

Fig. 3.

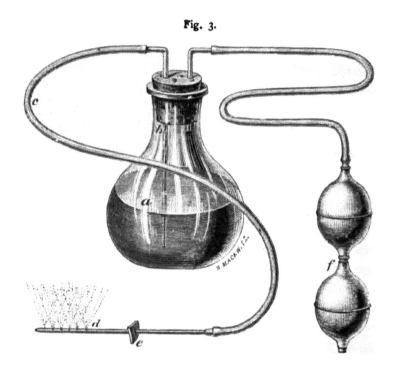

Fig. 3.—*a* represents the reservoir in which the medicated fluid is placed, *f* the air bulbs for forcing air into
the vessel, causing the liquid to flow up the tubes *b* and
c, and out of the holes in the catheter *d*, which is inserted into the nostril treated, nearly up to the shield *e*.
It will be noticed that the tube which reaches nearly to
the bottom of the reservoir, has a small hole in the side
at *b* : this is to allow air to enter while the water is also
going out, causing the latter to escape in an intermittent stream, resembling a very coarse spray. A slight
turning of the catheter will cause the spattering stream
to *wash* and *blow* the secretions away from their
lodging place. This stream of air and liquid is milder
and more efficacious than that of a steady stream. The

cleansing process may be greatly assisted by the patient closing the opposite nostril and giving a smart blow out of the one treated, sending the liquid and everything loose out with great force. The shield *e* on the catheter is to prevent the fluid from running on the hand of the operator.

Fig. 4.

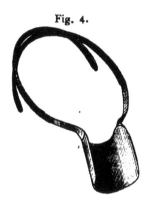

Fig. 4 is a Nose Spout to prevent the liquid and muco-purulent secretions from falling on the lips and chin, and from soiling the clothes of the patient while blowing the nose.

1205 Washington Ave.

Hospital Reports.

CITY HOSPITAL.

Notes by T. F. PRUITT, M. D., in charge.

A case of Chronic Pericarditis, with a large collection of pus in the pericardium, complicated by Pleuritis and Thrombus of left iliac vein.

Joseph Graf, German, age forty-nine, occupation that of a waiter, admitted to hospital Dec. 7th, 1872.

Previous history :—Patient had typhoid fever and acute rheumatism in 1866, chronic diarrhœa during the war and since,—lasting altogether two or three years. Has never had good health since the war, thinks army life was the foundation of his ill health. About two months ago, after exposure, was taken with pain in left chest and a severe cough, which confined him to bed one month. After this his health improved, though has had hæmoptysis several times since. Spat some blood when entered hospital, and complained at times of pain in the lungs. Has been losing flesh and strength rapidly since attacked. Knows of no tuberculous diathesis in family. Pulse 92; tempt. 99½° F. Urine contains neither albumen nor sugar.

Dec. 24th.—After two weeks of convalescence was attacked yesterday with pleuritic pain in left side; friction sound most marked in mammary region.

25th.—Pain increased; friction sound continues; tenderness on percussion.

26th.—Pulse 124, and somewhat weak; the above symptoms all aggravated.

30th.—Is again greatly relieved; eats and sleeps moderately well; no very marked effusion observable.

Jan. 5th, 1873.—Is sufficiently improved to walk around ward.

10th.—Is somewhat indisposed, keeps his bed continually.

12th.—Has been stupid for past two days, though troubled with insomnia and cough at night. Bowels constipated.

13th.—Bowels moved to-day after enema, stools consisted of scybala, and were followed by prolapsus.of rectum to the extent of two or three inches.

15th.—Some swelling of left foot, and cyanotic condition of same noticed this A. M.; complains of pain in foot, which is œdematous; pitting on pressure. Prolapsed portion of rectum presents a bluish, congested appearance, which, although returned, will not so remain.

16th.—Œdema and cyanosis of leg extends to knee. Pulse rapid and feeble. Complains more of pain in leg.

17th.—Thigh is also involved, purpuric spots on same, very thick. Pulsations of left femoral artery imperceptible, those of right very feeble. The right foot is beginning to assume the appearance of left when first attacked, pits on pressure, and presents a bluish appearance. Heart sounds very indistinct and muffled. Complains continually of excessive pain in leg. Sensation in leg is but little impaired.

18th.—Left groin swollen and greatly indurated, presenting almost the appearance of a large bubo. The case was examined to-day by Dr. Robinson, in connection with resident physician and assistants. The above symptoms exist in a much more aggravated form. The feebleness of heart and lung action was one of the most salient points in the case, remarked by all. Pulsations of left femoral artery still imperceptible, those of right growing more feeble. Right foot still œdematous and cyanotic, though morbid action is not taking place so rapidly as in left. The question arose as to the cause of the œdema and other morbid conditions of the leg. All agreed that the œdema was caused by obstruction to the returning circulation, or in other words by a thrombus in left iliac vein; Dr. Robinson going so far as to say that it extended up as high as the bifurcation and slightly beyond, giving as his reasons for same that the right foot was slightly involved, and that it must have been caused by the thrombus extending partly across right iliac vein at bifurcation, and obstructing returning current in same.

Patient died on the night of the 19th. The treatment was warm applications to limb (bottles filled with warm water and changed every hour), stimuli, etc.

Post Mortem.—On opening the chest a considerable amount

of pleuritic effusion was found in left side. The left external surface of the pericardium presented a rather corrugated appearance, with a projection resembling the appendages of the auricles. The left lung was quite firmly attached to the pericardium by old adhesions. The pericardium was seen to contain more or less fluid, and on making an incision into it about a pint of purulent fluid escaped. The lining membrane of the pericardium showed evidences of the old pericarditis, while the surface of the heart itself was roughened by deposits of plastic lymph, and presented a worm-eaten, ragged appearance, or that condition referred to by Niemeyer when two plates of soft butter had been put together, and drawn suddenly apart.

The abdominal viscera were apparently healthy. Communicating with the pericardium from below was an abcess within the abdominal cavity, the walls of which were made up by the diaphragm above, the liver to the right, the spleen to the left, and the stomach below, with the adhesions between these parts. This abscess contained about two or three ounces of yellow pus, and communicated with the pericardium, through the diaphragm, by two openings sufficiently large to admit an ordinary lead pencil. The lungs contained a small amount of tuberculous matter only. On cutting down over the femoral vessels, the iliac vein and artery of left side were found bound down by inflammatory products, while posterior to the vessels, and about midway of their course, was found a small accumulation of pus.

The iliac vein was found distended, while its contents presented some resistance. On laying it open a thrombus was found which extended from a little above the bifurcation to the profunda vein, into which it dipped. Below this point the femoral vein contained no clot as far as examined,—two or three inches.

The iliac artery contained a considerable amount of fluid blood. The tissues of thigh were greatly infiltrated with serum, which exuded freely through the cut surfaces. The tissue of the heart upon incision presented the appearance of fatty degeneration, which was subsequently confirmed upon microscopic examination by Dr. Robinson. The endo-cardium and valves of the heart presented no abnormal appearance.

ST. LUKE'S HOSPITAL.

Amputation of Hip-Joint—Death.—Dr. Everingham, of Butler, Bates Co., Mo., observed about the first of February, 1873, his son, aged twelve years, limping, complained of pain about and above the right knee. No redness or swelling, pain increased on using the limb. The boy was provided with crutches and directed not to use the limb. At the end of six weeks it was found that the limb could not be used without great pain. Soon after, perhaps about the 1st of April, a little enlargement was observed; this increased together with pain. Had intermittent fever from which he had suffered before ; his general health, which had never been robust, became more and more feeble.

On the 5th of August he was presented to me with above history. I found the limb measuring fifteen inches in circumference the swelling and extending to middle of thigh from knee ; superficial veins large and tortuous ; parts sensitive, a vascular thrill could be felt, skin stretched but not shining or inflamed.

On examination told the father it was malignant, and suggested amputation at hip, as affording the best hope. Dr. Everingham wished farther advice and took his son to see Dr. Gross.

August 15th.—Returned from Philadelphia, the boy had suffered a little from diarrhœa and had one or two chills, but had been put promptly on treatment by his father and was better.

We continued quinine and waited until the 19th. At this date his general health seemed fair, for a delicate boy ; he was cheerful and wished the amputation.

3.40 P. M.—Was given brandy.

4 P. M.—Dr. W. A. Barret administered chloroform, and under its influence he was taken to the operating room. Dr. Prewitt compressed the femoral artery at pubis, Dr. Gregory manipulated the limb, and as the catlin was passed through the limb, Dr. Lankford compressed the abdominal aorta with the heel of his hand. The anterior flap completed, Dr. Prewitt drew it forward. The capsule was divided; Dr. Gregory dislocated the head of the bone forward, the ligamentum teres was severed, and the knife passed behind the head, separating the remaining part of the capsular ligament, and formed the posterior flap which was at once secured by Dr. McDowell. Except the hemorrhage from the limb removed, the operation was almost bloodless.

The small vessels in the posterior flap were secured by Dr. Mudd and myself as Dr. McDowell released them one by one. The larger vessels in the anterior flap were secured before Dr. Prewitt released the flap. Other small branches now ligated as blood made their sites known. The femoral vein and one other were ligated, it being found that these vessels discharged too much bright blood to be left without ligature.

The flaps were left open, the boy was now weak; pulse feeble; the body covered with a profuse perspiration. ¼ grain of morphine was injected hypodermically, and the patient removed to his bed. Half an hour later he was still weak and pulse feeble, though improving. Ordered beef essence and ice.

6 P. M.—Pulse good.

9 P. M.—Pulse 100 and good; patient cheerful and not suffering. A little bloody serum discharging from cut surfaces. Beef essence continued; passed a comfortable night.

Aug. 20th, 6 A. M.—Pulse not so good; more frequent and less full; ordered brandy and gave ½ gr. morphine. No tossing or restlessness; no hemorrhage. Some bloody serum had exuded, but only a trifling amount; sick at stomach and vomiting occasionally.

9 A. M.—Pulse feeble and sometimes imperceptible; had vomited. Gave brandy and beef essence per rectum, and repeated every hour. Continued to sink and died at 2 P. M.—twenty-two hours after the operation.

A section of the limb showed a tumor involving the entire thickness of the bone in its lower half; well defined in its outline; exceedingly vascular with large blood spaces, with others filled with medullary matter and a radiating arrangement of illy developed bone.   JOHN T. HODGEN.

Reviews and Bibliographical Notices.

THE MINERAL SPRINGS OF THE UNITED STATES AND CANADA, with Analyses and Notes on the prominent Spas of Europe and a list of sea side resorts. By Geo. E. Walton, M. D., etc., New York: D. Appleton & Co. 12 mo. pp. 390.

[For Sale by the St. Louis Book & News Co.]

Physicians generally confess to a neglect of the critical study of therapeutics as related to the use of baths, and mineral waters. This attractive little volume, illustrated by maps and wood cuts, contains a description of the various mineral springs and sea side resorts, also the known facts concerning our mineral waters. The author informs us in the preface that he has consulted other authors, whose conclusions were drawn from hundreds of years of laborious investigation of the spas of Germany, France, Switzerland, and Italy. The portion relating to the springs of the *United States* is the result of a selection of credible evidence regarding them, gained by correspondence and personal observation. The work includes an account of all the important mineral springs at present known on the North American Continent; the medicinal properties of each, thus being suggestive in the selection of the particular springs which best fill the indications of each individual case. A copious index adds to its value for a busy practitioner. The book may be recommended as a valuable guide to these resorts, rules for bathing, etc.

CIVIL MALPRACTICE. A Report presented to the Military Tract Medical Society, January 14, 1878. By M. A. McClelland, M. D. Chicago: W. B. Reen & Co. Price, $2.00.

Malpractice is defined on the 8th page to be an "improper discharge of professional duty, either through want of skill, or through negligence." The subject is farther divided into civil malpractice, in which patients bring suits for damages which they have, or think they have, sustained; and criminal malpractice, in which the people or State, is made the plaintiff. This report is limited to the former. Numerous adjudicated cases are collated, illustrative of the usage of courts, and ability of the *average jury* at this time; and so much of the charge of various judges to juries, as may indicate the legal responsibility of physicians.

The remedy for the misfortunes of the profession in this regard is thought by the author, to be more thorough instruction of students in medico-legal jurisprudence, in the schools; while this may be well, we must differ with the reporter as to its being the remedy.

If malpractice consists in an " improper discharge of professional duty " as stated above, then those guilty of malpractice lack *knowledge* or *attention* to their duty as surgeons or physicians, and not a knowledge of *jurisprudence.* The remedy would be more thorough instruction in the duties of the profession, and in *bone-surgery* in particular; errors in which become monumental, and incite prosecutions. If prosecutions are instituted where no error of practice can be shown, no harm can result to the profession, or its members, but rather benefit; for in such case the prosecuted party improves his reputation by proving his competency, and the costs fall on the prosecutor.

Dr. McClelland has rendered a valuable service by collecting and arranging, in form convenient for reference, the various suits, and decisions of courts during the past few years—putting the profession on their guard toward evil disposed persons. We have long made it a rule to have an intelligent witness always present when we reduce or dress a fracture, dislocation, etc., also at each subsequent dressing, and on the final removal of dressings; which we think the best way to avoid suits of civil malpractice, where no malpractice exists.

FISTULA, HÆMORRHOIDS, PAINFUL ULCER, STRICTURE, PROLAPSUS, AND OTHER DISEASES OF THE RECTUM, THEIR DIAGNOSIS AND TREATMENT. By Wm. Allingham, F. R. C. S. Eng.; Surgeon to St. Marks's Hospital for Fistula, etc.; late Surgeon to the Great Northern Hospital. Second Edition, revised and enlarged. Philadelphia: Linsay & Blakiston, 1873.
[For sale by the St Louis Book & News Co ; price, $2 00]

A careful perusal of this little work of 265 pages, makes us believe that Mr. Allingham has placed the profession under debt to him for the eminently satisfactory manner in which he has treated the subjects considered. His extensive experience in the observation of rectal diseases, renders him eminently capable of speaking knowingly of these affections, and the practical, rather than the theoretical or disquisitorial manner in which he has imparted his knowledge, renders it an excellent book of the hour for the busy practitioner. Though the author's composition is not always smooth, nor his English the most elegant, still,—as he pertinently suggests—that has not absolved him from what he believed to be his duty.

Pictorial or photographic illustrations would very much assist the text, and we trust the next edition will, by such valuable aids, be rendered more complete. If the fear of rendering the book too expensive weighs as an objection, the illustrations could be published separate, so that at least those who desired and could afford, might possess them, while the text still retained its present cheap form.

Owing to the *delicate* location of rectal diseases, the general practitioner is not as well informed in regard to them as he should be, nor is he sufficiently careful in his diagnosis, so that what often is a slight matter easily rectified in the beginning, becomes through the inefficiency of the physician, a serious, and it may be an irremediable affection. No false delicacy, either on the part of the patient or of the medical attendant should prevent thorough examinations.

It is really gratifying to observe how amenable to proper treatment are these rectal diseases; cancers, lupoid ulcers, and some old cases of procidentia are exceptional, but fortunately, these are very rare.

Our author's Introduction tells of the importance of rectal diseases among the physical ailments, and of their comparative frequency to each other, and further as to the proper manner of examining the patient and of exploring the rectum.

We are pleased to find Mr. Allingham treating *fistulæ* by laying them freely open, on a grooved, probe-pointed director. He has no confidence in other kinds of treatment, unless in very exceptional cases indeed, and he very properly insists that the entire fistula with any or all off-shoots, or burrowing tracts, whether running upwards or laterally, must also be freely incised, as otherwise trouble will ultimately be had. Better err on the side of cutting too much than too little. In regard to the old question of operating in cases of phthisis, or tendency thereto, he does not believe in wholesale indiscrim-

inate operations upon tuberculous patients, but if care is taken
in the selection of proper cases, avoiding interference if possible with *rapid advancing* phthisis, and the operation be performed discreetly, at the right time of the year, and with favorable surroundings, the patient will generally do well, be bene-
fited and not damaged by the cure of the rectal malady.
Explicit and careful rules of conduct are given for the management of such cases.   In short, he is more favorably disposed
to the operation than most authorities, and we believe, properly so.

Among the causes of *hæmorrhoids*, mention is made of the
use of printed paper as a detergent—especially the cheap papers,
from which the ink comes off on the slightest friction—also the
neglect of proper ablutions, many persons seeming to forget
that the anus requires quite as much washing as any other part
of the body.   Several full chapters give all that need be said
on the subject of hæmorrhoids; a few cases are amenable to a
treatment short of the knife, but mostly operative interference
is required.   Our author is devoted to the ligature, he says:
" excision is too dangerous, the application of nitric acid and
other caustics is very limited indeed; great improvement is
needed in the apparatus before the galvano-cautery is generally
applicable; the écraseur is barbarous and often unsuccessful,
besides permanent contraction of the anal orifice has followed
its use, the clamp and actual cautery operation has been followed by pyæmia, ulceration, annoying pain and hæmorrhage."
Thus he ligates the hæmorrhoid, each by itself, not by transfix-
ion tying it in halves, nor after having previously passed pins
through to prevent slipping of the thread, but the tumor being
drawn down is separated from the muscular and sub-mucous
tissue on which it rests, by the scissors; the cut is made in the
sulcus or white mark which is seen where the skin meets the
mucous membrane, and this incision is carried up the bowel
and parallel to it, such a distance that the pile is left connected
by an isthmus of vessels and mucous membrane only. The
pile being firmly drawn out, the thread is tied high up on the
neck of the tumor in the deep groove made by the cut.

We have uniformly been successful with the clamp and the
cautery, but will take the first opportunity to try the plan so

general at St. Mark's, and for performing which, many good reasons are given by our author.

In cases of severe after-hemorrhage, he plugs up or tampons the rectum, having previously passed up a male catheter or flexible tube through which the flatus may pass, and thus possibly avoid much of distress to the patient.

Many cases of *fissure* or *painful irritable ulcer* are cured without operation, but if the base of the ulcer be hard and gray, and if the finger detects the sphincter hypertrophic and spasmodically contracted, resort is had to the knife, an incision full length of the ulcer and not less than quarter of an inch in depth is made. Our own experience, like the author's, inclines to a free cut. To be obliged to resort to a second operation puts the patient to inconvenience and places the surgeon in bad odor.

Treatment of *polypus recti* is by clamp and torsion, the ligature is also advised.

In *ulceration* of the *rectum*, the disease extends above, and is frequently situated entirely above the internal sphincter; taken early may be amenable to careful and prolonged treatment, but being neglected, leads to conditions quite incurable. A most valuable chapter is given to this subject. Here, as also under *cancer* of the *rectum*, colotomy is fully treated of, which operation is in favor with and has been performed over thirty times by the author.

Stricture of the rectum is treated by gentle dilatation with a conical bougie, remaining but a minute, and immediately removed if pain is induced. Testimony is given in favor of galvanism to restore muscular tone to the colon and rectum.

Among the causes of *procidentia recti* in children, is given that of allowing the child to sit upon the chamber utensil for an indefinite period, as practiced by many mothers and nurses.

Space will not allow us to even hint at the many good and practical things said about pruritus, impaction of fæces, cancer, rodent or lupoid ulcer, neuralgia, and villous tumor of the rectum. In two cases the coccyx was removed with benefit, for pain in the sacro-coccygeal joints.

All the subjects treated of are fully illustrated with cases taken from practice, which aid greatly the understanding and interest of the reader.

Mr. Allingham has practiced his specialty to some purpose, and too strong words of commendation cannot be used in praise of this book which embodies his experience.   A. J. S.

HANDBOOK FOR THE PHYSIOLOGICAL LABORATORY. By E. Kline, M. D., and others, edited by J. Burdon-Sanderson, M. D., F. R. S. Philadelphia : Lindsay & Blakiston.

[For Sale by the St. Louis Book & News Co]

(Notice continued of this valuable book from page 457 of the August Number.)

Inflammation of Epithelium :—The examination of the cornea is made at various dates after abrasion and irritation of the surface. After suitable preparation sections are made in both directions, and from this method : " Evidence is thus obtained, (1) of the divisions of the nuclei of the epithelial cells, (2) of the overgrowth of the bodies of the cells, and (3) of their subsequent division."

Epithelium and Endothelium of Ovary :—" It has been recently shown by Waldeyer that the ovary is only partly covered with peritoneum.   *   *   *   The remainder of the surface possesses a cylindrical epithelium." p. 147. Also, reference is made to this fact in the April number of this JOURNAL, page 211.

In Inflammation of bone, " the lacunæ are seen to contain groups of young cells instead of the ordinary branched cells."

Fibrin :—" Although the circulating blood contains either in its colored corpuscles or plasma, both the fibrin factors (paraglobulin, and fibrinogen), *i. e.,* the immediate principles necessary for its coagulation, it does not coagulate. In other words, the blood, so long as it forms part of the normal living body, contains no fibrin.   *   *   *   It can be proved experimentally : (1) that blood does not coagulate in the living heart or in a living bloodvessel, even when the circulation is arrested ; (2) that although normal blood ordinarily coagulates as soon as it is withdrawn from the body, there are certain circumstances under which the act of coagulation either does not take place or is accomplished in so imperfect a manner, that the clot is scarcely recognizable as such."

Vasomotor Nervous System :—The vascular nerves together with the *automatic centre* from which they radiate constitute the vasomotor nervous system. " That there is a vasomotor centre, and that it is intracranial, we learn by observing first, that if the medulla is divided immediately below the cerebellum, all the arteries are relaxed, and, that a similar effect is produced if certain afferent nerve fibres, which lead to the intracranial part of the cord, are excited. Its position has been lately determined with great precision in the rabbit by Ludwig and Owsjannikow, who have found by experiments, to which further reference will be made, that it is limited towards the spinal cord by a line four or five millimetres above the *calamus scriptorius*, and extends towards the brain to within a millimetre of the *corpora quadrigemina*.

"That the vasomotor centre is in constant automatic action is shown by the paralysing effect of section, whether of the spinal cord or of any nerve known to contain vascular fibres. If the action of the centre were not constant, division could not produce arterial relaxation. In relation to this constancy of action the word *tonus* is used. Arterial tonus means that degree of contraction of an artery which is constant and normal. It is maintained only so long as the artery is in communication with the vasomotor center." p. 244.

Vasomotor functions of the Splanchnic Nerves:— "When one of the splanchnic nerves is divided in the rabbit, the arterial pressure sinks; on electrical excitation of the divided nerve, it rises to a height which far exceeds the normal limits. * * * The reduction of pressure after section is attended with *increase*, the elevation of pressure after excitation, with *decrease*, of the frequency of the pulse." "The following numerical results are derived from one of Ludwig and Cyon's experiments: Previous arterial pressure, 90 millimetres; after division of left splanchnic, 41 mil.; during excitation of peripheral and of divided nerve, 115 mil.; after division of right splanchnic, 31 mil. After division of both nerves, the vessels of all the abdominal viscera are seen to be dilated."

Incompetency of the Tricuspid Valve:—" The most important of these conditions (which render the valve incompetent) is over-distension of the ventricle by which the ostium becomes too large to be covered by the valve. When this occurs during life, the phenomenon known as venous pulse presents itself. The right ventricle being still in communication with the ven-

33

ous system at the moment that it hardens, blood is injected by it backwards. When in the human subject this condition is permanent, it leads, first, to dilatation of the great veins, and, second, to similar incompetence of the vein-valves nearest the heart. In such persons two large swellings are seen on either side of the neck—the distended jugular veins—which pulsate nearly synchronously with the heart." p. 268.

Endocardial Pressure:—The introduction of an India-rubber bag, or ampulla, with a long stem, into one or other of the cavities of the heart, of the horse for instance, "can be effected in the horse, as I can testify from my own observation, without occasioning the animal the slightest suffering or inconvenience —a fact easily enough understood when we reflect that the internal surface of the vascular system is not supplied with sensory nerves." M. Chauveau "has shown that in the horse the interval between the hardening of the auricle and that of the ventricle is just about one-tenth of a second, and that the duration of the ventricular systole is about three-tenths, whatever be the number of contractions per minute; so that frequency of the pulse depends not on the time taken by the heart to accomplish each contraction, but on the interval of relaxation which separates one systole from its successor." The *relative* values of pressure in the horse is about 128 millimetres in the left ventricle, and 25 millimetres in the right.

Apnœa :—"When the blood is saturated with oxygen, respiratory movements cease, and the animal is said to be in a state of apnœa." The heart beats regularly, the eye answers to stimuli, but there are no respiratory movements. This term was first applied to this condition in 1864, by Rosenthal.

Dyspnœa is dependent on defect of oxygen :—It has been found "that the blood of an animal which before breathing nitrogen contained 18.8 per cent. per vol. of oxygen (at 760 millim. and 0°C.), contained after breathing nitrogen for one minute *a mere trace of oxygen* (0.8 per cent.); during the same period the carbonic acid gas had diminished from 47.2 per cent. to 39.4 per cent. These experiments are referred to here on account of their fundamental importance. They are much too difficult for repetition."

Animal Heat :—The temperature of the body· is dependent upon the relative activity of two processes, viz: heat producing and heat destroying. "The subject admits of being correspondingly divided into two parts—the study of the processes, and the study of the resulting state. The former is based on the measurement of the quantity of heat set free at the surface during a given period (calorimetry); the second on the measuremont of the temperature existing in the circulating blood and the tissue at the moment of observation (thermometry)." Frankland has found "that one gramme of albumen, in undergoing complete combustion into water, carbonic acid and ammonia, produces heat enough to raise 4998 grammes of water one degree centigrade. This fact we express by stating that 4998 is the heat value of albumen. In like manner Frankland has found the heat value of lean beef to be 5103, and of the fat 9069.

Tetanus.—The cure of Tetanus:

Obs. I.   *   *   * "Tetanus from an ordinary interrupted current is a continued contraction rapidly reaching a maximum, continuing (within limits) in that condition so long as the current is passing, and followed by a gradual relaxation upon the current being cut off." "Tetanus really consists of a series of simple muscular contractions fused together." pp. 371-372.

Obs. IV.—   *   *   * "By contraction, especially by tetanus, irritability of a muscle is diminished; after a period of rest the irritability returns even in a muscle removed from the blood-current."

Obs. X.—"During contraction, muscle becomes acid."

Obs. XI.—"During contraction, the temperature of the muscle rises."

The experiments in detail are given in each of the observations.

Digestion. Peptones:—Albumen is absorbed in very minute quantities, because "it will hardly diffuse through animal membranes. The peptones into which the albuminous substances are converted, on the contrary, diffuse very readily, and are thus easily absorbed. The gelatinous substances in the food are also changed somewhat by the gastric juice, so that after they have been acted on by it they no longer gelatinize." The change of starch into sugar continues. (Digestion in the stomach, p. 475.)

There are several kinds of peptones, with various reactions.

Pepsin :—"The strength of acid with which albuminous bod‑ ies are most quickly digested by pepsin varies with the nature of the body, and also with the amount of pepsin present."

"There seems indeed, to be a definite relation between the amount of pepsin and the strength of the acid, though what this is has not yet been determined. * * It can be shown that digestion is hindered when the acid is either too weak or too strong." "*A stronger acid is required for digestion if the pro‑ ducts of digestion are present in quantity in the solution.*"

"The stomach is not digested during life, because the alkali‑ nity of its walls is preserved by the circulation of blood in them."

Bile Pigments :—"The yellow color of fresh bile in man and carnivora is due to a coloring matter termed *bilirubin* (bilifulvin, biliphain, colepyrrbin, hematoidin, $C_{16}H_{18}N_2O_3$); the green color possessed by bile in herbivera, or acquired by the bile of carnivora after standing is due to *biliverdin*, a product of oxidation of the former." Bile appears to aid the absorption of fat, and emulsionizes it. "It is doubtful, however, whether it is to this property (emulsionizing) that the absorption is due."

Actions of Pancreatic Juice:—" 1, It emulsionizes fat; 2, it decomposes fats, liberating fatty acids; 3, it converts starch into sugar; 4, it digests fibrin, forming peptones, and afterwards decomposes them—leucine and tyrocine being produced."

Actions of Intestinal Juice :—1, It converts starch into sugar; 2, it converts cane sugar into grape sugar."

The secretions, milk and urine are treated in the XXXVIII chapter; and the last chapter is composed of "Practical Notes on Manipulation." Such is a very imperfect notice of some of the facts set forth (nearly all of which are accompanied with the methods of demonstration) in this very valuable, and to the practical physiologist, indispensable work. It is emphatically *a work of facts* and *demonstration*. Very few typographical errors are found. The publisher's work is well done with the exception mentioned above.   H. Z. G.

THE PRACTICE OF SURGERY. By Thomas Bryant, F. R. C. S., Surgeon to Guy's Hospital. With over five hundred illustrations. 8 vo., pp. 976. Philadelphia: Henry C. Lea.

[For Sale by the St Louis Book & News Co.]

In the Introduction we have a chapter devoted to the general principles of Diagnosis, in which there is also given, at the close of the chapter, special points for observation. These latter are well selected and arranged, either for reference or commitment.

Chapter I is on Repair and Inflammation. The doctrines set forth on these subjects being common to other late works it is unnecessary to farther notice them here.

The second chapter treats of Traumatic Fever, Septicæmia and Pyæmia, and is well arranged and written. We are glad to see among other remedies recommended, under the head of Treatment, quinine in large doses, for pyæmia and septicæmia.

Chapter III is on Trismus and Tetanus. Here again quinine in large doses is favorably mentioned; and we may take this occasion to remark that our English brethren are learning to appreciate quinine in much larger doses than has heretofore been practiced by them: they are moving in a direction in which it must be conceded we have been the leaders.

Chapter IV treats of Delirium Tremens. Opium in some form is with the author still at the head of the list of remedies; Hydrate of chloral is mentioned as giving promise of usefulness We had supposed its utility in this direction demonstrated.

The next department of the work is devoted to the Surgery of the Nervous System, which we are not allowed the space to review in detail. It is full and complete in subject matter, excluding, very properly, such specialties as the eye, ear, and dental surgery. There are many new illustrations introduced, which the author informs us were obtained principally from Guy's. They are generally good. The arrangement is well designed for easy and speedy reference. The style of composition is in many respects excellent, the gravest criticism upon the work being that it is not sufficiently authoritative for a text book: the author's opinion not being expressed in sufficiently definite and positive language.

We find but few inaccuracies. On page 600 the credit of bringing the operation for *vesico-vaginal fistulæ* to its present state of perfection is divided between Sims and Bozeman, in America; and Simpson and Brown, in England. Again, of the duck-bill speculum, "by some author's it is known as Bozeman's, by others Sims'." We think this attributable rather to inadvertance than a disposition to distribute the credit justly due J. Marion Sims to others. The work is an aequisition to our literature on the subject, on account of the many original observations and illustrations it contains. The mechanical execution of the work is excellent.

MANUAL OF CHEMICAL ANALYSIS, as applied to the examination of medicinal chemicals. A guide for the determination of their identity and quality, and for the detection of impurities and adulterations, for the use of pharmaceutists, physicians, druggists and manufacturing chemists. By Frederick Hoffman, P. H. D., Pharmaceutist in New York. D. Appleton & Co., 549 and 551 Broadway. 1873. pp. 498, 8 vo.

[For Sale by the St. Louis Book & News Co.]

The work before us is one especially convenient for reference; brief, yet sufficiently full and clear for most of the analyses necessary to detect the quality as to purity of nearly all the substances used by the pharmaceutist. The methods are generally uncomplicated; and numerous tables are supplied for reference. A number of the figures are duplicated, 48 and 47 being the same; also 51 and 60, and 55, 58 and 71, and others several times repeated. Of course this is, as we think, unnecessary. It is gotten up in good style.

ON STRICTURES OF THE URETHRA, results of operation with the dilating urethrotome, with cases. By F. N. Otis, M. D., Clinical Professor of genito-urinary diseases, College of Physicians and Surgeons, New York. A pamphlet of twenty pages. New York: D. Appleton & Co. -

In this *brochure* the author claims that the slightest abnormal encroachment upon the calibre of the urethra, and even such slight plastic infiltration as interferes with the suppleness of its walls without diminishing its calibre, may perpetuate existing urethral discharges and even excite them *de novo*.

He justly, we think, claims that the bougie à boule is the only instrument capable of detecting strictures of large calibre or a number of strictures in the same urethra. The divulsing instruments of Thompson, Holt, and Voillemier are incapable of rupturing these strictures; the urethrotome of Maisonneuve passes through them without cutting them completely, if at all, yet they keep up a urethral discharge.

Dr. Otis has devised a dilating urethrotome, with which he dilates the stricture to No. 26 English scale if necessary, passes the bulbous sound, which is part of the instrument, and, ascertaining the exact site and length of the stricture, divides it.

The Doctor was surprised to find that strictures divided in this manner were *cured.* He had a committee of experts to examine his cases with the bulbous sound and they were unable to detect any abnormal condition of the urethra. Though formerly a friend of the endoscope, he now regards it as a mischievous instrument in the treatment of chronic urethral discharges. He has found that the granular condition seen with the endoscope depends upon bands of stricture which may be permanently relieved by division only.

He believes that the divulsing and cutting instruments in common use do not completely sunder the stricture, hence its return.

In the cases operated upon the sound was occasionally passed till the incisions healed, and then discontinued.

The Doctor thinks the stricture tissue is removed in the following way: When the stricture is so completely sundered, and by subsequent dilatation a space is filled with new material, when contraction takes place, it does so at the expense of the new material, producing a greater separation of the sundered ends. "Hence the reënforcement of the stricture, by additional plastic material, diminishes until, by the natural tendency to absorption of foreign or surperfluous tissue, the stricture tissue gradually and completely disappears." T. H. H.

BOOKS AND PAMPHLETS RECEIVED.

CONTRIBUTIONS TO PRACTICAL SURGERY. By George W. Norris, M. D. Philadelphia: Lindsay & Blakiston. For sale in St. Louis by the new Medical Book Store of Gray, Baker & Co., 407 North 4th st. Price $4.

DICTIONARY OF PHARMACEUTICAL SCIENCE, containing a concise explanation of the various subjects and terms of pharmacy. Designed as a guide for the pharmaceutist, druggist, physician, etc. By H. V. Sweringen. Philadelphia : Lindsay & Blakiston. For sale by Gray, Baker & Co., 407 North 4th st., St. Louis. Price, cloth $6; sheep $7.

STATISTICAL REPORT OF TWO HUNDRED AND FIFTY-FIVE CASES OF DISEASES OF THE EAR. By H. N. Spencer, M. D. A reprint from the Transactions of Medical Society of Missouri. St. Louis : R. P. Studley Company, Printers.

CLINICAL NOTES ON NERVOUS DISEASES OF WOMEN. By Wm. B. Neftel, M. D. New York: G. P. Putnam's Sons.

TRANSACTIONS OF THE MEDICAL SOCIETY OF CALIFORNIA, for 1872 and 1873. Sacramento: T. A. Springer, State printer.

REFRACTION AND ACCOMMODATION. A Review of Dr. D. S. Reynold's Critique. By C. S. Fenner, M. D. A reprint from the *American Practitioner*, Aug., 1873. Louisville : John A. Morton & Co.

TETANUS AND TETANOID AFFECTIONS, WITH CASES. By B. Roemer, M. D. Reprinted from the ST. LOUIS MEDICAL AND SURGICAL JOURNAL, St. Louis: E. F. Hobart & Co. pp. 96 Price $1.00. To be obtained at the bookstores.

TRANSACTIONS OF THE ACADEMY OF SCIENCES OF ST. LOUIS. Vol. III. No. 1. R. P. Studley Company. Price $1.00.

TRANSACTIONS OF THE MEDICAL SOCIETY OF WEST VIRGINIA, for 1873. Wheeling: Frew, Hagans and Hall.

OPHTHALMIC SURGERY, Recent improvements in. By D. S. Reynolds, M. D. Louisville : John P. Morton & Co.

INFANT'S MANAGEMENT, Special rules for. During the hot season. By the Obstetrical Society of Philadelphia. Philadelphia : Collins.

MERCURY, Therapeutic effects and uses of. By Wm. H. Doughty. Atlanta, Ga.: W. R. Barrow.

MEMORIAL OF THE AMERICAN MEDICAL ASSOCIATION, concerning the rank of the Medical Corps of the U. S. A. To Congress.

CHILDREN, Proper Treatment of. Being the annual discourse before the Mass. Medical Society, June, 1878. By Charles E. Buckingham, M. D. Boston: A. Williams & Co.

A REVIEW of Dr. Fenner's pamphlet on Accommodation and Refraction. By Dudley S. Reynolds, M. D.

AN EYE CASE IN THE COURTS. By O. A. Robertson, A. M. (Harvard), M. D., etc., etc. Albany: Argus Co., printers.

BRAITHWAITE'S RETROSPECT OF PRACTICAL MEDICINE AND SURGERY. Half yearly part for July. For sale by the St. Louis Book & News Co. Price 1.50.

OSSICLES OF THE EAR, MEMBRANA TYMPANI, Mechanism of. By H. Helmholtz ; translated by A. H. Buch, M. D., and Normand Smith, M. D. New York: Wm. Wood & Co. For sale by Gray, Baker & Co., 407 North 4th street, St. Louis.

SKIN DISEASES, Their description, pathology, diagnosis and treatment. By Tilbury Fox, M. D., London. Second American from third London edition. Re-written and enlarged. New York: Wm. Wood & Co. For sale by Gray, Baker & Co., 407 North 4th st., St. Louis.

URINARY ANALYSIS, Guide to. By Henry G. Piffard, M. D. New York: Wm. Wood & Co. For sale by Gray, Baker & Co.

LAW AND INTELLIGENCE IN NATURE, and the improvement of the race in accordance with law. By A. B. Palmer, A. M., M. D., etc.

THE MEDICAL REGISTER AND DIRECTORY OF THE UNITED STATES, systematically arranged by States. By Joseph M. Toner, M. D., and S. W. Butler, M. D.

Of this work we have received advanced leaves for Alabama, including a brief sketch of the history and geography, mineral springs, medical institutions, hospitals and infirmaries, the medical laws of the State, also the medical societies, then follows the names of the physicians of the State in alphabetical order. Every physician should facilitate this invaluable enterprise by filling out and returning to Dr. Butler, a circular as soon as the same may be received.

Extracts from Current Medical Literature.

What is Cincho-Quinine?

This question is often asked by physicians who have not been made acquainted with the nature of this important agent, and therefore we republish the following article, which appeared in the JOURNAL in June, 1869, and which presents in a clear and explicit manner its nature and uses:

The chemical manipulation of the Cinchona or Peruvian barks reveals the presence in them of quite a number of most remarkable, complex bodies. No vegetable production, except the poppy, affords such a marvellous combination of valuable medicinal principles as the *loxa* and *calisaya* barks, and no substances have been studied with greater care or more intense interest by chemists. Nothing short of the subtle chemical forces controlled by the Infinite One, could construct from the elements of the earth and air a bitter principle like quinia, or those other agents associated in bark, so closely allied to it physically and chemically. A handful of the finely comminuted fibres of the yellow-bark, which resembles physically a dozen other varieties, is made to yield by the chemist, when treated with aqueous and alcoholic liquids and acids, a dark, bitter solution, unattractive in taste and appearance. If the process is skilfully conducted, or exhaustive in its results, there remains, beside the solution, a portion of woody fibre, inert and almost tasteless. It holds considerable coloring and some waxy matter, together with a little tannin; but the active chemical or medicinal principles have been removed, and are held in the dark liquid. The exhausted bark is not entirely worthless, for it may be dried and used as fuel. But what of the dark liquid? From this the chemist obtains, besides other substances, a portion of beautiful, white, silky crystals; not wholly of one distinct kind, but of several, all of which possess about equal chemical and therapeutical importance. No wonder it seems to the uninitiated in chemical manipulation a difficult work to perform. It is, however, quite easy to the thoroughly instructed. The first principle isolated may be the quinia. This is not held in the bark in its naked alkaloidal condition, but locked up, in the form of a salt, with another principle called *kinic acid*. In the bark it is *kinate of quinine*. We isolate the quinia, tear it from its embrace with kinic acid, throw that away, force it into a kind of matrimonial alliance with sulphuric acid, and in this condition of *sulphate of quinia*, use it as a medicine. This kinic acid marries into several other families resident in the bark, prominent among which are *cinchonia, cinchonidia, quinidia*, etc. Precisely how many of these alkaloidal principles the different kinds of barks contain, is unknown; but it is safe to assume that there are as many as four others which, although not distinctly pointed out, are tolerably well recognized. These *kinates* are all *kindred* in nature, and all labor to the same end, when isolated and set to work as therapeutical agents in the human system.

In one hundred ounces of good yellow bark, we obtain about two and three-fourths ounces of quinia, and two ounces of cinchonia, with variable amounts of the other principles, but less than the two named. It is to be regretted that we cannot remove the different families of kinates from the bark in their natural state of saline combination. It seems reasonable to suppose their action upon the system would be more salutary than in other forms. It is easy to isolate the kinic acid, and having the alkaloids, the kinates of quinia, cinchonia, etc., can be re-formed; but in these chemical changes so much disturbance to natural organic combinations is made, that, practically, we realize no marked advantages. It seems unnatural to force a natural alkaloidal base out of its association with an organic acid, and re-combine it with a mineral acid. This we do in the preparation of the sulphate of quinia. However, as it has served so good a purpose for many years, it is not best to quarrel with the theory.

All the alkaloids of bark possess about equal febrifuge and tonic properties, when isolated and administered in that condition. This has been proved over and over again by all competent chemists and physicians, from Drs. Gomez, Duncan, Pelletier, Caventou, down to the time of Liebig's researches, a quarter of a century ago, and from that time to the present by a hundred careful chemical and medical observers.

How the one alkaloid, quinia, came to supersede the others,

and drive them into the background, is easily understood, when we remember that it was about the first that was distinctly eliminated, studied, and experimented with; and the *éclat* it acquired caused everything else to be neglected. The natural bark, holding all the alkaloids, the quinia, cinchonia, quinidia, etc., has always been observed to produce more efficient and prompt results, both as a tonic and febrifuge, than the quinia, or either of the other principles in themselves; but holding also, as it does, tannin, gum, starch, fibrine, and coloring matter, all of which are medicinally interfering or inert, its use is rendered inconvenient and inadmissible in many cases. Besides, it is apt to produce disturbance of the gastric functions of an unpleasant character. Acting upon the idea that the natural alkaloidal principles of bark, in their simple, unchanged condition, separated from the gross, woody, and other matters, would better subserve all therapeutical ends than the barks themselves, or *any one* of the alkaloids separately employed, Cincho-Quinine has been prepared.

The Ophthalmoscope in Mental and Cerebral Diseases. Mr. Aldridge. Also, *The Sphygmograph in Lunatic Asylum Practice.* Mr. Thompson. *West Riding Reports.* 1872. By T. W. Fisher, M.D.

Passing by all questions relating to home, cottage or hospital treatment, for the sake of abbreviation; also, the subjects of mechanical restraint and separate asylums for habitual drunkards and criminal insane, we come at once to the strictly medical treatment of insanity. The above subjects will be found fully discussed in the first two documents mentioned. That important part of treatment which consists in the personal moral influence of the physician over his patient, hardly admits of consideration in this place.

Dr. Blanford believes thoroughly in the efficacy of medical treatment in insanity, and is supported by the great majority of practical alienists. This belief has a sure foundation in the fact of the physical basis of all mental disorder. Dr. Blanford treats very satisfactorily of diet and bathing. He advocates forcible feeding for patients who refuse their food because of supposed dyspepsia, with a foul tongue, fœtid breath and loaded bowels. Dyspepsia is almost always the *result*, and not the *cause* of nervous depression. The fullest diet, with stimulants, often effects a speedy cure. (See page 206.) That a full diet is required in most cases might be inferred from the impoverished state of the blood, as shown by examination. (See *Lancet*, May 3, 1873, on the Histology of the Blood in 143 Insane.) The proper method of forced alimentation is discussed at length (pp. 215 to 224). Dr. Moxey, in *Lancet*, May 31, 1873, defends his "Nasal Method of Enforced Alimentation." It is a pity such methods cannot be availed of for the thousands of patients, in ordinary practice, who slowly and persistently starve themselves. For a very able analysis of the most common form of voluntary starvation, see the paper of Dr. Lesé- gue on Hysterical Anorexia (*Archives Générales*, April, 1873.) It is beyond question that patients are constantly allowed to die of simple starvation through a slipshod expectancy in treatment. In hospitals, the much-dreaded bugbears of mechanical restraint and enforced feeding save more lives than any other single agencies.

Of bathing, Dr. Blanford speaks in qualified praise. He thinks there is risk of too great depression from hot baths of long duration, as used by the French. He prefers, in mania, a bath of 92°, and suggests allowing it to cool while the patient is in it, thus avoiding shock. Dr. Lockhart Robertson strongly advocates the wet sheet in recent mania, frequently applied and long continued. Dr. Blanford intimates that a large part of the benefit derived is from the very efficient mechanical restraint it affords. Dr. Wilkins comes to the conclusion, in his report, that baths are over-estimated, and perhaps abused, in France, and too much neglected in this country. Dr. Skae, of Edinburg, and Dr. Blanche, of Paris, have, after years of experiment, discontinued the warm bath in acute mania, on account of occasional fatal results.

Tonics, stimulants and laxatives are required in most cases of insanity. The underlying diathesis should be medically treated also. On the use of sedatives, some difference of opinion exists, though most alienists rely on them largely, and with good results. No doubt, they are open to great abuse, as Dr. Maudsley affirms, especially when the chemical restraint of drugs is substituted for a rational use of mechanical restraint, as is the case in some English hospitals under the pressure of popular feeling.

Opium must still retain the first place in the treatment of melancholia of the subacute form. It has a directly curative effect which chloral has not. Dr. Wolff bases its use on sphygmographic indications, which show that a full dose, after a short period of irritation, acts by paralyzing the vaso-motor nerves. Its use is followed by general relaxation, cessation of agitation, diminish painful nervous sensations, and by psychical and corporeal calm. The dose should be carefully individualized, and should be small when the pulse is already slow and venous system relaxed, as in old age, paralysis, fatty heart, etc.

Chloral is universally employed as the most valuable known hypnotic. It is better suited to cases where excitement exists, though it produces sleep in cases of depression. It may be given to advantage by the rectum. Dr. Madden prefers it to opium in puerperal mania, in doses of from ten to thirty grains. (*Brit. and For. Med.-Chir. Rev.*, Oct., 1871.) Mr. Aldridge examined three patients under the influence of chloral, and found, first, increased vascularity of the retina, followed by anæmia, the condition characteristic of healthy sleep, thus confirming Dr. Hammond's observations (On the Physiological Effects and Therapeutical Uses of Chloral, *N. Y. Med. Journal*, Feb., 1870). Though the treatment of mania is assisted by chloral, the disease seems to run a definite though modified course in spite of it. Hence the objection to pushing the remedy to extremes, with a view to cut short the disease, as is often attempted in ordinary practice. I have good reason to know the frequency and danger of this error. Dr. Maudsley, in his address before the Royal College of Physicians, August, 1871, referring to the use and abuse of sedatives, says he is opposed to giving chloral every three or four hours, and reserves its use for bedtime.

Of the extreme value of the *bromides*, especially in epilepsy, perhaps enough has been said in the medical journals of late. For their physiological effects, the reader is referred to the papers mentioned and to Drs. Clarke and Amory's recent monograph.

Hyoscyamus is a valuable and reliable sedative; belladonna is less so, and cannabis indica least of all, though Dr. Clouston strongly recommends the latter in combination with bromide of potassium.

Conium has recently been largely experimented with, and its

effects on the temperature and pulse carefully noted. Dr. J. Crichton Brown finds it of great value in mania from its effect on the motor centres. He has observed that the corpora striata participate in the usual vinous staining in patches seen in death from exhaustive mania. He thinks it soothes the irritated and exhausted centres of motor activity, without affecting the mental excitement directly. He finds the average duration of treatment, in twelve cases of recovery from mania treated by conium, to be one hundred and two days; in twelve cases treated by other sedatives one hundred and fifty days. Dr. Kitchen demonstrates, by thermometer and sphygmograph, its effect in reducing the temperature and pulse, and gives cases showing its effect on muscular activity.

Ergot was found useful by Dr. Brown in (1) recurrent mania, (2) chronic mania with lucid intervals, (3) epileptic mania. Dr. Kitchen used it to advantage in headaches, both from plethora and anæmia of cerebral vessels, in mania, epilepsy and delirium tremens. He gave it in half dram doses of the fluid extract, or three to six grains of ergotine before meals. He found it did not effect the temperature, but increased the frequency and tension of the pulse. It was shown by Mr. Aldridge to contract the minute arteries of the retina when taken continuously for several days.

Nitrite of Amyl was found to increase the size of the small arteries when at the height of its action.

The use of the ophthalmoscope becomes more and more evident as observations accumulate. The work of Dr. Allbutt, noticed by Dr. Jeffries in his late Report on the Progress of Ophthalmology, will serve as a text-book for the general practitioner, to be supplemented by the more recent investigations of Dr. Noyes, Mr. Aldridge and other observers. No space is left to speak of electricity in its application to mental disease. All the text-books on electro-therapeutics, except that of Drs. Rockwell and Beard, give a chapter to this subject. Electricity is certainly valuable in treating such complications as neuralgia and paralysis, and as a general tonic. Its direct application to the head, with a view to definite effects upon the brain, must be considered as rather empirical at present.—*Boston Medical and Surgical Journal.*

Infant Mortality in England. '

On the occasion of opening a new hospital for children at Pendlebury (Eng.), the Bishop of Manchester gave some curious statistics on this subject. In the North of England only 7 per cent. of children under one year die annually; whereas in Manchester and Liverpool, nearly 28 per cent., or nearly four times that number, die in the same period. Out of 41,805 deaths in Manchester in four years—1868 to 1871 inclusive—the number of deaths of children under five years was 20,025, or 48 per cent. "It was not," adds the Bishop, "for him to say, what he was not competent to say, to what extent—by the exercise of the powers entrusted to the municipal authorities of closing houses that were positively unfitted for human habitation—that infant mortality might be mitigated."—*Boston Med. and Surg. Jour.*

Use of Collodion in Erysipelas.

Dr. Broca recommends painting with collodion over the healthy skin, all along the edges of the inflamed surface, and over a space at least six to eight centimetres in breadth.—*Ibid.*

The Value of Oatmeal.

La France Medicale informs us that M. Dujardin-Beaumitz, having obtained a large quantity of meal from Scotland, has been experimenting with it, young children being the subjects of the experiments. He observes that without speaking of the *bouillies* (porridge?) and cakes which the Scotch prepare from the meal, it is employed by them as food for young children, although the form in which it is said to be so used appears somewhat novel to such of us as have been a good many years absent from "the land o' cakes," namely, a jelly prepared by macerating a tablespoonful of the meal in a glass of water for twelve hours, then straining through a sieve, boiling till the whole assumes the consistence of jelly, and adding sugar or salt according to taste. According to analysis, 100 grammes of the meal contain gr. 8.7 of water, 7.5 of fatty matters, 64 of starch, 12.2 of nitrogenous matters, 1.5 of mineral substances, and 7.6 of cellulose, dextrine and loss. Its nutritious value, therefore, as food for children, in regard to azotic or plastic elements, and such as are "respiratory," is analogous to human milk, or that of a cow. Besides these, it contains more iron than do most of the ordinary articles of food.

M. Beaumitz had fed four newly-born infants on the preparation just described, and in all of these with satisfactory results.
He considers that in addition to its quality as food, it acts
efficiently against colic and diarrhœa. It enters into the composition of the Syrup of Luther, which is said to be much used
in Germany. M. Gillette, surgeon of the hospital of Melun,
has also given oatmeal "combined with cow's milk," to six
chrildren, and his experiments have proved how that food may
be valuable in cases where the natural supply of milk is deficient.
He adds that the nearer the infant approaches its first year, the
more does alimentation by oatmeal appear to be profitable.—
Med. and Surg. Reporter.

Transmission of Cholera to Animals.

Dr. Leo Popoff has published (*Berliner Klin. Wochensch.*, Aug.
12, 1872) a series of experiments performed upon dogs with the
idea of demonstrating the possibility of inoculating these animals by means of cholera-excrementa. He first carefully observed the effect of introducing putrid animal matter into the
blood, and then demonstrated how these lesions differ from the
characteristic symptoms of cholera in the dog. This difference
is most striking in the *post-mortem* changes, consisting in hæmorrhagic inflammation of the stomach and intestines, and ulcerations
of the lymphatic glandular apparatus of the intestine. Where
the experiment employed was fresh, the disease produced corresponded perfectly to the symptoms of cholera. Where the
material introduced had been allowed to stand several days,
the symptoms produced were partly those of cholera, and
partly those following the introduction of putrid matter.

The conclusions arrived at by Dr. Popoff are :—

1. That cholera may be produced in animals through inoculation by means of cholera-excrementa, the vomited matter, or
even of the urine of patients suffering from this disease.

2. That when the excrementa have stood for some time, the
symptoms produced are not altogether pathognomic of cholera,
but resemble, in part, the effect produced by the introduction of
any putrid animal matter into the economy.

3. That the severity of the symptoms depends in a degree
upon the freshness of the excrementa.

4. The infection may take place from the introduction of

34

the *materies morbi* immediately into the blood, *i. e.*, without coming in contact with the intestine.

5. The characteristic symptoms of cholera poisoning in animals are produced, not immediately after the introduction of the poison into the economy, but only after the lapse of a fixed interval from one to three days.—*Boston Med. and Sur. Jour.*

Homœopathic Pilules.

The most careful chemical analyses have failed to demonstrate the presence of either aconite, atropia, or belladonna in pilules which professedly contained in one hundred parts one part by weight of the drug. Comparative experiments showed that $\frac{1}{8000}$ of a grain of aconite would have been detected with certainty. This corresponds to about $\frac{1}{160}$ of a grain of the extract of aconite; while the quantity which should have been present is from $\frac{1}{4}$ to nearly one grain, or more than one hundred times more. Similarly, $\frac{1}{8000}$ of a grain of atropia would have been discovered,—twenty-four times as much was supposed to exist in the preparation.

We would certainly be obliged to place cures, should there be any following the use of such pilules, entirely to the credit of the imagination.—*The Medical Times.*

Nature of Mumps.

In a note on the above, read to the Academy of Sciences by Claude Bernard, the author, Dr. Bouchut, states that parotitis is simply a salivary retension due to catarrhal inflammation of the excreting canal of the parotid.—*London Lancet.*

Night-Sweats of Phthisis.

In some valuable notes of practice in the Bellevue Hospital, New York, published in the *Medical Record* of that city, we find that for the relief of the above exceedingly troublesome symptom some patients are taking $\frac{1}{80}$ of a grain of sulphate of atropia in solution *ter in die*; some are taking $\frac{1}{160}$ of a grain at bedtime, and the success of this mode of treatment has already been sufficient to entitle it to further trial. Another plan of treating these night-sweats is also practised. It consists in taking the patient out of bed, if found sweating profusely in the night, sponging him with water as hot as he can comfortably bear, and, after being wiped dry and having his flannels replaced, putting him back to bed. It is stated that sometimes a single sponging will arrest the sweating for two or three days. In the French hospitals, according to a recently published thesis of M. Finot (*Rev. des Sciences Med.*), agaric, tincture of aconite, phosphate of lime, etc., are employed for the same purpose. The reporter in the latter periodical, M. Rabuteau, speaks highly of the efficacy of phosphate of lime.—*Med. Times.*

Battle-Field Surgery.

According to M. Langenbeck, the intervention of the military surgeon should begin immediately after a battle, and at the latest before the end of the second day, whether for amputation or conservation—operations should be performed within twenty-four hours; immobilisation practised by means of apparatus. For gunshot wounds in the shoulder joint, elbow, and foot, secondary resections may be permitted, but for those in the hip and knee-joints, and all articulations much disorganised, prompt resection is necessary, care being taken by making a longitudinal incision to preserve the periosteum.— *The Doctor.*

Obituary.

Dr. James W. Clemens, Professor of Physiology in the St. Louis Medical College, died August 7, at Arcadia, Mo. Our readers of 1866 and 1867 will well remember that the late Dr. Clemens was one of the *associate editors* of this journal during those years. Not alone his colleagues in the college, or the St. Louis Medical Society, of which he was a highly esteemed member, but the profession of the city and country at large sustain a loss in the untimely death of Dr. Clemens, which will be deeply felt and earnestly deplored by all who knew him.

At a meeting of the St. Louis Medical Society (and other
members of the profession) the following expressions of appreciation of the deceased, and condolence with his deeply afflicted
family, were adopted:

On motion of Dr. McPheeters, Dr. J. B. Johnson was appointed
Chairman and Dr. J. S. B. Alleyne, Secretary. The Chairman
alluded to his intimate acquaintance with the deceased, paying
a high tribute to his culture, in point of noble, amiable traits of
character, as well as scientific attainments.

As the Doctor's remarks were entirely extemporaneous (as
was the case with Dr. Prewitt and others who heartily concurred) we cannot give them in full.

Dr. Thomas Kennard submitted the following:

"MR. PRESIDENT—After a long, painful and most trying illness,
our friend and fellow-member, Dr. James W. Clemens, has been
relieved from his suffering. With a constitution gradually
undermined by physical suffering, and a mind over-taxed by
study, he succumbed to the laws of nature, and at last found
rest, but sad to say, that rest is death, and it is painful for us
and for all those who were near and dear to him, whom he has
left behind, to realize the fact that for him every tie of friend-
ship, of family and kindred, has been broken, and that we, who
have known him so well, and have been so intimately associated
with him, will in future know him only by his deeds, for, my
fellow-members,

'We live in deeds, not in years; in thought, not in breaths;
In feelings, not in figures on the dial.
We should count time by heart-throbs.
He most lives who thinks most, feels noblest, acts the best '

"Our deceased friend was born in the profession. His father
was an eminent and successful practitioner of medicine, in
Wheeling, Virginia, and the son, from his boyhood, knew the
trials and troubles of a physician, but when he grew up, so
devoted was he to science, that he determined to make medicine
his life-study. He soon became zealously devoted to the study
of the profession of his choice, and dedicated to it all of his
intellectual energies, and finally sacrificed his life in its pursuit.
He was a diligent and faithful student, a hard worker, an original and accurate thinker, and, by his perseverance and mental
acquirements, has already attained a high position in the ranks

of his profession. His ability has been recognized and duly acknowledged by his appointment to the chair of Physiology in the St. Louis Medical College, which had been once filled by such an original thinker and able man as our deceased friend, Dr. John H. Watters. Dr. Clemens was a very modest man and of retiring disposition, and it was with much difficulty that his true character could be understood. He, perhaps, had fewer intimate associates in the profession than any one in our city who had attained the same degree of eminence. It is to his credit, however, that those who knew him best appreciated him the most. He was a good and devoted husband, a kind brother and an indulgent father; and whatever faults he may have had, they were not those of the heart, but of the head. His place will be very difficult to fill in the ranks of his profession, and although he was carried off in the beginning of his usefulness, he has left a name with those who knew him that will never die. He has gone to a better and a happier home; then why should we mourn his death, for that which is our loss is his gain, and we too will soon follow him to the silent grave.

> ' Our time is fixed, and all our days are numbered,
> How long, how short, we know not This we know:
> Duty requires we calmly wait the summons ' ' '

RESOLUTIONS.

On motion of Dr. Hodgen, the Chair appointed a Committee on Resolutions, consisting of Dr. Gregory, Dr. Baumgarten and Dr. Prewitt.

After an interval, Dr. Gregory reported the following resolutions, which were adopted unanimously.

WHEREAS, It has pleased an inscrutable Providence to remove from among us a professional brother of much promise, Dr. James W. Clemens, who had already attained an enviable distinction in his profession, had worked earnestly but quietly, till appreciative associates marked him as a rising man, and but for his early death was destined to reach a high position in the profession of his choice,

Resolved, That in the death of Dr. Clemens we mourn the loss of an able member of our profession, devoted to the science of medicine with an earnestness and a spirit of research characteristic of the true student, of a noble gentleman, with genuine sympathies and warm attachments.

Resolved, That we will attend his funeral in a body.

It was ordered, on motion of Dr. Kennard, that the resolutions be published in the daily papers and the medical journals of the city.

The meeting then adjourned.

The following resolutions were passed by the Faculty of the St. Louis Medical College on the occasion of the death of Prof. J. W. Clemens:

WHEREAS, By the inscrutable dispensation of an All-Wise Providence, the Faculty of the St. Louis Medical College is called upon to mourn the death of Dr. J. W. Clemens, one of its most worthy and zealous members, therefore,

Resolved, That in the death of Dr. Clemens, the medical profession has lost one of its most ardent votaries, one who, if life had been spared, would have been among its brightest ornaments and most valued members;

That as a teacher he was peculiarly efficient in his special branch of medicine, and a most useful member of the faculty from which he has been so peremptorily removed;

That as a man he was an example of all that was true and good.

Resolved, That the Faculty tenders to the family of the deceased its heartfelt sorrow at their irreparable loss.

Resolved, That these resolutions be spread on the records of the College, and that a copy be sent to the family of the deceased and published in the ST. LOUIS MEDICAL AND SURGICAL JOURNAL. J. S. B. ALLEYNE, M. D.,
Sec'y of the Faculty.

WM. TYLER SMITH, M. D., F. R. C. P., died June 2nd, of apoplexy, aged fifty-eight years.

PROF. ROMBERG, the distinguished author of the famous work on "Diseases of the Nervous System," died at Berlin, on June 16th. (*New York Med. Journal.*)

Meteorological Observations.

METEOROLOGICAL OBSERVATIONS AT ST. LOUIS, MO.

BY A. WISLIZENUS, M. D.

The following observations of daily temperature in St. Louis are made with a MAXIMUM and MINIMUM thermometer (of Green, N. Y.). The daily minimum occurs generally in the night, the maximum about 3 P M. The monthly mean of the daily minimum and maxima, added and divided by 2, gives a quite reliable mean of the monthly temperature.

THERMOMETER FAHRENHEIT.

JULY, 1873.

Day of Month.	Minimum.	Maximum.	Day of Month.	Minimum.	Maximum.
1	67.0	84.0	18	70.0	88.5
2	67.0	82.0	19	65.5	79.0
3	72.0	93.5	20	61.5	84.5
4	75.0	95.5	21	65.5	85.0
5	67.5	90.0	22	67.0	89.5
6	63.5	85.0	23	68.5	92.5
7	69.5	86.5	24	72.0	94.0
8	63.0	80.0	25	73.0	96.5
9	62.5	83.0	26	72.0	78.5
10	69.0	85.0	27	66.0	90.0
11	59.0	78.0	28	71.0	92.5
12	63.5	90.0	29	70.0	87.0
13	73.5	97.0	30	70.5	89.0
14	77.0	97.5	31	70.0	82.0
15	78.0	98.5			
16	77.0	97.5	Means	69.2	88.7
17	78.0	98.5	Monthly Mean 78.9		

Quantity of rain : 5.88 inches.

NOTICE.

INFORMATION WANTED.—Circulars calling for information for the MEDICAL REGISTER AND DIRECTORY OF THE UNITED STATES are being rapidly sent out, and this portion of the labor will soon be completed. It is earnestly desired that the responses be as prompt and as full as possible. *It is important to physicians, who have any education or standing, that they appear properly on this record*, as the work will be one of permanent value, and will be constantly referred to. The forms containing the Directory of the first set of eleven States and Territories (Alabama to Georgia, alphabetically, inclusive), are now in the hands of the printer, and there are but a few days in which informat on can be inserted in those pages.

Officers of public medical institutions of *all kinds*, hospitals, asylums, dispensaries, colleges, medical societies, etc., are particularly requested to furnish us with lists, catalogues, announcements, etc., in order to give brief histories of these institutions, and for use in perfecting the REGISTER AND DIRECTORY in all its parts.

It is intended that the work shall be exhaustive, and as nearly *correct* as may be, and it will be issued as speedily as possible; but the labor is immense, and the work is delayed by the want of promptitude in receiving replies to circulars and letters.   S. W. BUTLER, M. D.,

115 S. Seventh Street, Philadelphia, Pa.

Mortality Report.

FROM JULY 19th, 1873, TO AUG. 23d, 1873, INCLUS.

DATE	White.		Col'd		AGES.											TOTAL.
	Males.	Females.	Males	Females	Under 5 yrs	5 to 10	10 to 20	20 to 30	30 to 40	40 to 50	50 to 60	60 to 70	70 to 80	80 to 90	90 to 100	
Saturday 26	137	103	6	6	136	14	13	20	17	18	12	16	5	1	...	252
" 2	110	92	9		116	12	9	17	24	21	6	4	2		...	211
" 9	138	92	5	1	114	9	13	32	21	19	16	8	3	1	...	236
" 16	110	88	3	5	106	3	21	24	17	11	7	4	2		...	206
" 23	102	84	4	3	102	12	8	14	18	14	16	4	3	1	...	193
Total,	597	459	27	15	574	50	64	107	97	83	57	36	15	3		1098

Disease		Disease		Disease		Disease	
Alcoholism	2	Cyanosis	1	Hydrocephalus	14	Poison	1
Apthæ	1	Cystitis	1	Hypertrophy	1	Pyemia	3
Asthenia	1	Debility	15	Hydrocardia	1	Scald	1
Abscess	1	Delirium Tremens	4	Inanition	8	Scarlatina	1
Abscess of Liver	2	Diarrhœa	18	Inflammat'n Brain	1	Scrofula	1
Anemia	1	Dropsy	10	" Bowels.	5	Softening of Brain.	1
Apoplexy	7	Drowned	7	Intussusception	1	Small Pox	7
Asphyxia	1	Dysentery	30	Injuries	2	Shot Wound	2
Atrophia	10	Colitis	2	Lockjaw	13	Spina Bifida	1
Bright's Disease	1	Eclampsia	2	Marasmus	43	Summer Complaint	51
Bronchitis	2	Enteritis	17	Measles	2	Syphilis	1
Burns	1	Erysipelas	2	Meningitis	46	Tabes Mesenterica	1
Cancer	7	Fever, Cong	3	" cereb-spin	16	Teething.	7
Catarrh	2	" intermittent	6	Morbus coxarius	1	Trismus	3
Chill, conges	4	" puerperalis	5	Metritis	1	Uterine Uremia	1
Cholera	80	" relapsing	1	Nephritis	1	Unknown	1
" Infantum	147	" typhoid	7	Noma	1	Worms	1
Cholera Morbus	109	Fracture	1	Old Age	11		
Conges. of Brain	26	Gangrene	2	Peritonitis	10	Total	1098
Conges of Lungs	12	Gastritis	4	Pertussis	2	Stillborn	58
Consumption	55	Hæmoptysis	1	Pleuritis	2		
Convulsions	58	Hepatitis	9	Pneumonia	20		

Long Island College Hospital,

BROOKLYN, NEW YORK.

THE REGULAR COURSE OF LECTURES,

In the Long Island College Hospital, will commence on the fourth day of March, 1874, and end the last week in June following.

FEES.—Matriculation, $5 00. Professors' Tickets, $100 00. Demonstrator's fee, $5.00. Graduation fee, $25.00. Hospital Ticket gratuitous.

SAMUEL G. ARMOR, M. D., Dean,

Brooklyn, New York.

1y—sept

THE SAINT LOUIS

Medical and Surgical Journal.

OCTOBER, 1873.

Original Communications.

ON EXCESSIVE VOMITING DURING PREGNANCY.

By M. M. PALLEN, M. D.

In the September number of this Journal I related a case of excessive vomiting during pregnancy, in which the patient was placed in a hazardous condition, and who was promptly relieved by the induction of abortion.

Of the fatality of such cases I cited statistics, and of the necessity of action at the proper time. But to decide when is the proper time is a question of much consideration. Every conscientious physician would desire to carry his patient through to the full term of utero-gestation, but if this cannot be done, it is his duty to sacrifice the embryo to save the life of the mother.

The rules which guide me are these: if she cannot retain anything on her stomach whatever, vomiting up even cold water; if she is daily losing flesh, showing that she really does not retain any portion of the food taken, and all the known remedies in such cases have

been tried and found inefficient ;* if there be insomnia
and restlessness, and if the pulse is under 100, then
the operation ought to be performed. But if the pulse
is 120 or more, and there are tinnitus-aurium, delirium,
and dimness of vision, it is too late to perform the operation—she will die. I have done it five times at the
request of others, but every one of them, as I anticipated, died.

What is the cause of such excessive vomiting? Most
women have nausea and vomiting in the early months
of pregnancy, some during the whole period of utero-
gestation, and some in the latter months only. It is
rather a physiological than a pathological condition.
But this excessive vomiting, yielding to no known remedies, attended by severely distressing symptoms and
hurrying the patient to the grave, must have some exciting cause.

Dr. Grailly Hewitt's idea of its being owing to a
retroverted uterus is not tenable, because a retroverted
uterus in pregnancy is not of common occurrence, and
when it does occur it produces other symptoms.

Years ago I published in this Journal my belief, and
always taught in my lectures, that it was produced by
some disease of the womb itself—not displacement. I
have had no occasion to change my opinion. Such disease may be granular erosion of the cervix, simple congestion of the neck with enlargement, or endo-cervici-
tis. This shows how important it is, if any of such
conditions exists, to cure it before conception. The
difficulty is, that the female does not know it, nor is
the physician apprised of it. But when it does occur,

[* Including *electricity* which has promptly relieved cases which resisted all
other remedies ; also quinine in gr. x doses per rectum.]

and her life is saved by the procuring of abortion, a recurrence of the accident ought to be obviated by the removal of the cause.

Having decided about the necessity of the operation, the question arises how it is to be done. One waits until the faintest glimmer of hope of carrying her on to the full period of utero-gestation has passed, and then he must act promptly. If the excessive vomiting occur in the earlier months, say within sixteen weeks after impregnation, it is important that the entire ovum should come away without rupture of the membranes. If the membranes are ruptured, and if the embryo escape and the membranes remain, the patient may have irritative fever, or alarming and even fatal hemorrhage. To two cases, in one night I was called, of alarming hemorrhage produced by the introduction of a knitting-needle by the ladies themselves, who had no excuse whatsoever for so doing, except that they did not want any more children. They were both married.

To secure the expulsion of the entire ovum, a small probe or uterine sound ought to be passed into the cavity of the womb and carried *around* the ovum so as to detach it from the decidua. Let one beware of passing it within the membranes. Afterwards give the tincture of ergot in such doses as can be retained. If the sixteenth week be passed, it is better to rupture the membranes and trust to the action of the uterus afterwards; but be it remembered, that one cannot define the time to a certainty. Every case must be treated on its own merits, and the physician must use his own judgment. Excessive vomiting does occur after the seventh month. Whatever may be said to the contrary, the rupture of the membranes is attended with almost immediate relief, and the child is born alive and will as likely live as in any other premature labor.

ANENCEPHALOUS MONSTER.

By R. W. ERWIN, M. D., Athens, Ohio.

On the 10th of June I was called to attend Mrs. H., *æt.* 38, in her sixth confinement. She had been in labor about 30 hours. The pains were frequent and of short duration. The bag of waters was presenting at the vulva, and distending the vagina by the considerable quantity of fluid it contained. The child could be felt, but the touch would immediately drive it beyond reach in the liquor amnii, it not having engaged in the pelvis. This fluid on the giving away of the sac was discharged so rapidly as to render syncope imminent. There must have been from three to four gallons. It ran through the bedding upon the floor, and then across the room, forming quite a pool. The escape of the water brought the child's head into the inferior straight. A drachm of Squibb's fl. ex. ergot was given immediately, which in 15 or 20 minutes began to arouse the uterus from the atony present, and the labor proceeded to a natural termination. The *Pseudo-encephaliens,* such it proved to be, was a girl weighing about nine pounds with a body plump and well-developed. The face was small with just enough integument above the eyes to allow attachment of the lids. The frontal bone, including its supraorbital plates ; with squamous portion of the temporal, parietal, and occipital to basilar part ; with cervical vertebræ excepting their bodies in front, were entirely absent. Resting on the sphenoid were the rudimentary cerebral lobes, symmetrical and about as large as hickory nuts. The corpora quadragemina undeveloped, formed part of the mass. Covering the brain substance, was a membrane, firm and fibrous, that ran back over the base of the skull and down the channel for the spinal-cord. In the region occupied by the medulla oblongata normally, was contained about a drachm of liquid that could be pushed up or down. There was not the slightest appearance of any part of the cerebellum, medulla oblongata, or spinal cord, in the cervical region present. The small rudimentary cerebral mass had no connection below except what the dura mater afforded. Notwithstanding the absence of all these, the child breathed in a gasping manner for about four minutes, and its heart beat about ten minutes after birth—death resulting from apnœa. The action of the heart during the time that respiration continued, was regular and strong. Its failure was gradual. This is an example of respiration being established and continued without the existence of nerve centers and nerves which are supposed to preside over that function. The sympathetic nervous system would seem from this case to be able to exercise some control over the circulatory and respiratory acts. From the almost instantaneous death following injuries to the medulla, we may conclude that this power is not ordinarily exercised. The external parts of the ears were stubby and bent down upon the neck on both sides, just as if pressure had been long made upon them.   The malformation of the ears I think gives a clue to the whole.

In Sir James Simpson's Obstetrical Memoirs, by Priestly and Storer, placental inflammation is reckoned among the causes of monstrosities.   A few cases are cited in proof of the statement.   The embryo from the placentitis is bound fast.   The disturbance in development will be in ratio to the degree and extent of placento-fœtal adhesions, and pressure induced thereby. In the cases recited by Simpson, the adhesions were present at birth.   The instance here recorded affords no such positive proof, unless it be in the flattening of both ears, and the bending of them down upon the sides of the neck.   Their position impresses the mind at once of the existence of pressure at some time in intra-uterine life.   That such a malformation was due to adhesion of the head of the unfolding embryo to its enveloping membranes I do not doubt.   It could not have been produced otherwise.   The absence of the other organs and parts had the same cause.   The subsequent hyperamniotic secretion floating the fœtus with the bodily motion of the mother ruptured the adhesions and left it in the condition found at delivery. Had the after-birth been critically examined, I have no doubt but that the remains of an old placentitis would confirm this explanation.   Simpson says, " M. Brachet enumerates as causes of placentitis, blows upon the belly, falls, violent succussions, sudden and great movements, frights, emotions, all kinds of lively and profound sensations, and diseases of the mother, particularly metritis, and other inflammatory complaints, etc."

NEW INSTRUMENTS FOR THE EXAMINATION
AND TREATMENT OF THE THROAT,
NOSE AND EAR.

By THOS. F. RUMBOLD, M D., St. Louis, Mo.

The Warm Spray Producer (Fig. 1) is used for treating the nasal cavities from their anterior openings.

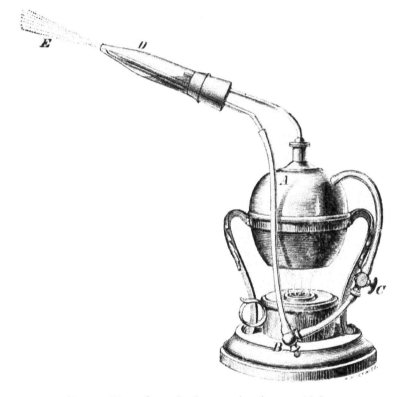

FIG. 1.—Warm Spray Producer, (reduced to one third)

A is the reservoir into which the water is placed, this is to be heated only to about 112° F. by the lamp under it, and 'may contain a little iodine, ammonia, or other volatile agent when required; the medicated fluid to be

made into a spray is placed in the large glass tube or
container (*D*), the air bulbs (seen attached to the
Catheter Nasal Douche Fig. 3, p. 480, September
number,) are fitted on the India rubber tubing at *B*;
the faucet (*C*) is turned so as to admit the required
amount of air from the air bulbs, to force the heated air
from the reservoir into the container (*D*); to produce
the proper temperature of the spray at *E*, the other
branch of the India rubber tubing connects with the
spray producer in the container. As the point of the
container (*D*)—which is to be inserted into the nostril—
will become too warm by the heat, a common India
rubber nipple shield should be slipped over it; this
also prevents any spray from escaping, except from
the opposite nostril.

This instrument—which I have employed since 1868
—is very useful in treating those cases affected with
chronic inflammation of the mucous membrane of the
nares that have but little secretions, also, for some cases
of sub-acute catarrh of the nares and Eustachian tubes
of children: they need only to close the nostril not
treated, when the force of the warm spray will inflate both
middle ears, sometimes without the act of swallowing,
but more frequently the child will make an involuntary
act of deglutition, at the time of closing the nostril;
then of course it is forced in in greater quantities. It has
also proved very beneficial in myringitis and furuncle.

With but little expense, any steam spray producer
may be made into a Warm Spray instrument, as it is
seen that this is but an addition to the "Siegle-Bergson"
apparatus, with no alteration except the opening into
the steam boiler.

C

A

FIG. 2.—Soft Palate Retractor, (reduced to one-third.)

In the early part of 1867, I had a large tumor or polypus to, remove from the superior wall of the pharyngo-nasal cavity, which gave me a great deal of trouble, because I could not retain the soft palate sufficiently forward. A narrow hook could not give as extended a view as a wide one; but frequently as soon as this was placed behind the soft palate, an involuntary contraction of the levator and tensor palati muscles took place, the consequence was that the edges of the hook injured the velum, thus rendering the toleration of the hook impossible. This led me to devise the spreading Soft Palate Retractor as represented in Figure 2, which obviates this difficulty, as the " spring" of the two limbs of the instrument will yield sufficiently to the contraction of the muscles to prevent any injury to the soft palate. Pressure on the lever (*A*) causes the hooks to separate, stretching the soft palate to the utmost lateral extent, while traction on the handle increases the antero-posterior diameter. The uvula is prevented from dropping by the small piece of thin India rubber tubing (*B*), that is slipped on over the hooks. The instrument may be maintained in its expanded condition by the retainer (*C*), which is operated on by a spring.

If the posterior nares, or the pharyngo-nasal cavity is to be inspected, it will be more convenient for the operator, more pleasant for the patient, and secure a better examination, to request the patient to hold

down his own tongue.   I have found a long handled
tongue depressor (Fig. 3) the most suitable for this

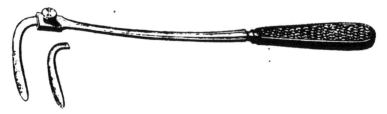

FIG 3 —Long-handled Tongue Depressor, (reduced to one third).

purpose, as it puts the patient's hand that holds it out
of the physician's way.   A long or short tongue-piece
can be fitted into the shaft adapted to the length of the
jaw of the patient.   These tongue-pieces being made of
nickel-plated German silver, can be bent to any angle, so
as to depress the base of the tongue as much as is desired
for each case.

FIG. 4.—Acou-Otoscope, (reduced one-half.)

The more of the senses the physician can employ in
the examination of the Eustachian tube, and middle ear,
the more certain is he of the correctness of his diagnosis.   Since 1869 I have been greatly assisted in the examination of this canal and cavity—especially in patency
of the tube—by what I have called the Acou-Otoscope.
(Fig. 4.)   This instrument is for auscultating the ear
while inspecting the membrana tympani during the in-
flation of the middle ear.   It resembles a Gruber ear
speculum with the smaller half cut off;   the larger end
is covered with plain glass; a metal tube, five inches

long, is attached to it, to allow the sound formed in the Eustachian tube and middle ear, to reach the examiner's ear through an India rubber tube, from a Camman's stethoscope, that is slipped on the stem or handle, the beveled extremity is slipped into one of Gruber's speculums, and this is placed in the ear to be examined. The patient can hold the instrument by the long extremity in his hand, keeping the speculum in proper position for the physician to see the membrana tympani, while the latter is inflating the middle ear by Politzer's method, or other means. Thus, the practitioner is enabled to hear if air passes through the Eustachian tube, note the characteristics of the sound, and see the movements of the membrana tympani at the same time.

It will be observed that this instrument is similar to Siegle's Pneumatic Aural Speculum—which is used for a very different purpose—also that his speculum may with but little expense be altered, and then employed for the purposes just described, without injuring its use for a pneumatic speculum.

1205 Washington ave.

PRINCIPLES OF TREATMENT FOR CROUPOSE PNEUMONIA.

By Prof. Th. Jürgensen, of Kiel.

(Volkman's Clinica. Lectures.—Translated from the German by Dr. Henry Kirchner, St. Louis, Mo)

Gentlemen, to-day I unfold before you a leaf from the every-day life of medical practice. An old one,

covered with writings, and yet one, upon which decade after decade registers its knowledge and ability.

How is a physician to act at the bedside of a patient
with pneumonia? Not—how is the physician to treat
pneumonia? In so choosing the position of the question, I would like to define by it my standpoint from
the beginning.

Any one who has seen a great number of patients
suffering from inflammation of the lungs, knows that
in spite of the apparent similarities in the main features,
nowhere are to be found so manifest deviations, again
in the main features. "Croupose pneumonia"·—this
is more an anatomical diagnosis, based upon definite
physical signs, than a pathologic, even approachingly
constant complex of symptoms. Think of the pneumonia of the aged ones, and remember the picture exhibited by a man in the vigor of life. Is there a
greater difference in the form of appearances and yet
the anatomical knife shows often enough the same alterations.

It is therefore necessary above all, that we require
emphatically in pneumonia, *not to treat the disease, but
that the patient be the object for treatment.* The justice
of this demand is in a theoretical point of view, as a
matter of course not to be discussed; but look into
practice, and even into many works upon the subject,
and you will agree that I head my discourse with something belonging to A. B. C.

You know how ready I am to separate, clinically,
from the traditional picture of the "acute," "genuine," "primary," pneumonia, the smaller groups belonging to the same category. But from the standpoint we occupy to-day, that of the therapeutist, we

not only must give up this separation, but also draw the secondary pneumonias, as far as they are "croupose," into the line of our discussion.

Croupose pneumonia as anatomically defined (not how or where originated, or as it may appear clinically) is the object of our consideration.

Much refers to the other forms, but not all. What are the deviations from the normal, constantly called forth by pneumonia? A definite answer to this simple question we may expect. But we must know, that at present we can only discuss in broad outlines and we are necessitated to leave the search after an exhausting definition to another time.

Acknowledging this restriction, without reservation we answer:

Pneumonia calls forth—

1. A restriction in the function of the lungs.

2. Fever.

Whatever else is observed is to be deduced from these alterations from the normal, or it does not essentially belong to the nature of pneumonia. The disease is hardly entirely without fever. The intensity of it admits the greatest fluctuations. In marastic aged, the temperature is elevated, if even the fever not in itself, yet a reliable criterion for the same, often only a little above $38°$C.—there has been observed already $42°$C in some cases of the disease.

That the function of the lungs is diminished, teaches the anatomical knife. The extent and quality of the exudation at least show the same variations as the fever. The second question is above all in refer-

ence to the danger created by pneumonia for the diseased individual.

What is the cause of death in pneumonia?

Is the disease of the lungs itself, or is the fever sufficient in the concrete cases to be the undeniable necessity of death? We must emphasize *no*.

Imagine a man of 20 years who has pneumonia, with
an infiltration of the whole lower left lobe, and a temperature of 40°C., on the sixth day of the disease; then a
few hours later, nearly well, after the natural crisis has
set in and his temperature lowered to 37°C. Who will
insist, or with a shadow of probability contend, that in
the lungs something worth speaking of is altered, and
with just as little propriety can you put a mortal œdema
that appeared a few hours before the crisis, upon the
alterations of the lungs *as such*. Take further what is
known from experience, that a chronic pneumonia ending in cirrhosis, or a pleuritis with compression of the
lung and flattening of the thorax, produces a much
more considerable disturbance in the activity of the
lungs, and that this is borne with comparative little inconvenience for a number of years. On the other
hand, as to fever; compare the pneumonic with a typhus patient, after the same lapse of time. If the fever
alone was a sufficient explanation for the deaths in
pneumonia, there would have to be within the same
time, the same number of deaths from both diseases,
as soon as the temperatures were the same. According
to communications from the disciples of Liebermeister,
there were in the first week 31.8 per cent. deaths by
typhus, but in the first week by pneumonia 75.5 per
cent. of the whole number of deaths by either of these
diseases. These statements, in the absolute height of

numbers, may only have a local bearing. But the proportion of the two is surely an agreeing one everywhere. From this fact there is no justification to deduce the deaths in pneumonia from the intensity of the fever alone. There will be an abundance of points to reject this view.

In order to avoid the censure of dogmatizing, I will expressly admit, that in some cases pneumonia may prove fatal in the beginning by the height of the fever alone; even before a considerable alteration of lung tissue is accomplished. This not very frequent occurrence has no influence on the principles of our explanation, it is secondary. But when, allowing this exception, neither fever nor the affection of the lung each in itself suffices to bring danger to the pneumonic, what then? Are we to look for a hypothetic third, or venture to explain with the given conditions? I think the latter.

Each of these two factors alone, does not suffice to endanger the life of the patient, but the disturbance in the function of the lung as well as the fever, are both obnoxities. There lies nothing nearer than the thought that both combined may accomplish what they cannot do singly.

There are, therefore, two possibilities.

The affection of the lungs and the fever may each have a peculiar point, where it may be attacked, or both have a common one.

I hold this latter to be the correct view and the view to be proven. I therefore set up the doctrine:

The danger of croupose pneumonia threatens in first instance the heart. The patients die of insufficiency of the heart.

Now for the proving of the assertion.

1. *The pneumonic exudation effects an increased resistance to the lung circulation and therefore imposes a greater demand for work upon the right ventricle.*

The pneumonic exudation exercises a pressure upon its neighborhood. According to the laws of impermeability of space, it demands room for itself. Its propulsive powers being sufficient, it displaces the former occupants * These are—the air that filled the bronchi and alveoli, the blood that filled the vessels of the diseased lung section. The displacement of both is possible only to a certain degree. For there are other powers in opposition to the pressure of the exudation, those that move the blood as well as the air in the lungs. The propulsive power of the exudation on one hand, and on the other the muscular power expended by the heart and respiration, combat each other. The magnitude of displacement depends upon the effect of the three factors against each other.† One thing is sure, as soon as an equilibrium is established, the quantity of blood to be forced through the diseased portion, meets with greater resistance. Then, of course, is the same accomplished for the portion extraneous to the diseased lung vessels, what occurs when in a connected system of pipes, a portion of the waste pipes are closed, and you demand that within the same time an equal quantity of fluid to be transmitted as by an

---

* The increase in volume of the diseased portion of lung in every pneumonia may find a place here to complete the proof. In larger infiltrations there are often found depressions from the ribs upon the inflamed portion.

† The conditions during exudation must in reality become very complex, as a considerable portion of it has its origin from the blood vessels, subject therefore, to the same propelling agency as the blood. The solidification of the exudation forms a definite chapter, and to this point refers the here stated conclusion.

open system. This can only be accomplished by an increase of propelling power. That means for our case; the right ventricle requires more power to propel the blood through the lungs, when by an infiltration of that part, that is affected by pneumonia a retardation of its circulation is to be prevented. The left ventricle has also to bear the increased difficulty, produced by the pressure of the exudation on the equally difficult nutrition (bronchial arteries) of the inflamed part of the lungs, as slight as the same may be.

2. *The alterations by pneumonia ⁚in and upon the lungs, cause a lowering of the propelling power established by the aid of the organ for the blood.*

By the respiratory muscles the lungs are put into condition to facilitate the circulation. The lungs themselves are, in this instance, a purely passive organ. But in order to use this living force of the respiratory muscles for the maintenance of circulation, the lung must be able to alter its volume—expand and contract. If a portion of the lung is infiltrated, it is not in the condition any more to alter its volume, yet the relation of the motors for the section involved remains the same. The proportion of power of the motors—the muscles of respiration must remain the same, as they act on the *whole* thorax. But as, by the ability of the lung to expand, the living force produced by these muscles is mostly used for the circulation, therefore must be so much lost for the circulation as the infiltrated. portion needs during normal function.

The diminishing caused by the altered physical condition is rendered still more considerable by a never-wanting physiological moment.

In most cases, pneumonia is accompanied with in-

36

flammatory conditions of the corresponding pleura. Pain therefore is felt as soon as the respiratory gliding of the corresponding pleuras upon each other causes an irritation. From the beginning a desire exists to make this gliding as slight as possible. In opposition to this, the necessity to breathe sufficiently is urgent. This is accomplished by fixation of the diseased side, while the sound one moves. The execution of this theoretically justified procedure is done instinctively; most frequently so that the patient lies on the diseased side. By it he causes the muscles that move this half of the thorax to lift a part of the weight of his body. The force necessary thereto has no effect on the half of his body upon which he lies. The other methods used by pneumonic patients, such as tying, holding on to something, curving the spine to approximate the ribs, have all the same effect, only different in quantity. But as on the side upon which he lies, the whole lung, and not only the diseased portion, becomes less expanded, the living force of the respiratory muscles for the aid of the heart's action, is lost. In how far, by an increased labor of the muscles of respiration, the normal task of circulation can be accomplished is *a priori* not to be decided. The more active the muscles are, the greater are the demands upon the force of the heart. For the harder laboring muscles require blood, in the contracted muscles the vessels are compressed, during contraction exists a greater resistance. This increase of labor falls upon the left ventricle, and is therefore of lesser importance.

3. The diminishing of the surface, produced by the pneu-
    monic exudation, on which blood and air come in contact

in the lungs, causes increased labor for the propulsion of blood and air in order to effect a complete exchange of gases.

Where a pneumonic exudation fills the bronchi and alveoli no exchange of gases can take place. It is therefore the maximal effect of each breath, be it superficial or deep, to be of necessity so much diminished, as normally takes place in the at present diseased portion. If now in a given time a complete ventilation is to take place, the forces by which blood and air are carried to the place of interchange must increase. Therefore the heart and muscles of respiration have to perform more work. As mentioned before, the greater labor of the respiratory muscles falls upon the heart.

4. The fever gives expression to the local disturbance created by pneumonia.

The fact itself needs no comment. Every critically ending pneumonia, that shows a falling off in temperature of 2° or 3° C. distributed over the space of a few hours, teaches that only by the fever, is caused the dispnœa, and the forced activity of the heart. The disease of the lungs surely has not retrograded to such an extent, within so short a time, that the complete alteration should be deduced from a lessening of the same. But if some one should not accept this proof as convincing, there is still another that cannot be upset. The same reduction of pulse and respiration, the same euphoria takes place, when a cold bath reduces the temperature to the normal standard, but it disappears as soon as the effect of the bath passes off, and the temperature rises again.

The question may be asked, in what manner is the actual disturbance brought about?

This is not difficult to answer. It is to the point in the following sentence :

5. *The fever causes a greater labor for the heart, which is directly obnoxious to the same.*

The most prominent symptom of fever is the increased temperature. With the rising of bodily heat rises the frequency of the pulse (Liebermeister) ; that is, the number of systoles increase within a given time ; from which follows, in other words, that, at the same time the duration of diastoles diminishes,* the laboring time of the heart is increased and the time of rest lessened—it is required to perform more work than normal. During fever the formation of carbonic acid is increased beyond the normal (Liebermeister, Leyden). If an increase within the organism is to be avoided, it must be eliminated quicker than in health. This can only take place by an increase in the force of the heart and of the respiratory muscles, as explained before.

The fever leads to a degeneration of the muscular fibres of the heart (Zenker, Liebermeister). As the quantity of force produced by the contractions of the heart is proportional to the number of its constituting primitive fibres, any loss of them must be equivalent to a diminishing of its force. The same holds good for every single primitive fibre. Their force is dependent upon the contractile element contained therein. It is anatomically proven that, by the fever the primitive muscular fibres are diminished (destruction of a definite

---

* The theoretically given possibility, that by an increase of the number of systoles, the duration of every single one is shortened, does usually not take place in any remarkable degree. It is only necessary to feel the pulse to convince one's self.

quantity) and also the contractile element of the remaining ones (fatty degeneration and detritus) ; therefore the fever leads to a lessening of the power of the heart as a whole. The same thing is effected, that the inert mass originated by the transformation of the contractile substance, by reason of its inertia, and its elasticity causes an intrinsic resistance, to overcome which, a part of the living force, set free by the contractions of the heart, is absorbed. Without overcoming this, a contraction is impossible. The indirect obnoxity is to be mentioned, that the fever exercises upon all organs of the body. The lessening of nutrition, amounting to almost complete cessation in highly febrile states, but noticeable to a certain degree in every febrile condition, will touch those parts most heavily, whose expenditures are the greatest. These are the constantly laboring muscles—heart and respiratories. You see thereby how all center upon the heart and how it is the heart, which suffers in the last instance.

As a simple consequence of the foregoing, I formulate the duty of a physician at the bed-side of pneumonia thus :

The physician must make the heart capable, during the existence of pneumonia, of accomplishing the extra work imposed upon it by the disease.

This general demand has two sub-divisions :

1. Prophylaxis against debility of the heart.

2. Subduing the already existing debility of the heart.

Do we succeed in overcoming the disturbance in the function of the lungs by getting rid of the local affection? Some physicians are of the opinion that by a timely "energetic" interference the "inflammation of the lungs " can be moderated, or even brought to a conclusion. But how is the proof for this assumption? Opinions based upon one's own authority or upon the dogmas of another, you find plenty—hardly any other disease has been the baby, so much fed upon the dogmas of the reigning " school." But proofs you may ask for this dogma with just as little propriety as for any thing else. By a little closer observation, you will easily notice that behind this "sometimes," "once in a while," "often," etc., that introduce such recommendations, indeed only a subjective view or a repeated tradition, without a thorough examination is hidden. It is always to be remembered, that conditions, resembling a pneumonia in the essential points may have vanished within 24 or 36 hours, and that the duration of many a fully developed pneumonia, only last a few days. I will touch here a question of principle. Is the anatomical alteration of the lungs, that you find in pneumonia, the most prominent in the picture of the disease, or something secondary, that only has an eventual significance? In other words: Is pneumonia a local disease in which the inflammation of the lungs (no matter in what manner it originated) conditions all consequences, or does the inflammation of the lungs and its sequelæ depend upon the fever as one common cause? According to my opinion the latter is the case, and I will refer to it later. In this case, the attacking of the local alteration has only significance from the standpoint that was developed before, stands therefore in the same line with the intestinal lesion in typhus abdominalis. This view may be accepted or rejected, the fact is this, there are no remedies against the local disease of the lungs— or they are not known to us up to this time.

*So the fever remains the therapeutic points of attack.
That it is th s in first line, points out most emphatically the repeatedly urged fact, that in spite of lasting local disturbances,
generally with the cessation of the fever, also the power of
the disease is broken.*

In the present state of our knowledge, the prophylaxis against debility of the heart in pneumonia corresponds with the treatment of fever. But some circumstances should especially be mentioned.

I formerly advanced the doctrine, and hold on to it
with tenacity, for the treatment of *typhus abdominalis*
to be: *sine thermometro nulla therapia.* That is, in this
disease the heat of the body as such predominates to
such an extent, that every exceptional something (intestinal hemorrhage, perforation, etc.,) has to be taken
care of besides. Therefore the heat measurable with
the thermometer is the unconditional guide for the
physician. This is different in pneumonia. Here the
sentence sound: *sine pulsu nulla therapia.* And if you
ask me if I rather treat a severe pneumonia without the
thermometer or without the observation of the pulse, I
would say without reservation: away with the thermometer!

It is necessary to express this definitely, and to take
the same standpoint of our predecessors in our time
adducted to measure. It is necessary so much the
more, the thermometer being so much a simple instrument, that you can explain its therapeutical use to the
most stupid nurse. The judgment of, or even the observation of the pulse requires a definite dexterity, which
is only to be acquired by long practice. All honor to
the sphygmograph, but external to the clinic, it is no
instrument for the sick bed. If the pulse shows by

something in any way—and together with its frequency
there are many things to be noticed, that it stand well
with the heart, the temperature is *not* determining, if
even it should go over 40°C. On the other hand, can an
absolute low temperature, if in the concrete case the
heart suffer at the same time, demand our interference?

We have next to discuss the method of attacking the
fever.

Is it allowed to bathe a pneumonic patient, in order to
reduce the heat of fever?

It cannot be denied that here *a priori* objections
might be raised, that awaken doubts just from the
standpoint of my view. You may point out, and with
justice, that every bath, from the moment that the vessels of the periphery contract under the influence of
cold, brings on an increased resistance to the blood current and with it an increased labor for the heart. The
next question is whether there could not take place a
complete paralysis of the heart overloaded with blood.
In the same direction operates the heat, increased by
the bath itself, on the increased demands upon heart
and respiratory muscles, produced by the increased generation of carbonic acid. But experience enables us to
quiet these doubts. I must state that I and my hearers have never had any reason to regret the application
of cold—although with my knowledge nobody has employed the bath so frequent, so cold, and with so untir-
ing energy as I have. That during the bath a fatal collapse may ensue I do not doubt in the least, and the
bath may have been the cause of the collapse. But the
collapse must be avoided, by observing a very simple
caution. By the bath is imposed a greater labor upon
the heart transitorily. Should it therefore not be pos-

sible to put the heart transitorily in the condition to perform such increased labor, to heighten its force? Certainly, we can accomplish this always. Only you must not take anybody in the last moment of his life as an object for trials with the bath, whereby I emphasize the "last." For if it be not the last we may hope sometimes in pneumonic patients to sustain life—what is to be done, I will explain hereafter. Another impediment to cold baths—one for carrying through the treatment in practice generally with physicians and laymen equally impeding is—the belief that the patient takes cold therefrom. The fear that such might occur makes otherwise rational men as timid as children to whom you tell the tale of the black man. And yet this scapegoat of taking cold in already existing pneumonia (the influence of cold as cause that may have called forth a pneumonia I admit,) is an objective indifferent something. So, to remove this spectre, restlessly moving about for hundreds of years, I will develop my experience and my views based upon an abundant material proof in a different direction.

The pneumonic needs above all fresh air : If you can have it without causing draft, all right. But if I have to choose between fresh air and draft, I choose the draft and my patients do well. If I can not do better I let them bathe under these conditions and let them expose their skin to a current of air when they come out of the bath. How often do the unfavorable circumstances of my polyclinical patients compel me to help myself with such primitive measures, when ventilation has to be accomplished by a broken pane of glass or an open window, and I see more seldom the "school shaped" complications such as bronchial catarrh, pleuritis, pericarditis, etc. Just as seldom have I noticed an influence on the origin of sequelæ, that often develop from the local affection, such as chronic pneumonia, phthisis, etc. I would therefore not hesitate, in those cases where an abstraction of heat is required and no water to be had, to expose my patients to cold air until the necessary measure of cooling was accomplished. This would subjectively be a harsh procedure in a greater measure than the cold bath, but be surely of advantage to the patient. My experience justifies the declaration in opposition to the theoretical objection and contrary to the undue prejudice, that abstraction of heat is admissible in pneumonia. I am happy to have herein the *weighty authority* of Liebermeister,* who with a purely antipyretic method, brought down the mortality from 24.4 per cent. to 8.8 per cent., but holds the remark as sufficient: "That the results obtained in the treatment of croupose pneumonia by cold baths, are encouraging enough to proceed in the same direction."

The next question here, is the *extent* of cooling. Here the maxim is my guide, *that the abstraction of heat has the significance of a prophylaxis for the heart, and that the fever is the most dangerous enemy of the heart.*

With strong individuals and not too severe disease, without complications, you can follow the rule that is generally followed in the treatment of typhus. Here a bath is given of the temperature that well-water generally has, as often as the temperature in the rectum reaches 40° C. The duration of the bath is taken according to its effect. It is between 7 and 25 minutes. It is here given a simple formula in which the individ-

---

* Méjor über die Behandlung d. crupösen Pneumonie und kühlen Bädern.— Basel, 1870.

ual factors—size of body, adipose tissue, those from the disease, intensity of fever, with external circumstances, temperature of water—are contained. But this is not sufficient for pneumonia. There are occurring cases, as is known, especially in aged people, as also in especially fat people, finally in debilitated ones, in whom the temperature never or very seldom rises to 40°C, but where it runs between 38.5° or 39.5°C. These require special care. I like to avail myself of the advantage, that is given by the rise and fall of temperature over a period of twenty-four hours, parallel to the normal—that is hardly wanting in the common febrile diseases. Lukewarm baths of 20° to 24° R. in the early morning hours, (4 to 7 o'clock) used for 20 to 30 minutes, bring down the temperature for a relatively considerable time in these cases. A dose of quinine at the same time makes the effect of the bath more lasting. While the low temperature lasts, the heart has time for rest. This, of course, does not exclude a repetition of the bath at some other time of the day: whoever makes it a rule to observe the pulse carefully, will soon know the exact measure of interference. With younger children you can use the wet sheet, only do not be satisfied to wrap the thorax exclusively in a wet cloth. The reduction of heat is hereby a small one, that at most suffices for children at the breast. The thermometer must be consulted diligently of course. I do not like these "packs," as they cause much more trouble and inconvenience for the attendants and the patients than baths, and accomplish much less. On the other hand, there are pneumonias in which the intensity of the fever—not alone measurable by the absolute height of temperature, but also by the resistance of the same against antipyretic measures, that are only broken by the most energetic abstraction of heat *coup sur coup.* . There is no choice, either you leave the fever free play and then the patient is generally lost, or you use force without fear and carry through with perseverance your views accepted as true. Of course, you run the risk in case of an unfavorable issue, to be pointed out by the public as the originator of such an end. The choice will not be difficult for a conscientious physician, who is convinced of the truth of his views.

How far you can go, I have experienced when several years ago my little daughter aged nineteen months got a severe pneumonia at short intervals for the third time. The temperature rose to over 41° C. and returned to this height after baths of 16° C., so that I was forced to reduce their temperature to 5° and 6° C. and use them for ten minutes at a time. My child got well and not a single time I noticed the slightest sign of collapse during the space of several days during which the extreme reduction of temperature had to be kept up. Some time later I had the opportunity several times to treat patients in this wise. I never had cause to regret my persevering. But one caution I impress upon you : *Do not let a pneumonic be bathed without first giving him a stimulant and increase the same when the temperature of the bath has to be very low or the bathing time is to be extended.* Why the heart before the bath has to be sustained I have mentioned before. The definite cooling that comes to its maximum ¼ to ½ hour after the bath also might call forth, in feebleness of the heart's action, signs of collapse. On the other hand it appears to me that by the stimulant the temperature of the body is sooner equalized. I generally allow before the bath one to two tablespoonsful of claret. But as soon as the slightest sign of an imperfect heart action occurs, port wine or madeira is to be used, and when necessary, even champagne. In employing perfectly cold baths I give, say five minutes before, during the bath and immediately after, every time one to three large table-spoonsful of wine; this always must be a large table-spoonful of a stronger wine. To children proportion-ately.less. In severe cases I take for children relatively more wine than grown persons. Absolute rules can not be formulated. And again it is the pulse that decides the more or less. Once more I express emphatically : *Who wants to treat pneumonia without unpleasant interludes with cold baths must not spare stimulants.* The pneu-monias that are to be treated with warmer baths are to be judged from this point also. Here the heart's action is mostly low from the beginning and you have to look for a prolonged course of the disease. It would be very wrong to employ the stronger stimulants from the beginning. If you are compelled to take the baths *cold*, of course you cannot spare them. Some experience suffices to act with decision in the given case.

With the direct abstraction of heat I regularly em-ploy the quinine. It has the invaluable preference before other antipyretics, that it diminishes the tem-perature without harm to the heart, and as I have shown, by diminishing the production of heat. Tartar emetic and its younger brother veratria diminish the temperature only at the expense of the heart,—both produce collapse. In the employment of digitalis the effect comes very late, you lose the control of the heart when you most need it. Who, that employed digitalis and used active doses, has not met with cases in which the collapse called forth by digitalis came at the same time as the defervescence of the fever? Whoever saw such a condition does not feel much desire to repeat it. I am very willing to admit that in many cases in individuals with vigorous heart the above named remedies can be borne without harm and as far as they lower the temperature are employed with some utility.

But is it justified to employ a remedy that might eventually bring harm to the patient, when you can obtain a better result in a way that does not endanger him?

The antifebrile effect of venesection is trifling and unsafe. Whoever makes a venesection on account of the fever, resembles the wise man who cuts down a tree in order to get its fruit. The adherents to this indication for venesection give the very best proof for its rejection by their own statistics. Especially at present when we have at command remedies acting with more certainty. This indication at least should be stricken from the text-books. It is a most welcome plaster for the conscience of the weak man, whom destiny has made physician for the punishment of mankind, when he gives in to the pressings of his clients and opens a vein for the fortification of his position. *Credite experto!*

[To be Continued.]

Hospital Reports.

CITY HOSPITAL.

Reported by Isaac N. Love, M. D., Assistant Physician.

Fracture of the base of the skull.—William. W., aged 24 years, by occupation a *brass finisher*, a native of the United States, during the night of July 29th, 1878, received injuries.

July 30th, 1. A. M.—He was brought into the surgical ward completely insensible; breathing labored; pulse weak; pupils dilated; surface of body cool. Examination reveals a lacerated wound over the left frontal eminence, exposing the skull, but the continuity of same is unimpaired. There are some contusions of face and head. A sero-sanguinolent fluid exudes from the left external ear. A minute examination reveals no other external injuries than those above mentioned. No injury to skull so far as can be ascertained.

Treatment :—Rest.

July 30th, 8 A. M.—From the left ear the sero-sanguinolent fluid still discharges, and the "night attendant" states that this has been constant since last visit. No material change in condition as regards sensibility, respiration, pulse, etc. Considerable echymosis around both eyes, but more especially the left one.

Treatment :—Evaporating lotions applied to contusions of face and scalp. Hydrarg. chlor. mit. gr. iij every 3 hours upon tongue until 12 grains shall have been used.

July 30th, 4 P. M.—Bowels moved freely half an hour ago; skin is warmer and pulse a little fuller than this morning; pupils somewhat contracted and not responsive to light. Is becoming delirious. Serous discharge continues from left ear.

July 31st, 8 A. M.—Patient has been wildly delirious during the past night, but is more quiet this morning. Is entirely oblivious of all around him; taking cognizance of nothing; pulse 60. Takes nourishment in the form of fluids when urged to do so.

Treatment :—Brom. potass. gr. xx, quin. sulph. gr. ii, ext. ergot (fl.) gtt. x, every three hours.

August 1st, 8 A. M.—Passed a pretty good night and is quiet this morning. Is perfectly rational, having recognized friends who have called to see him, and also answered questions satisfactorily, but the same have to be written, as he is unable to hear a single vibration of sound. Complains of some pain at posterior part of skull, and is unable to use his *maxillæ* in chewing food, owing to pain it creates or excites in temporal regions. The right pupil appears normal this morning, responding to light, but left pupil is closely contracted and does not respond. A close examination reveals entire loss of vision in left eye. Fluid still exudes from ear, but in smaller quantities.

Treatment :—Two or three drops of a three gr. sol. of atropia put in left eye. Other treatment continued.

August 1st, 4 P. M.—Patient continues rational. Pulse good. Pupil of left eye—in which the atropia was dropped—is dilated to its fullest extent. The presence of a single ray of light cannot be appreciated by it. Is this loss of vision dependent upon extravasation of blood into posterior part of orbit? Complains of no headache, but a dull dead sensation prevails in the head. All questions have to be written as he continues totally deaf.

Treatment :—Bromide and ergot discontinued. Quinine sulph. gr. i, three times daily.

August 4th.—Echymosis around eyes and face is disappearing, and at no time has there been any evidence of inflammation in either eye. Wound over left frontal eminence is healing quite kindly. Serous discharge from ear has been gradually growing less until now it has entirely ceased. Pupil of left eye still continues greatly dilated

Treatment :—Quinine sulph. discontinued. Nothing further save perfect quiet.

August 5th, 4 P. M.—Suffering with very acute pain in head this evening.

Treatment :—Brom. potass. gr. xxx every three hours.

August 6th, 8 A. M.—No pain this morning and patient is feeling pretty well. Stopped brom. potass.

August 6th, 4 P. M.—Again suffering with pain in head, but not so much as last night.

Treatment :—Resumed bromide and prescribed a little quinine to be given during the night.

August 7th, 8 A. M.—No pain in head nor elsewhere; is feeling *"first-rate."* Can hear no sound as yet. Can see nothing as yet with left eye; pupil continues dilated; right eye normal.

August 8th.—Patient is doing well, and his friends are anxious to remove him to his boarding house where he will be in more retired "quarters." Deeming his removal safe with proper care, consent is given, with directions to keep him quiet for some time, and feed with good nourishing food but nothing stimulating.

Remarks :—Was this a case of *fracture of base of skull?* Many of the attendant symptoms certainly point to that lesion. The complete insensibility; disturbed respiration; feeble pulse; dilated pupils, with absence of external fracture, would not necessarily indicate fracture of *base.* But the serous discharge from the ear (the source of this discharge probably being the cerebro-spinal fluid, and its evacuation through the ear being effected by the rupture of the *cul-de-sac* of the arachnoid membrane which surrounds the auditory nerve as it passes along the auditory canal in petrous portion of the temporal bone,) strongly favored that conclusion. Another strong point in its favor, was the symptoms of *intraorbital extravasation* in left eye and complete loss of vision in same.

" *Ashhurst,*" in his late work on surgery, says : " Hemorrhage into the orbit and areolar tissue of the eye-lids, constituting in the former case what is known as *intraorbital echymosis* may be considered as presumptive evidence of the existence of fracture of the anterior fossa." He adds : " Yet this symptom *may* be due to the giving way of a blood vessel without lesion of the bony structures." He also remarks : " A *discharge of thin watery fluid* from the ear is very significant of *fracture.*

" *Robert,*" who is considered good authority, having given much attention to this subject, says, that cases of fracture accompanied by discharge of cerebro-spinal fluid are always fatal. " *Ashhurst*" thinks this is a mistake, for several well authenticated cases are on record in which recovery has ensued in spite of the occurrence of these discharges, though of course in any case which recovers there is always the possibility of an error having been made in the diagnosis.

" *Gross* " says, great stress is laid—and justly—upon an escape

37

of serosity from the ears as a diagnostic symptom of fracture of *base.*

Drs. Hodgen and Lankford, consulting surgeons, saw the case from time to time, and were of the opinion that there was fracture of the base.

The only argument that could be suggested against the above case, being that of *fracture of base of skull,* would be that the patient recovered.

Dr. Hodgen was called to see the case some two weeks after he left the hospital. He complained of headache from time to time, said he felt more comfortable in a dark room. Dr. Hodgen recommended good nutritious diet and rest in the darkened room if more agreeable. Believing his services to be unnecessary as the patient was during well, he did not again visit him.

August 27th (29 days after receipt of injury).—The writer called to see the patient from motives of professional interest and found him doing well; appetite good; sense of hearing returning slowly; no vision in left eye; occasionally a little headache, but said he was gradually improving from day to day and expected to return to the East soon where his family reside.

Reviews and Bibliographical Notices.

Surgical Diseases of Infants and Children. By M. P. Guersant, Honorary Surgeon of the Hôpital des Enfants Malades, Paris, etc., etc. Translated from the French by Richard J. Dunglison M. D. Philadelphia: Henry C. Lea; 1873. pp. 351. 8vo.

[For sale by the St. Louis Book and News Co.]

It is probably owing to national differences in rearing children, clothing and feeding them, as well as to differences in climate and constitution, that the reading of foreign works on the treatment of their diseases is found to be so unrenumera•

tive. Having in view also the better results of American surgery, and the independent advances of its recent activity, it was with no great interest that we took up the work whose title is given above ; but an examination disclosed unexpected merits.

The author has been long connected with the Hôpital des Enfants Malades of Paris, which was transformed from a religious institution early in this century. It is situated beyond the Latin quarter and about' midway between the gardens of the Luxembourg and the grounds of the Hôtel des Invalides. The nurses are sisters of charity, and it contains some seven hundred beds for children of between two and fifteen years. About four thousand children are estimated to be treated there yearly.

At this hospital M. Guersant delivered clinical lectures between the years 1840 and 1860, and now, being still its honorary surgeon, he sums up in this book his views on many of the surgical disorders so frequently brought to him, treated and lectured upon.· In seventy-three brief chapters, the longest of but sixteen pages, he goes over extensive ground, discussing subjects of every degree of importance from crushed fingers to lithotomy.

He is doubtless correct in his statement that surgical operations upon children are more difficult than those upon adults ; less space requiring more delicate manipulations, while the rapid succumbing of children to pain and loss of blood requires greater speed. His epigram, " before an operation we must be physicians, surgeons in its performance, and at last physicians again," applies to surgeons for children. In young patients subject to hemorrhage, he recommends a course of perchloride of iron for several days previous to the operation. With regard to anæsthesia he speaks well of chloroform, without speaking of the vitally greater advantages of sulphuric ether. In his after-treatment it has been his practice to lift the lint from the wound on the second day, in order to treat promptly any threatening complication. He has had good results from the use of elastic collodion in erysipelas, and in " an unpromising character" of the wound, which expression appears to refer to commencing sloughing,·from applications of pure lemon juice.

From another source we learn that the general rate of mortality of the hospital is one in thirty-eight. It would have been interesting, if in many of the chapters the rate of mortality had been given for the separate operations. Here and there occur hints of the prevalence of the fatal hospital scourge of erysipelas. Thus we find page 75: "we have employed, especially for the treatment of erectile tumors and nævi, the actual cautery and caustics, powerful remedies to which we resort in all surgical diseases in which they are applicable." In speaking of wens on various parts of the head he says p. 79: "We do not hesitate to say that as the bistoury sometimes induces erysipelas, we have relinquished the use of the cutting instruments in extracting these cysts, and we apply to all, indiscriminately, even those of the eyelids, the Vienna caustic, unless they are seated on the inner surface of the lid."

Although the patients in this hospital are in the lower ranks of society, disfiguring results of operations are carefully avoided. As an example, under the head of cervical adenitis, "which so often leaves frightful traces of its invasion," he greatly prefers treatment by setons of three or four silk threads, the scars of which in a little while entirely disappear.

In the article on coxalgia, a rough apparatus is described on account of its cheapness, but it contains not much else to repay the study of the American surgeon. In the related chapter on chronic arthritis, however, is a short summing up of the surgical pathology of inflammation of the joints, which seems to be based upon original dissections, and, although it cannot be called deep or exhaustive, it is fresh and interesting.

Tracheotomy he dwells upon at length, thoughtfully giving the very important after-treatment and manipulations. He has performed it more than three hundred times, but he does not give his ratio of success. He objects to the operation upon patients under two years of age. We must not omit mentioning his instrument for washing and making applications to the pharynx. It may be briefly described as a hollow tongue-depressor, perforated upon the upper surface of the extremity, the fluid being introduced through the handle by syringe or tube.

The chapter upon vesical calculus is very practical and instructive. During his twenty years at the institution, one hundred and forty cases occurred. We quote the following because it supplies statistics from cases of children alone:

" 1. From lithotomy performed in a hundred cases, we lost fourteen, * * * eight of these deaths dependent on the operation, being from inflammation of the cellular tissue of the lesser pelvis, and even from cystitis accompanied with nephritis; and six of intercurrent affections. * * * Of three rectal fistulæ, following the operation, two were cured; and, so far as we know, two perineal fistulas still remain uncured, while three of our little patients continue to be affected with a certain amount of incontinence of urine.

" 2. In forty operations for lithotrity—thirty-five boys and five girls—seven deaths occurred, four of them produced by intercurrent diseases, such as croup and scarlatina, and only three as the result of the operation. In one of these latter cases death was due to cystitis, consequent on pinching of the bladder, and in the other two also to violent cystitis, complicated with inflammation of the ureters and kidneys. The results of lithotrity performed in cases in which the calculi were so large as to require four, five, and six applications of the instrument, were such as to give us great uneasiness, on account of the supervening inflammatory symptoms, and from the difficulty often experienced in the extraction of calculi lodged in the urethra. We have not met with incontinence of urine as a result of our lithotriptic operations and our little patients were shielded from all danger of urinary fistula.

" We are, therefore, of the opinion, as the result of our practice, that it will be best to encourage the use of lithotrity in children, restricting it to the circumstances already referred to,* but that we must still resort to lithotomy by preference, when the calculus is very large and inflammation of the urinary apparatus exists as a complication.

The book, in its literary style, possesses the charm of brevity and clear statement. It may not, however, be hypercritical to call attention to some blemishes in the translation, as on page 222, where occurs the phrase : " we will have only the tendo

---

* That is to say, cases where the health is good, the calculus not over two-thirds of an inch in diameter, not very hard, nor mulberry shaped, adherent nor multiple, and he would use lithotrity in children fifteen or eighteen months old without regard to sex.

Achillis to divide,"—a use of "will" for "shall," which is a provincialism of certain portions of the United States. On p. 73, we are told that one class of tumors "may strictly be confounded" with another. Is this English? If so, what does it mean?

But in general the translation is in remarkably good idiomatic English, doubly satisfactory after reading some of the recent medical translations from the German.

We are convinced that surgeons and general practitioners desirous of obtaining an insight into this branch of the best French conservative practice will do well to obtain this book.

C. E. B.

CLINICAL ELECTRO-THERAPEUTICS, MEDICAL AND SURGICAL. A Hand-book for Physicians in the treatment of nervous diseases. By Allan McLane Hamilton, M. D. 8vo., pp. 184. New York: D. Appleton & Co

[For Sale by the St Louis Book & News Co.]

We have read this work with much interest, and consider the author eminently successful in the execution of his design, as made known in the Preface, namely, to supply a simple guide in the use of electricity for the general practitioner, rendered as *practical* as possible by avoiding as many of the confusing theories, technical terms, and *unproved* statements as possible. He endorses electricity only as a "very valuable remedy in certain diseases, not as a specific for every human ill, mental and physical;" but invaluable as a therapeutical means in nearly all forms of nervous disease.

New modes of application (in our author's opinion) not sufficiently tested, have been omitted. The work is sufficiently illustrated with cases.

The increased attention given to *electricity*, as a remedial agent, prompts every physician who desires to keep up with the advance of science, to seek the latest discovered, and most reliable facts concerning this subtle agent possible. Many ingenious and scientific artisans are busy projecting and supplying the most durable and convenient apparatus to utilize this agent, so long known but little used; description of which, with directions to keep the same in order, are given in a chapter at the conclusion of the work. Dr. Hamilton's book is opportune, and will be highly prized by busy practitioners who have

not time to study the subject critically, and trace all the refine-
ments attempted in more elaborate works.

A TREATISE ÒN THE PRINCIPLES AND PRACTICE OF MEDICINE; de-
signed for the use of Practitioners and Students of Medicine.
By Austin Flint, M. D., etc. *Fourth Edition*, 8vo. pp. 1070.
Philadelphia: Henry C. Lea, 1873.

The popularity of Prof. Flint's *Practice of Medicine* as a text-
book is likely to be maintained, as each new edition is thoroughly revised, and re-written, where needed to bring the work
up to the times. By incorporating the latest reliable contributions from Europe and this country to this department of medicine, and re-writing many sections, the author has given this
edition the freshness and interest of a new work.

The labor bestowed by the author on this edition cannot fail
of appreciation.

The general plan of the book is not materially altered.
Diseases of the nervous system and of the kidneys, have received special attention, making these chapters of particular
interest to the physician who wishes to be informed of any
progress on these subjects.

General pathology, etiology of tubercle, and carcinoma;
causation of contagious and infectious diseases being *sub-judice,*
will also be read with much interest.

The author's treatment being tempered by a large experience in hospital and private practice, is happily free from hob-
bies, and much to be commended. As a text-book it is without
a rival.

A GUIDE TO URINARY ANALYSIS, for the use of Physicians and
Students. By Henry G. Piffard, A. M., M. D., Physician to
the Charity Hospital, to the New York Dispensary for Diseases of the Skin, etc., etc. New York: William Wood & Co.,
27 Great Jones Street. 8vo. pp. 88.

The object of the work before us is to encourage in general
practice a more frequent examination of the urine, and especially in the clinics; and to simplify the methods now in use so
far as to make them sufficiently easy, yet accurate and simple
for every day application.

The motive is laudable, for we know that few practitioners

examine the urine as frequently as they should, or become as familiar with the information furnished by this secretion as they should, and as they might easily and profitably. An exhaustive analysis, in every case in which we desire to have certain information respecting a specimen of urine, is simply out of the question both as to time and expense, but in the vast majority of cases, but a few minutes are required by one of experience, to give the information desired. In a few cases the microscope is indispensible; but this book, if followed closely, will give the desired information in most cases, in private or hospital practice.

It is especially for the student, to make him familiar with the easy details of examinations, that the work is valuable; and it should be in the hands of every student who is attending clinics. The importance of taking specimens of urine passed at different times in the twenty-four hours, is shown by a case mentioned page 9. "A patient recently sent us a number of specimens of urine passed on going to bed, which all contained sugar, while the urine passed the following morning contained none. This naturally led to a more favorable prognosis (justified by the result) than if we had been obliged to form an opinion from an examination of specimens of the mixed urine, which would have constantly responded to the test for sugar."

The type is clear; paper of excellent quality, tinted.

INSANITY IN ITS RELATIONS TO CRIME. A Text and a Commentary. By William A. Hammond, M. D., etc. New York: D. Appleton & Co., 1873, pp. 78.

The author first recites three typical cases which occurred in France; also the judicial proceedings had in each case. The object in selecting cases in a foreign country being "to secure entire absence of all disturbing factors." Then follows a commentary in which the principles are set forth on which a judgment may be founded as to the responsibility or non-responsibility of the accused, in like cases. The author considers it highly absurd to hold that just before and just after, the commission of a *homicide* the accused may be *sane*, and give no evidence of disease of the brain except the homicidal act, and that at that moment, disease did exist. The author holds that an insane person who has committed a murder should never again be allowed to go at large on account of the great danger of relapse;

that the insane should never be confined in ordinary prisons, but in penitentiaries especially for insane criminals; and finally with all our care injustice to some extent, will attend upon every legal process.

The subject is treated in an interesting manner, and the suggestions timely, and important.

AN INTRODUCTION TO THE STUDY OF CLINICAL MEDICINE. Being a guide to the investigation of disease for the use of students. By Octavius Sturges M. D., Cantab., etc. Philadelphia: Henry C. Lea.

[For sale by the St. Louis Book and News Co.]

The author does not dwell tediously on details, but credits the student with some knowledge and common sense.

The author believes it "less by the use of subtle arts, and intricate instruments, than in the exercise of common observation guided by *method*, that the phenomena of disease are revealed." Both student and practitioner will find the book eminently suggestive.

CONTRIBUTIONS TO PRACTICAL SURGERY. By George W. Norris, M. D., late Surgeon to the Pennsylvania Hospital, etc., etc. Philadelphia: Lindsay & Blakiston. 1873. Price $4.00.

[For sale by Gray, Baker & Co., 407 North Fourth Street, St. Louis.]

We here have a work of 318 pages, made up of the following subjects: Fractures, Dislocations, Amputations, and Ligaturing of Arteries, not treated of in detail or exhaustively, but only in certain directions, as they have been investigated by or have fallen under the observation of the author. The articles have mostly already appeared in print in the *American Journal of Medical Sciences,* but new matter has been added to them, and two of the essays appear for the first time.

A service of thirty years in the Pennsylvania Hospital has given Dr. Norris a surgical experience entitled to great regard, and his laborious researches as embodied in this present collection of his papers makes it exceedingly valuable to those interested in surgical subjects. We could have wished that the statistics and investigations had been brought down to the present time, that they might be more, in fact, quite complete. Still, because it has not been done, and though more might have been said on some of the subjects considered, the value of what is given is not marred thereby.

The chapter on *non-union after fractures* is already favorably known to the profession, and it is very complete up to the time it was written. It proves that non-union is comparatively a rare occurrence; delayed union is more frequent. The various causes, both constitutional and local, are given at some length. Though cases do occur which cannot reasonably be explained, in which, as Paget says, there seems to be simply a "defect of formative power." The various expedients of resort to induce union are fully reviewed. A partiality to the seton is manifest and strong argument given in its favor. It has been more or less of a pet resort in this country, and especially in Philadelphia, ever since Physick many years ago brought it forward. Compression and rest are properly recommended as the first means of resort, and "where pressure directly over the seat of fracture is made use of, the tourniquet is preferable to the roller, as by means of the screw a more equible degree of pressure can be kept up," etc. We would suggest that what is true of the tourniquet is more especially true of Malgaigne's screw apparatus, as devised by him for the tibia. A modification or improvement of this, but the same in principle, has been employed by the editor of this journal in two cases of delayed union with most excellent result. It is applied externally to the splint, thus no undue constriction of the limb can take place as happens with the tourniquet. Resection is the last resort advised, as it is so serious and often so unsuccessful. A most valuable table of one hundred and fifty cases of non-union, with mode of treatment, result, etc., is given.

One of three resorts may be employed for the relief of "deformity following an unsuccessfully treated fracture:" First—"pressure and extension of the limb may succeed," if the union is not already too firm. Second—the "callus may be ruptured." Third—"resection" may be resorted to. These different plans are fully considered and cases given in which each expedient was successfully resorted to.

Statistics of the fractures and dislocations treated in the Pennsylvania Hospital during the twenty years preceding 1850, with extended remarks on the mode of treatment, results, etc., are given. These statistics, though imperfect in some important particulars, are valuable as showing hospital cases and practice, which differ always from the proportion of cases and the results to be found in private practice   Since the period included in this report of cases, such great improvements have been made in the treatment of many fractures, that we must believe a better showing of results could now be had.   But it is a significant fact that out of the 2,109 cases treated, not a single case of non-union occurred.

We are pleased to note that our author calls attention to the fact, that fracture of the neck of the thigh bone within the capsule, may, and does occur without being recognized, until after certain use of the limb the sensible signs of this lesion, shortening, evertion, etc., are suddenly made manifest.   From what had fallen under our own observation, we several years since called the attention of the profession to this matter.   Its importance is enhanced by the fact that if thoroughly understood, useful limbs may be saved to those who otherwise become lifelong cripples   Dr. Norris suggests as a solution to this anomaly that the fragments become "interlocked," but we now know positively that in these obscure cases the force which fractured the bone did not rupture certain *retinacula,* or offshoots of the capsular ligament, which hug the femoral neck and are in some instances quite prominent, thus the fragments were held closely together, until use of the part caused these figmental ligaments or thickenings of the periosteum to give way, when shortening and the other signs appeared.

Some of the difficulties encountered as shown in the report of fractures and dislocations would have been greatly simplified and easily overcome had chloroform been in use at that time. Resection of the head of the bone in compound dislocations is very properly advocated, especially if difficulty is experienced in the reduction or retention.

A most worthy article follows on compound fractures. Scarcely sufficient value in these cases is attached to suspension of the limb both as regards the comfort of the patient and ease of dressing, as also the more excellent results that may thus be attained.

Statistical tables are given of two hundred and twenty-eight amputations done at the Pennsylvania Hospital, also a table of results, etc., after ligation of arteries, compiled from all sources, with extended remarks and valuable conclusions.

A case of varicose aneurism at bend of arm, with treatment

etc., closes the work. The book is nicely gotten up, well printed on heavy paper, tinted. The leaves should have been cut before leaving the bindery, and an alphabetical index added would greatly enhance its value. Having derived both pleasure and instruction from its perusal we realize that it should be found on the shelves of every surgeon's library. A. J. S.

CHEMISTRY : General, Medical, and Pharmaceutical, including the Chemistry of the U. S. Pharmacopiæ, a Manual on the general principles of the Science, and their applications to Medicine and Pharmacy. By John Attfield, Ph. D., F. C. S. Fifth edition. Revised from the Fourth (English) edition by the author. Philadelphia: Henry C. Lea, 1878, pp. 606.
[For Sale by the St. Louis Book & News Co]

Better evidence of the popularity of this work with students of chemistry, could not be asked than the fact that it has reached the *Fifth Edition*, in the short period of five years. This extensive demand for the book has afforded the author repeated and ample opportunities to revise his work, and supply such additions as this rapidly advancing department of science may have developed to the present time.

The author has been eminently successful in his design, viz : "To write for the pupils, assistants, and principals engaged in medicine and pharmacy, yet the book is found equally useful for persons having no opportunities of attending lectures, or performing experiments, while its index of *six thousand* references, fit the work for consultation in professional practice. The book contains tables for the convertion of the troy and metric systems of weights and measures, and formulæ for the convertion of the degrees of the Fahrenheit, Centigrade, and Reaumur thermometric scales into each other." We commend this text-book to students advisedly.

HANDBOOK OF PHYSIOLOGY. By William Senhouse Kirkes, M. D. Edited by W. Morrant Baker, F. R. C. S., etc. With two hundred and forty-eight illustrations. A new American from the eighth enlarged English edition. Philadelphia : Henry C. Lea, pp. 656.
[For Sale by the St Louis Book & News Co.]

As it is clearly out of the power of any student to be absolutely thorough, in all departments of science connected with the medical profession, it is a question of the first importance to decide how much he will try to master, in the time alloted to his pupilage. If he is confronted with the most elaborate and complete works as text-books, in each department, perceiving the utter impossibility of a thorough study of each and all, he becomes discouraged and disgusted ; neither is he competent to select the most important themes to be studied and facts to be treasured in the memory, but must depend more or less on those who have been over the ground. The author seems to have appreciated these facts in the preparation of this handbook, and we think him particularly happy in the selection and arrangement of the most useful material for the student of medicine, who is too often crowded and overborne with a multitude of studies during the term of lectures. The book is of convenient size, clear type, on good paper, most of the illustrations are excellent. This edition should increase its former popularity.

BOOKS AND PAMPHLETS RECEIVED.

CLINICAL ELECTRO-THERAPEUTICS, Medical and Surgical. A hand-book for physicians in the treatment of nervous and other diseases. By Allan McLane Hamilton, M. D., with numerous illustrations. New York : D. Appleton & Co., 1873.

[For Sale by the St. Louis Book & News Co.]

PHYSIOLOGY, Handbook. By Wm. Senhouse Kirkes, edited by W. Morrant Baker, F. R. C. S., M. D. With two hundred and forty-eight illustrations. A new American from the eighth enlarged English edition. Philadelphia : Henry C. Lea.

[For Sale by the St. Louis Book & News Co.]

PROSTATE, Diseases of, their pathology and treatment, com-prising the Jackson Prize Essay for 1860. By Sir Henry Thompson, F. R. C. S. Fourth edition. Philadelphia : Henry C. Lea.

[For Sale by the St. Louis Book & News Co.]

CEREBRAL CONVULSIONS OF MAN, According to original observations, especially upon the development of the fœtus. Intended for the use of physicians. By Alexander Ecker, M. D. Translated by Robert T. Edes, M. D. New York: D. Appleton & Co.

[For Sale by the St Louis Book & News Co.]

HIGH ATMOSPHERIC PRESSURE, Including Caisson Diseases. By Andrew H. Smith, M. D. Prize Essay.

CHOLERA AT NASHVILLE. By W. R. Bowling, M. D. 1873.

TYPHOID FEVER, Treatment of. By Joseph F. Montgomery, M. D. Sacramento, Cal.

EPIDEMIC OF MALIGNANT CHOLERA. By Alfred Stillé. Reprinted from the *Philadelphia Times.* Philadelphia: J. P. Lippincott & Co.

[For Sale by the St Louis Book & News Co]

Extracts from Current Medical Literature.

Observations upon the Treatment of Yellow Fever. By Joseph Jones, M. D., New Orleans, La.

1. Yellow fever is a self-limited disease, and can not be arrested by drugs. The poison of yellow fever, as well as the deleterious products resulting from the chemical changes which it excites, are eliminated mainly by the skin and kidneys. Black vomit is the *result* of the action of the yellow fever poison upon the blood and upon certain organs. It should neither be regarded as the active cause nor be treated as *the disease.* Black vomit must be viewed as a *result* and not as a *cause* of diseased action. Therefore the functions of the skin and kidneys should be promoted by suitable means during the progress of the disease. During the early stages the physician should employ those measures which are best adapted to equalize the

circulation and promote the regular and free exercise of the functions of the skin and kidneys. Stimulating diuretics should, as a general rule, be avoided, as they tend to increase the irritation and congestion of the kidneys. A favorable impression may be made upon the circulation and upon the skin by the free use of the hot mustard foot-bath, by the vapor-bath, and in certain cases by the warm-water bath. The action of the skin and kidneys may be promoted by draughts of lemonade and of warm decoctions of mild diuretics, as orange-leaf and sage-tea, and water charged with carbonic acid.

2. The diet should be light but nutritious. Beef-tea, chicken-tea, corn and rice gruel, and barley-water are the best forms of nourishment, and should be continued at regular intervals throughout the active stages of the disease. Solid food, and even bread, should be avoided. In many cases the preceding measures, accompanied by absolute rest in bed and the careful and continuous attention of an experienced nurse, will be all that is required. Alcoholic stimulants should be used with caution, and their effects noted. They have proved beneficial in certain cases attended with great prostration in the stage of febrile excitement. Champagne, when pure, is perhaps one of the best forms of alcoholic stimulants, from the presence of the carbonic acid with which it is charged.

3. Efficient but gentle purgation in the *early part* of the *first stage* of active febrile excitement may prove beneficial in relieving in a measure the congestion of the kidneys and liver, and in removing fecal matters from the bowels. If mercurials are employed, they should be used in the early part of the first stage, not later than the second day of the disease. For an adult from eight to twelve grains of calomel or blue mass will be sufficient. Purgatives should not be administered in the second stage of calm.

4. Quinine may prove beneficial in the *earliest stage* of the disease by its effects upon the nervous system, and by its power of diminishing the temperature and equalizing the circulation; but this drug has no such curative effect in yellow fever as it has in paroxysmal malarial fever. Yellow fever will run a definite course, and pass through a definite series of changes, whether quinine be administered or withheld. After a careful examination of the statements of Blair and others, we have

failed to discover any facts or cases by which the power of
large doses of quinine to *abort yellow fever* can be fully and une-
quivocally established.   It is very evident, from his own statements, that the action of Blair's favorite compound of calomel
and quinine, having the symbol 20×24, was very uncertain ;
and questions may be raised as to whether the cases said to
have been aborted were yellow fever at all, or whether they
may not have been some form of malarial proxysmal fever, or
whether they may not have been the milder forms of yellow
fever, which would most probably have progressed regularly
to convalescence after the hot stage of febrile excitement.
Our own experience, as well as that of many others, has not
accorded with the statement that after yellow fever has been
established it *can be aborted*.   Of course it would be entirely
unnecessary to argue the question with those whose diagnostic
powers are so acute that they are able " to detect a case of yellow fever before the supervention of the hot stage."

The power of quinine not only to arrest but also to ward off
paroxysmal malarial fever is undoubted ; and it has been used
extensively, not only in the treatment of yellow fever, but
more recently as a prophylactic.   Dr. Newkirk, who was at
Asuncion during the recent severe epidemic of yellow fever,
assured Dr. Wm. Nathaniel Hiron, of Buenos Ayres, that the
mortality was small, and that quinine was very generally and
extensively used ; and he expressed his belief that quinine was
prophylactic, and that its continuous use in a healthy person
during an epidemic caused any disease that showed itself to be
mild and tractable.

Dr. Hiron, in his account of the recent severe epidemic of
yellow fever in which Buenos Ayres, with a population not
larger than that of New Orleans, lost, according to the most accurate estimates, nearly twenty thousand of her citizens, records
the additional fact, illustrating the prophylactic properties of
quinine, that " of eleven *practicantes* (dressers) of the Hospital
de Hombres eight took quinine in doses of three grains daily.
All of these had fever of a benign form.   Three took no
quinine; these had the fever very severely, and one died."

While the facts relating to this important subject are too few
to warrant any decided conclusion as to the propriety and
necessity of using quinine as a prophylactic by those exposed

to the yellow-fever atmosphere, at the same time there are facts which indicate that quinine acts not so much as an "antidote" to the poison, but as an "antidote" to the *effects* of the poison, in the system, by preserving the integrity of the blood, regulating and promoting excretion, equalizing the circulation, and fortifying the nervous system against the action of the poison. According to Binz, quinine has the power of arresting putrefacation and fermentation, and is an active poison for all low organisms, animal and vegetable; and Dr. Grace Calvert has confirmed the observations of Binz, and announced the power of quinine to prevent the development of fungi.

These facts have been applied to the explanation of the effects of quinine upon the process of inflammation. Thus according to Conheim's views, pus being mainly a collection of white blood-globules which have passed through the walls of the vessels—quinine having the power of arresting the motions of the white corpuscles, hence preventing their exit from the vessels—the alkaloid arrests, or at all events diminishes, the formation of pus during the course of inflammation. The well-established effect of quinine in producing a *decrement of temperature in fever* has been referred to its power of destroying the ozonizing power of certain substances; and as the red corpuscles have this power, quinine in the blood is supposed to diminish the oxidation of tissue, and thus to lessen the production of heat. Thus Ranke and Keener found that the tissue changes were diminished under the action of large doses of quinine. Zuntz has recorded the observation that quinine, in ten-grain doses, lessens the daily excretion of urea by one third or more; and Unruh has found the same to occur when quinine is administered in fevers. Harley added quinine to blood, and found that it took up less oxygen and gave off less carbonic acid than blood which had not been thus treated. Zuntz and Schute have employed the changes in the alkalinity of the blood for the determination of the same fact. Thus, if fresh blood be drawn, a development of acid begins in it, and continues, at first rapidly, then more slowly, till putrefaction sets in; and as this acidification depends on oxidation, the diminished alkalinity of the blood thereby produced furnishes a test of the rapidity with which oxidation proceeds; and it has been determined by the experiments of Zuntz, Scharæubroich,

38

and Schute that quinine, bebeerine, cinchonine, and picrate of sodium lessen, in different degrees, the production of acid, and consequently prevent the oxidation of the blood.

The experiments of Binz are especially important in their bearing upon the question of the direct action of quinine upon the chemical changes of the blood, or of its indirect action through the nervous system, which show that when putrefying liquids are injected into the circulation the temperature of the body rises; but if the fluids be previously mixed with quinine, whereby the putrefactive processes are arrested or destroyed, the rise in temperature is either entirely arrested or considerably diminished. Such experiments not only throw light upon the therapeutic action of such alkaloids as quinine, but they also illustrate, as it were, the very nature of the processes of those diseases, the effects of which they modify or counteract, by the peculiar chain of chemical actions which they induce in the blood.

5. While local blood-letting may be beneficial in the first stage, when practiced chiefly for the relief of local congestions of the stomach and kidneys general blood-letting is injurious on account of its depressing effects upon the heart and nervous system. Cut cups should be employed with caution, and in the majority of cases they are unnecessary. The circulation will best be influenced by dry cups, sinapisms, and hot mustard foot-baths. Blood-letting, either in large or small quantities, repeated at intervals, is injurious, because it permanently reduces the pulse, prostrates the powers of life, and quickens the fatal termination.

6. The employment of the mineral acids internally, as the nitro-muriatic, from its supposed beneficial effects upon the jaundice, as well as of the tincture of the sesquiohloride of iron, from its supposed power of arresting or preventing black vomit, is of very doubtful propriety. If the view be correct that black vomit intimately associated with and even dependent upon impairment if not complete suppression of the functions of the kidneys, and if to a certain extent it be an effort of nature to relieve the blood of certain poisonous constituents, such agents can have little or no remedial power, and they are in many cases directly injurious by their irritant action upon the congested, irritated, and softened gastric mucous membrane.

7. While opium and its preparations may, in certain cases attended with sleeplessness and great restlessness in the first stage, produce favorable results, at the same time they possess no power of arresting or curing the disease; and should be used with great caution, as they may act with great energy and even poisonous effects when the function of the kidneys is impaired or arrested. This observation applies equally whether opiates be administered by the mouth or by subcutaneous injection.

8. The maintenance as far as possible of absolute rest in the recumbent posture. This precaution appears to be indicated by the results of experience, as well as by the *lesions of the heart,* which I have shown by careful post-mortem examinations to be characteristic of this disease. The central organ of the circulation is structurally altered and enfeebled in yellow fever. The muscular structures of the heart present alterations similar to those observed in the liver and kidneys. Oil and granular albuminoid or fibroid matter is deposited within and around the muscular fibrillæ, and the organ after death presents a yellow, flabby appearance. In some cases time is required for the restoration of its free and vigorous action, and this result is impossible without absolute and continuous rest in the recumbent posture.

Every case of yellow fever should be regarded as *serious,* however slight the symptoms may appear; and on account of the profound structural alterations of the heart, liver, and kidneys, and the profound alterations of the blood, the closest medical attendance and the most careful nursing is demanded.

9. The maintenance of free ventilation, and at the same time the avoidance by proper coverings of sudden changes of temperature.

I have shown by numerous careful analyses of the urine, and by microscopical examinations of the kidneys after death, that in fatal cases the lesions of these organs are profound. The results of these investigations afford an explanation of the fact that sudden changes or depressions of temperature often cause sudden and fatal changes in cases of yellow fever. By sudden depressions of temperature the function of the skin is diminished or arrested, internal congestions promoted and augmented in the enfeebled state of the circulatory and nervous systems which characterize the second stage of calm and depression, and the already crippled kidneys have an additional amount of work thrown upon them, while at the same time they are still further incapacitated for the performance of this work by the increased congestion.

10. The sudden fatal termination of many cases of yellow fever is to be referred chiefly to the sudden arrest of the function of the kidneys. Complete suppression of urine in yellow fever is of more fatal import even than black vomit, which it often accompanies and precedes. In cases of suppression of urine in yellow fever the malpighian corpuscles and tubuli-urin-ifiri are filled with granular albuminoid matter, oil-globules, and detached epithelial cells. If the cessation of the excretion of urine was due simply to capillary congestion or defective enervation, it might be met by appropriate remedies; but the results of my chemical and microscopical examinations have placed in a clear light the reason of the impotency of all measures heretofore proposed for relief of this fatal symptom. The tincture of ergot has been said to have restored the excretion of the urine, but this powerful agent has failed in my hands. The careful physician endeavors to promote the regular action of the kidneys, as indicated in section 1, from the very inception of the disease. As long as the kidneys excrete urine freely, we may entertain hopes of recovery, even though black vomit and jaundice may have supervened.

As a general rule, suppression of the urinary excretion is speedily followed by restlessness, delirium, and coma, and in some cases convulsions. It is folly to expect any good results from sedatives and the various preparations of opium in such cases. Counter-irritants to the surface and the prolonged use of the hot and warm baths alone promise any good.

11. Yellow fever is a self-limited disease, occurring, as a general rule, but once in a life-time. The constitution of the blood and even the textures of the body are altered. The most important organs, as the heart, kidneys, and liver, as well as the most important nutritive fluids, are profoundly impressed. These changes of the blood, heart, kidneys, and liver, and perhaps also of the nervous system, may be compared to the profound changes induced in the blood and organs, and especially in the integument, by the small-pox poison. I have shown by

careful analyses that when the kidneys cease acting in yellow fever, urea and carbonate of ammonia and bile accumulate in the blood, brain, liver, and heart. Many of the nervous symptoms characteristic of yellow fever are referable to the retention of the bile and the constituents of the urine in the blood.

If this view be correct, we can not by *drugs arrest* or *cure* yellow fever any more than we can arrest or cure by drugs smallpox, measles or scarlet fever. If drugs accomplish the effect of promoting the free and regular action of those emunctories through which the poison and the products of its action are eliminated, and if, further, they tend to preserve the integrity of the blood, and to sustain the action of the circulatory and nervous systems, they will, without doubt, achieve much good, and perhaps all that we are justified in looking for in the present state of our knowledge.

By judicious treatment, and by proper attention to ventilation, diet, and rest, we place the patient in that condition best adapted to the successful elimination of the poison and the products of its action ; but we do not arrest or cure the disease, as we certainly may do in paroxysmal malarial fevers, by the proper administration of quinine.—*American Practitioner.*

Sick Headache.

In a report on the treatment of this distressing affection, Dr. Wilks recommends three remedies. To cut short an existing attack, he gives bromide of potassium in doses of gr. xv. to xx. One dose is often sufficient. As a prophylactic he uses the cannabis indica. Of guarana, he says : "Thirdly, guarana has been introduced to our notice as a remedy for sick headache, and here again, we have a very valuable addition to our Pharmacopœia. In many instance, especially those of ladies, I have had the most positive assurance given to me of the power of this drug in arresting headache, so that not the slightest doubt can be entertained of its immense value. A dose is usually taken when the headache is approaching ; and if this is not quickly successful in arresting it, a second powder is swallowed ; after an hour or so, if the remedy is to be useful, the headache has disappeared. I know of several cases in which the greatest enthusiasm is expressed by patients as to its merits. At the same time, I am constantly hearing of cases where it has failed.

I am now trying it in smaller doses by daily administration. I feel certain that these three drugs—bromide of potassium, cannabis indica, and guarana—constitute a most important addition to our nervine medicines, and that in them we have remedies against a terrible complaint which, a few years ago, constituted the opprobrium of medicine. I might say that I know of cases where galvanism has very speedily cured a pain in the head; and I can call to mind the case of a lady, where the application of the bisulphide of carbon invariably relieved the most severe headaches." *Nashville Jour. of Med. and Surg.*

Specialties.

Dr. Barnes says, "I have recently been honored by a visit from a lady of typical modern intelligence, who consulted me about a fibroid tumor of the uterus; and lest I should stray beyond my business, she was careful to tell me that Dr. Brown-Sequard had charge of her nervous system; that Dr. Williams attended to her lungs; that her abdominal organs were entrusted to Sir William Gull; that Mr. Spencer Wells looked after her rectum; and that Dr. Walshe had her heart. If some adventurous doctor should determine to start a new specialty, and open an institution for the treatment of diseases of the umbilicus—the only region which, as my colleague, Mr. Simon, says is unappropriated—I think I can promise him more than one patient.—*London Lancet.*

LINTON DISTRICT MEDICAL SOCIETY.

The semi-annual session of this society will be held in Montgomery City, Missouri, at 2 o'clock P. M., on Tuesday, November 4th, 1873, and continues in session two days.

The officers are, President, Dr. S. N. Russell, of Mexico; Vice Presidents, Drs. W. T. Lenoir, of Columbia, and W. B. Adams, of Danville; Secretary and Treasurer, Dr. H. H. Middelkamp, of Warrenton.

Meteorological Observations.

METEOROLOGICAL OBSERVATIONS AT ST. LOUIS, MO.

By A. Wislizenus, M. D.

The following observations of daily temperature in St. Louis are made with a MAXIMUM and MINIMUM thermometer (of Green, N. Y.). The daily minimum occurs generally in the night, the maximum about 3 P M. The monthly mean of the daily minima and maxima, added and divided by 2, gives a quite reliable mean of the monthly temperature.

THERMOMETER FAHRENHEIT.

AUGUST, 1873.

Day of Month.	Minimum.	Maximum.	Day of Month.	Minimum.	Maximum.
1	70.0	89.0	18	61.0	87.5
2	70.0	80.0	19	65.0	91.0
3	75.5	80.5	20	67.0	92.0
4	61.5	79.0	21	67.0	89.0
5	63.5	83 0	22	67.5	92.0
6	64.5	87.5	23	68.5	93.0
7	68.0	89.5	24	73.0	97.0
8	70.5	91.5	25	76.0	99.0
9	74.0	92.0	26	73.0	98.0
10	73.0	95.0	27	70.0	88.5
11	75.0	95.5	28	67.0	86.0
12	75.0	90.5	29	64.5	87.5
13	73.5	90.0	30	67.5	95.5
14	67.0	86.5	31	73.0	101.5
15	67.5	86.0			
16	68.0	82.0	Means	68.9	89.5
17	60.0	80.0	Monthly Mean 79.2		

Quantity of rain : 0.04 of an inch.

Mortality Report.

FROM AUG. 22d, 1873, TO SEPT. 20th, 1873, INCLUS.

Date	White.		Col'd.		Ages.											Total.
	Males.	Females.	Males.	Females	Under 5 yrs.	5 to 10	10 to 20.	20 to 30.	30 to 40.	40 to 50.	50 to 60	60 to 70.	70 to 80.	80 to 90.	90 to 100	
Saturday 30	116	83	2	3	120	7	4	17	13	20	10	6	4	3	...	204
" 6	109	72	3	1	96	2	8	16	18	17	15	8	4	1	...	185
" 13	108	65	9	3	99	4	8	20	13	17	12	7	2	3	1	185
" 20	68	68	4	3	81	4	3	14	14	12	8	6	1		...	145
Total,	401	288	18	10	396	17	23	67	58	66	45	27	11	7	1	717

Accident	 2	Debility	20	Hepatitis	 3	Peritonitis	 4
Atrophia	 6	Diarrhœa	26	Hydrocephalus-....	4	Pneumonia.	18
Bright's Disease...	3	Disease of the Heart	2	Inanition	8	Premature Birth....10
Bronchitis	9	Dropsy	2	Inflammat'n Brain	7	Rheumatism........ 2
Burns...	1	Drowned	3	" Bowels.	7	Scarlatina 2
Cancer.............	6	Dysentery ..	30	" Liver	7	Small Pox ... 6
Cerebritis	2	Entero-colitis.	2	" Stom	1	Septicæmia 1
Chill, conges	2	Enteritis 14	Injuries....	2	Softening of Brain. 1
Cholera	12	Erysipelas..........	1	Intemperance	5	Suicide............. 5
" Infantum..58	Fever, Bilious	5	Jaundice	1	Summer complaint 5
Cholera Morbus	.50	" intermittent...	7	Laryngitis......	3	Tabes Mesenterica 23
Cirrhosis	. 2	" malignant...	2	Lockjaw...........	2	Teething. . . 17
Conges. of Stomach. 2	" remittent ...	8	Marasmus	48	Uteri Carcimona . 14
" Brain ..14	" typhoid .	10	Meningitis	34	Tetanus, ... 1
" Lungs	3	" congestive	6	Mening . cereb-spin	8	Tumor of Stomach . 1
Consumption	..38	Fracture of skull	2	Mania-a-Potu. . ..	1	
Convulsions . .	42	Hemiplegia ...	1	Old Age...	6	Total........717
Croup	3	Hemorrhage	8	Paralysis	2	Stillborn......... 42

Long Island College Hospital,

BROOKLYN, NEW YORK.

THE REGULAR COURSE OF LECTURES,

In the Long Island College Hospital, will commence on the fourth day of March, 1874, and end the last week in June following.

FEES.—Matriculation, $5 00. Professors' Tickets, $100.00. Demonstrator's fee, $5 00. Graduation fee, $25.00. Hospital Ticket gratuitous.

SAMUEL G. ARMOR, M. D., Dean,

Brooklyn, New York.

1y—sept

THE SAINT LOUIS

Medical and Surgical Journal.

NOVEMBER, 1873.

Original Communications.

DO THE MANIFESTATIONS OF VENEREAL DISEASE DIFFER IN THE MALE AND THE FEMALE?

By THOMAS KENNARD, M. D , St. Louis.

This question is one of immense importance not only to the practitioner but to the patient. It introduces at once the question of the unicity or duality of syphilis, and requires us to determine in our minds which is the correct theory. Whether there be in reality two entirely distinct venereal sores, each characterized by invariable and well defined lesions, which cannot be mistaken by the experienced surgeon ; the one reproducing its like with constancy and universally followed by constitutional syphilis, and the other a mere local sore which never, under any circumstances, infects the system, or whether there be but one kind of syphilitic virus, manifesting itself differently in different localities and different constitutions. This, I say, is a momentous question both to the surgeon and his patient, for upon its solution depends his prognosis and method of treat-

39

ment, and the sufferer's peace and happiness of mind. It is of the most vital importance to be able to say that any venereal sore, from the characteristics which it presents, cannot, by any possibility, be followed by constitutional infection, for upon the determination of that one point alone may depend marriage, or, what is far more important, the dissolution of the holy bonds of matrimony, and the destruction of the happiness of a whole family. Nor is it unimportant whether the sore be treated merely as a local affection or as the initial lesion of a series of serious constitutional complications. In the former case local treatment only would be demanded or justifiable, whilst in the latter, unless judicious specific constitutional treatment be resorted to, a lifelong taint, would be imparted to the system, the manifestations of which may harass the patient during his whole life; communicate the disease to his wife and transmit it to his children and children's children. Then, the all important question for every practitioner to determine is, whether the primary manifestations of this protean disease be such and so invariable as to enable him to say whether such and such a venereal sore will never be followed by constitutional infection, and whether another or other certain kinds will inevitably be followed by blood contamination. Again he must be able to say whether the primitive lesions are always the same in *both sexes*. The study then of the disease, in both the male and the female, is an absolute necessity to enable any one to draw correct conclusions in regard to this disease. The great mass of mankind unfortunately do very little thinking, and the majority of our profession are too ready to follow the teachings of dis-. tinguished authors and teachers instead of viewing every doubtful point as a problem to be worked out by themselves.

The doctrine of the duality of the venereal virus, that is, the existence of one kind, which will always manifest itself in the form of a hard chancre, after a certain period of incubation; which has its origin from a similarly indurated sore, or rather from one in which induration to a greater or less extent has existed, and been its typical characteristic; which is almost always single, never multiple except from simultaneous inoculation; one where the edges are sloping, hard, often elevated and adhering closely to the subjacent structures, with a surface presenting the appearance of having been hollowed or scooped out, which is smooth and secretes but little pus, the discharge being mostly serous, and not inoculable upon the same patient or upon any other person who has been previously affected by syphilis. A sore which has, as an invariable accompaniment, enlargement and induration to some extent of the inguinal glands on one or both sides, which are freely moveable and painless and which very seldom suppurates. This is designated the chancre, the hard chancre, the syphilitic sore, and is considered to be the only initial venereal lesion which can be followed by blood contamination and constitutional symptoms, and which will invariably be followed by secondary symptoms unless very promptly and properly treated.

The other kind of virus is that which also originates from a sore similar to the one which it produces, which acts much more rapidly in producing its external manifestations than the other, which has no period of incubation, but, a short time after inoculation, will give rise to one or many sores, or ulcerations perforating the

entire substance of the mucous membrane or the skin
as the case may be; having irregular abrupt, and well
defined edges, with irregular boundaries, and uneven
base, and secreting freely a ˙ purulent secretion—which
may readily reproduce its like upon the same individual
indefinitely—or at least for a great number of times.
Cases in which, if the glands be affected either by the
extension of the inflammation or the conveyance of the
poison by the lymphatics, they will invariably suppurate
and become open sores, secreting inoculable pus like
the original ulcer. This is considered a purely local
affection, and, it is claimed, cannot under any circumstances give rise to constitutional symptoms.

This doctrine of duality, then, claims that in every
instance we can form an infallible opinion of the nature
of the disease from the external appearance of the sore,
and be able to state in every case whether our patient
will have constitutional syphilis or not, and hence it has
captivated so many young men and general practitioners,
who have read just enough upon the subject to confuse
themselves, and have not enjoyed enough practical experience to have formed any opinion of their own, or
to dare to dissent from the prevailing views of the day.
This view, first originating on the Continent of Europe,
has now entrapped the majority of writers upon syphilis
throughout the civilized world, and yet, I am certain
that the exceptions to the rule are so numerous that we are
not justified in assuring any patient, and more especially
a *female*, that because they have a non-indurated sore,
or what we designate a chancroid, therefore it is impossible for them to have secondary syphilis. I am free to
acknowledge that in the male, a chancroid is very seldom
followed by constitutional disease, but in the female the

rule does not hold good, because the exceptions to the rule are too numerous. Ricord had observed that certain kinds of sores presenting uniform and peculiar characteristics and which were always indurated, were invariably followed by constitutional symptoms, and that another class of sores, having the property of reproducing their like, and capable of being transmitted by inoculation, but never indurated, were seldom followed by constitutional symptoms, but generally acted simply as local sores. That was the opinion which the great investigator arrived at.

In 1852, Bassereau examined carefully into this question suggested by Ricord, and came to the conclusion that there were two distinct kinds of venereal sore; the one, the indurated or true syphilitic sore, and the other, the soft or simple sore, or what we now designate as the chancroid. The former, the true infecting chancre, and the latter the non-infecting sore. He came to this conclusion from the confrontation of persons affected with the venereal disease with those from whom they had gotten it, and those to whom they had transmitted it, that like produced and transmitted like in every case. That is, that those who had hard chancre received it from a person who had hard chancre, and could only impart that kind of sore to another, whilst those suffering from soft chancre had been inoculated by one similarly affected, and could only transmit the same kind of sore to another. The former always being followed by constitutional symptoms, and the latter never. Three years later, another Frenchman, M. Clerc, advocated the same doctrine, and arrived at the same conclusions, namely, that there was a duality of the syphilitic virus; two kinds of virus, producing two entirely distinct sores; the one always contaminating the blood, the other only capable of producing a local sore.   M. Bassereau very learnedly contended that the soft sore was of very ancient origin, having existed long before syphilis was ever seen, and was, in reality, the contagious ulcer, which the ancients describe as being common among them, and that the hard chancre, the true syphilitic sore, was never known nor described until the memorable epidemic of the 15th century.   M. Clerc, on the other hand, maintained that the chancroid, or soft sore, was a modified chancre, originating from the inoculation of hard chancre upon a person at the time suffering from, or who had previously suffered from true syphilis, just as people have the varioloid, or modified small-pox, after having had vaccinia or variola, but very seldom had true variola under similar circumstances.   His idea was that the soft sore was a derivative of the hard sore, and hence he proposed the name of chancroid (clinically a very appropriate name).   Thus originated, or rather was revived, the idea of the duality of the syphilitic virus.   This view was not, however, a new one, for many of the early writers on venereal disease describe the hard or indurated chancre, and its accompanying induration of the inguinal glands, as the kind of sore that usually infects the system, and the soft non-indurated sore, with suppurating bubo, as the one which seldom gives rise to constitutional symptoms, and made the presence of induration the characteristic symptom of the true chancre; but they were too practical to contend that none but indurated sores were ever followed by contamination of the blood, but admitted that constitutional symptoms often followed soft sores, and even simple abrasions.   John Hunter, Carmichael, and many others, had noticed this difference between hard and soft chancres, and Carmichael even contended that each peculiar primary sore produced its peculiar secondary manifestations.

Now this theory is a very nice one, and if its truth was only borne out by the teachings of practical experience, would prove an extremely satisfactory one, and save both patient and physician a great deal of trouble and anxiety in regard to the future, but experience has taught us that the true Hunterian chancre is much more rare in the female than in the male, and is not the only kind of venereal sore in the female, which is a true chancre, and will infect the system. Infecting chancres of all kinds are, however, undoubtedly much less frequent in the female than in the male. The proportion in the latter being not more than one in ten or twelve, whilst in the former it is one in four or five, as stated by our best authorities. Chancroids are much more common in females than in males, that is, the soft sore has a much greater tendency or liability to become multiple in woman than in man, owing to the peculiar formation and functions of the female genital organs, and the greater amount of mucous surface exposed, and the close apposition of these sensitive parts. The female genital organs are more complicated in every way, and subject to many more sources of irritation: such as the abnormal discharges from the womb and vagina that often excoriate the delicate mucous membrane, and thus render the multiplication of sores much more easy. We often find from three to five, and sometimes more, chancroids on one woman, and it is very seldom that we find only one, if that has existed for a few days without treatment. These and all other venereal sores are situated, as a rule upon the external genitalia, on the labia majora, the labia minora, at the inferior commissure, and the extreme lower portion of the vagina, and more rarely involve the clitoris and meatus urinarius. In a very limited number of cases, they are seated high up in the vagina, in the urethra and upon the cervix uteri.

"In seventy-six cases of chancroid examined by M. Robert, of Marseilles, for the purpose of determining the relative frequency of seat, thirty were found about the inferior commissure, seventeen on the labia minora, eleven at the entrance to the vagina, seven on the vulva, four near the meatus urinarius, three on the inner surface of the labia majora, two on the clitoris, and two on the caruncula. In thirty-five cases, completing a series of 111, the soft chancres occupied different situations along the interior of the vagina."

My experience, which has been somewhat extensive, having made at least ten thousand examinations of females, confirms the statement of M. Robert in the main, but I have found a much smaller proportion of sores occupying the interior of the vagina than he gives. It has been very rare indeed to find a sore so far within the vagina that it could not be detected without the aid of the speculum, that is, by one accustomed to making examinations. We do find the soft chancre occasionally upon the neck of the womb, and then it has a roundish elevated appearance like the mucous papule.

The chancroid upon the female is much more irregular in shape than upon the male, unless it be upon the external parts, or on some portion of the labia majora. Thus situated, it presents the same appearance as in the male, whilst in other places, its shape may vary according to its seat, and the condition of the parts at the time of infection.

The chancroid is far more common in the lower classes than in the upper. In hospital practice we find it much oftener then we do the hard sore, but in private practice the proportion of hard chancres is much greater. Some authors give the ratio as three to one, and precisely the reverse among charity patients. This may be accounted for from the fact, that the lower order of men contract the disease from the lowest order of prostitutes, who like themselves, are not only extremely filthy and negligent in attending to their persons, and frequently perfectly oblivious to soft, painless sores that may exist, and allow them to multiply and repeat themselves indefinitely. Moreover most of these common women have been upon the town for a long time, and during the early part of their career, have suffered from true syphilis, and consequently are in a great measure proof against its repetition. On the other hand, men in the higher walks of life seek the society of the better class of courtezans, and the young or those who are recently initiated into the mysteries and miseries of harlotry, who pay very particular attention to their genitalia, and are very careful not to allow any sore to remain long unhealed upon their persons, but not only that, but never having had syphilis, they are more likely to get it, and communicate it to their friends, than those who have sunk to a more degraded position.

John Morgan, A. M., M. D., of the University of Dublin, Surgeon to the Westmoreland Lock Hospital, etc., who has written a work styled "Contagious Diseases," says that out of one thousand cases of females under his care at that institution, he saw only twenty cases of what could be called the typical indurated sore, and that the register of the Lock Hospital for many years back corroberates his observations. He also states that among 1000 cases he only saw one case of truly intra-vaginal sore, and it was not indurated at all, and more-over he had never met with a case where a male had contracted a venereal or syphilitic sore from a female who had no sore except a superficial erosion or ulcera-tion of the cervix, but that he had known gonorrhœa to be communicated that way frequently, and that this would account for men catching the gonorrhœa occa-sionally from a woman who, at the time of coitus, and afterwards, had no vaginal discharge or other symptom of the disease. The experience of medical examiners under the Social Evil Law, will confirm the statement of the great preponderance of the chancroid over the chancre, especially among the lower class of the women under their charge, and if they follow up the history of the cases that they commit to the hospital, they will not unfrequently find constitutional symptoms follow-ing the soft sores.

In patients suffering from gonorrhœal, or simple va-ginitis, or irritating vaginal discharge of any kind what-soever, excoriations of the mucous membrane are very liable to occur, and consequently a series of chancroids are often found on the inner surface of the labia majora, which sometimes run into each other, forming a large and irregular sore, and producing infiltrations of the cellular tissue, with great induration and swelling of the parts. Higher up and just within the entrance to the vagina, the same irregularity in the form of the chan-croid is likely to occur, and from the same causes. The upper two-thirds of the vagina is rarely ever the seat of a venereal sore, much more rarely so than the os tincæ or cervix uteri even, because the lips of the mouth of the womb become ulcerated very easily. Chancres in this region resemble superficial excoriations from non-specific causes, and present no special appearances which will enable us to distinguish them from simple erosions, and hence the necessity of attending to all abrasions and ulcerations of the cervix in prostitutes, whether we believe them to be venereal in their nature or not. Venereal sores of all kinds, but more especially those that are considered to be non-infecting, require prompt treatment and very careful attention in the female to prevent further inoculation and multiplication, and the severe pain which they are likely to produce.

The fact that more men suffer from hard chancre than women may, it is true, be in a measure accounted for from the fact that one woman may infect many men, whereas, a man suffering from such a sore, will rarely have the inclination or the hardihood to indulge in sexual intercourse at all. Hence the enforcement of the Social Evil Law, and the requirement of the immediate seclusion and prompt treatment of diseased prostitutes has done very much to diminish the frequency of infecting chancres in women, and thus tended very materially to check the spread of syphilis. It is stated that in the female Lock Hospital (Lourcine) of Paris, where about 270 beds are kept occupied by patients suffering from venereal disease, that the number of cases of infecting chancres does not exceed fifty annually, I mean the indurated or classical hard chancre, for that is the only kind of sore that the majority of authors claim can infect the system, and here is where I am

forced to differ with them.   My experience has taught
me that this is one of the false facts, which has been
taught medical students for many years, and which has
been taken for granted as true by the majority of practitioners, whose knowledge of syphilis has been gained
more from the books than from practical experience,
and is consequently in many instances very imperfect
and incorrect.   The nature and form of chancres is not
determined entirely by the nature of the syphilitic
virus, but depends upon the location in which it is developed and the idiosyncracy of the patient.

The dualists of the present day do not contend that
induration is an invariable symptom which may be
detected in every infecting chancre, and by this admission they really acknowledge the truth of what I am
contending for, viz: that we cannot always diagnosticate between the chancre and the chancroid.

Bumstead, one of the most enthusiastic advocates of
the dualistic doctrine, says, " Now the *question is not*
whether the initial lesion of syphilis always presents
well-marked characteristics, or whether it can always be
distinguished from a chancroid.   It is freely admitted
that aside from anto-inoculation which is often impracticable, diagnosis is in some cases impossible.   We may
go further, and assert that even were it never possible
to distinguish a true chancre from a chancroid, the
proof of their distinct nature would be just as strong
as at present.   *The question is,* whether a striking difference, a local character on the one hand, and a constitutional character on the other, which have long been recognized as pertaining to venereal ulcers, is constant in
successive generations."   This candid admission proves
clearly enough then, that we cannot positively diagnos-

ticate and prognosticate syphilis, for if we admit that
oftentimes the most striking symptoms arè wanting,
how are we to determine with absolute certainty into
which class to place a venereal sore. Induration is not
always present in the true sore, and is consequently not
an unvarying system of syphilis.

Moreover if a chancre be the same in every individual, and if syphilis be invariable in its external manifestations, why does the time of its incubation differ so
widely in different cases. In almost every other disease except hydrophobia, the so-called period of quies-
cence or incubation is uniform. In variola, scarlatina,
rubeola, etc., we can calculate the period for the
appearance of the eruption very àccurately, but in
syphilis the period of incubation differs very much.
From cases of direct inoculation on untainted subjects,
the period of incubation has been found to vary from
ten to forty-six days, giving a mean of twenty-four
days. Cases have been recorded, however, where the
period of incubation was 50, 70, and 72 days, and Dr.
Hammond gives one where the interval was only thirty-
six hours.

Dr. Gross says: " My observations would lead me to
infer that, while there are really two varieties of chancre,
the indurated and the soft, as described by the French
syphilographer, they do not by any means possess the
properties which he ascribes to them. The hard chancre is unquestionably most frequently followed by constitutional symptoms, but to maintain that it is so exclusively, is what, I am sure, no experienced practitioner
will admit. So far from giving my adhesion to such a
doctrine, I have had the most unequivocal evidence, in
numerous instances, of the infecting properties of the

soft chancre. Indeed, I am satisfied that some of the very worst cases of secondary and tertiary syphilis that I have ever been called upon to treat have been cases of this description; originating generally in very small sores upon the head of the penis or prepuce, perfectly soft in their consistence, very superficial, manifesting no disposition to spread, and soon completely disappearing."

"Such chancres frequently exist without the knowledge of the patient, their discovery being, perhaps, purely accidental. It is, doubtless, this form of ulcer which has given rise to the absurd notion, yet not entirely exploded, of the possibility of the formation of bubo, without the precedence or concomitance of chancre."

The differences in form and feel of chancres are many times of an accidental character, and not entirely dependent upon the nature of the syphilitic · virus, but the effect of the virus is modified ·by local and constitutional causes, and differs in its manifestations in different individuals, just as we find every other disease does There can be no reason why syphilis should always be uniform, any more than variola, scarlatina, etc., should.

Dr. Morgan says: "I am forced by the accumulation of evidence based on absolute observation of very many hundreds of cases, to conclude that, while in the male, the occurrence of an indurated sore is the usual harbinger of constitutional infection, in the female it is by no means so; and that with them constitutional infection as certainly, and even with greater gravity, follows the sore which is without induration; and in this city (Dublin) at all events, we might truthfully state, that while in the male the indurated sore, with its pleiad of enlarged glands in the groin, is the more certain index of an infected system, in the female it is by no means essential ; and a sore without the least similar evidence is, as a rule, also as correct an index of an infected system, and might, in fact, be in *them* styled the infecting sore. This observation arises from no inexactitude of examination. The records of the Lock Hospital prove this fact at the present day, and so long since as from 1843 to 1848. Mr. Egan, Surgeon to the same hospital, states that but twenty-nine of the indurated, excavated ulcers came under his notice in five years." "Nearly all the patients in the Dublin Lock Hospital suffer from non-indurated sores only, and yet are almost invariably constitutionally infected. Bœck, of Norway, reports the following case : "A very young girl, K. E., (whose sister was a *fille publique*,) intending to adopt this kind of life, presented herself for inspection, and received the usual certificate from Mr. Lund, the official surgeon, who noted at the same time that she had the *hymen intact*, and was therefore a virgin. In a few days afterwards she came to the hospital suffering from small non-indurated ulcers near the vulvo-vaginal glands. She was frequently examined with the greatest care, but no other affection could be found ; but in six weeks afterwards, constitutional signs appeared. Any inexactitude of examination in this case must be regarded as impossible, and this observation together with others, has made me certain that the non-indurated sore in women can produce constitutional syphilis."

"Cullerier," in speaking of the different names given syphilitic sores by different authors says : "In the actual state of science, none of these denominations are free from objection. The infecting chancre is not always indurated. I do not admit that the sad privilege of infecting the system is the exclusive property of one form of chancre alone, or that the chancre which is called simple, has no natural relationship nor affiliation with syphilis. I shall notwithstanding make use of the generally received names, the clinical value of which is universally known." One of the most insidious forms of infecting chancre, and that which is so much more often found in females than in males, is the simple erosion. The ulceration is then so superficial that its surface is on a level with the surrounding parts. It may be either round or irregular ; its dimensions are variable, and frequently when situated on a mucous membrane, it can only be distinguished by its color from the neighboring parts. The presence of specific induration would remove all doubts ; but this is often so slight and fugitive as to escape the notice of the physician himself. * * * Hence the great number of chancres that pass unnoticed by the patient, or the nature of which is not recognized. Such chancres simulate perfectly simple erosions." (Cullerier.)

We find not unfrequently, the cethymatous chancre, resembling a pustule, which occurs on the external integuments, and consequently is generally covered with a crust. It is sometimes indurated, or rather is surrounded by inflammatory engorgement, but does not present the typical induration, which is claimed as the characteristic sign of the true chancre, and yet it is often followed by secondary symptoms. It was probably this form of chancre that induced the early writers to describe syphilis as a pustular disease, commencing on the genital organs and gradually extending over the whole body.

Again a very large number of cases show no signs of

induration whatever, on the very portions of the body where induration most commonly is found, and yet they are true chancres, and most certainly will infect the system unless very promptly and properly treated. Contamination of the blood with syphilitic poison will often follow the most simple looking ulcerations, and even mere cracks, fissures and abrasions of the mucous membranes, without the slightest feeling of induration, or the most remote resemblance to the so-called classical chancre. The enlargement of the glands in the groin is the only symptom likely to excite suspicion, and to direct us to a correct diagnosis.

The indurated bubo is then of far more importance in forming a correct diagnosis of a venereal sore in a female than is induration of the base of the sore itself, for it is not so often absent, whereas the induration is by no means a constant accompaniment of the infecting chancre.

This absence of induration in the female, must, in my opinion, depend on the peculiar conformation of the female genitalia, on the nature of the tissues involved, and on the locality of the sore, and not on the difference of sex, for the infecting sore on the lips, mammæ, fingers, and any external portion of the body is as invariably and distinctly indurated as in the male, and there is no reason why mere difference of sex should cause any difference in the nature of the sore.

Another clinical fact, which would tend to substantiate the view that the form of the sore depends in a great measure upon its locality, is the early appearance and prevalence of the so-called mucous patch upon the female genital organs. More than half of the women who suffer from syphilis, have mucous patches on the inner side'of the labia majora, on the labia minora, just within the vagina, on the neck of the womb or around the anal orifice, and in every location, this very common affection differs in its general appearance, though one and the same affection in every instance. So, too, we find virulent bubo far more common in men than in women. Not more than one woman in ten, suffering from chancroids, has a suppurating bubo, whilst in men, one out of every four has it, which is probably due to the fact of certain anatomical differences in the distribution of the inguinal lymphatics in the two sexes.

Induration of the inguinal glands is then by no means so common, or so characteristic of true syphilis, in the female, as in the male. Nor do we find the suppurating bubo following the chancroid, near so often in the female, as in the male. Secondary syphilis, however, unfortunately follows the suppurating bubo in the female quite frequently, and the suppurating bubo is often cutaneous with marked constitutional disease. I might fill pages in illustrating the facts stated above, for the works are full of them, and my own individual experience has furnished examples enough to convince any one open to conviction; but I will not take up your time with such details—for tables of cases are not very interesting at best, and those who would be inclined to doubt my conclusions, would not be likely to give much credence to my report of cases, but, like the dualistic authors, would conclude that my mistakes had arisen from inexactitude of observations, or want of knowledge.

The dualists contend that there is in reality but one syphilitic virus, but that the venereal sores classed by the unitists as syphilitic, have no connection with true

syphilis at all. This is the view generally entertained
at the present day, and is in main correct, and, for clinical study and teaching, is a most admirable doctrine,
and far more useful and practical than the old confused
doctrine of the early writers; but I contend that its advocates have pushed the distinction too far, and attempted to draw the diagnostic lines too closely, for we
do not yet thoroughly understand the relations existing
between all venereal sores and constitutional syphilis.
Induration, either of the sore or the glands, is not a *"sine
qua non"* of every true syphilic sore, although the most
constant and reliable symptom to direct us in forming
a correct diagnosis. Constitutional symptoms do follow soft sores occasionally in men, and much more
often in women, and artificial inoculation from the
sore has produced the typical hard chancre in some
cases, as reported by Ricord, Cullerier, Melchior
Robert, Langlebert, Morgan, and others. Some reliable
authorities have even gone farther than this, as Melchior Robert, who states that he took the pus from a
perfectly soft chancre on the penis, and by inoculating it
upon the lip of the same person, produced a characteristic hard chancre. Others state that occasionally a sore
will have every appearance of a chancroid, and remain
so for a long time, and then, without any additional infection, present all the characteristic symptoms of a
chancre, as, enlarged indurated glands, etc. The dualists contend that this confusion originates from imperfect observrtions, and undertake to explain all these
cases are errors in judgment, and to get over the change
in the nature of one and the same sore, they had advanced the idea of the mixed chancre. That is, the existence at one and the same point of the chancroidal

and syphilitic virus, each running its own course, and consequently developing itself locally at different dates. It is very true that we are all liable to err in diagnosis, but I can see no reason why one school is any more liable to make mistakes than the other, or more likely to misunderstand or misrepresent facts as observed in the cases before them; and as long as the most experienced specialists differ in their opinions about duality and unicity, how is the general practitioner or the medical student to be expected to diagnosticate venereal sores correctly. The doctrine advocated by the dualists, clinically, answer our purposes far better, and leads to much the most rational treatment, but in their anxiety to establish their doctrine as infallible, and make their diagnostic rules apply to every case, they have mislead many inexperienced persons in forming a prognosis, and made them give unreliable assurances to the patient, in regard to his future immunity from disease.

THE DEBATABLE GROUND.

By Jos. ADOLPHUS, A. M., M D., St. Louis.

In the May number of the *Medical Archives*, my distinguished and learned friend, Prof. E. Montgomery, continues his able defense of his " Plea for the Antiphlogistic Treatment" of inflammations. Prof. Montgomery's ability to maintain his part of the controversy is undisputed. The courteous and affable manner in which he has treated me is duly appreciated. On the

score of politeness he has the advantage; but this is
in part owing to his superior culture and affability.
The Professor compliments my last article, in the February number of the *Archives*, by styling it a very able,
ingenious and argumentative article ; this is very flattering indeed, taking into consideration the fact that
Prof. Montgomery has not succeeded in invalidating
any of the facts and principles contained in the article
alluded to.

In regard to the intrinsic merits of the question in
controversy, I hold that Prof. Montgomery is still far
from successfully defending the doctrines and principles
he laid down and enunciated in his original " PLEA."
His paper in the May number of the *Archives* served
him only in the light of a codicil to an apology, rather
than an argument in defense of his original plea. This
Prof. Montgomery in part acknowledges, although he
charges me with having placed him "in a false position." I can assure my dear friend that he is entirely
mistaken in regard to this, and when he reviews
more closely my paper in the February number of the
Archives he will be ready to take back this charge.
Prof. Montgomery has several times quoted Rindfleisch
to sustain him in this controversy. I am not a little
astonished that my esteemed competitor should construe
Rindfleisch to mean by the words "antiphlogistic therapeutics," blood-letting. I shall quote from Rindfleisch and show the pith of his argument on this point,
and if Prof. Montgomery can obtain any aid or comfort from it, all right.

"It is manifest that if, by our medical skill, we could
succeed in removing again the cells which have wandered
into an inflamed organ, this organ would return to the

same condition in which it was before the inflammation, provided we deduct the modification of the connective tissue fibres mentioned in the previous paragraph, which meanwhile would likewise soon disappear.   The question of the possibility of a resolution of inflammation, and the means of inducing the same has, therefore, a highly practical interest.   It might at first occur to us, to send away the cells in the same way in which they came, that is to say, to let them wander farther.   In this, moist heat is applied with advantage.   Exaltation of temperature also accelerates, as is known, the movements of amœboid cells.   When, therefore, the inflammatory infiltration is not great, and the inflammatory irritant does not continue to act, one may hope, by locally increasing the temperature, to diffuse the already present wandering cells over a greater space, and gradually to convey them into the lymphatics.   A second mode of resolution of existing inflammatory infiltration becomes possible by the fatty degeneration of the cellular element.   We saw above how fatty degeneration converts all kinds of cells into a milk-like detritus, of whose immediate resorption naturally no hindrances stand in the way.   The presence of abundant amounts of fluid in the inflammatory focus appears to be a decided condition for the commencement of fatty degeneration.   Busch has made an interesting experience that under the influence of erysipelas, massy sarcomatous proliferations disintegrate, and I have most certainly convinced myself in one of his cases, that the sarcoma cells thereby fall into fatty degeneration.   Heat would also be appropriate for keeping down a lasting hyperæmia of this kind.   In spite of this double indication, the moment of time must be exactly considered in which

one may pass from the cold to the warm treatment of
an inflammation. The object of the cold treatment is
by an artificially induced contraction of the vessels principally to restrain exudation, with reference to prohibit-
ing the farther emigration of colorless blood corpuscles.
We would only pass to the use of warmth, either when
this indication has been fulfilled, or when it can no
longer be fulfilled ; for it is evident that heat is a two-
edged sword. Who will be surety that instead of a depression of the exudation which, indeed, we would first
of all desire, a stronger concentration of mobile cells
shall not occur at the heated point, that is to say, suppuration and formation of abcess? A certain amount
of heat evidently acts depressing, a higher degree irritating to the process of inflammation ; the former
causes the largely exuded colorless blood corpuscles to
wander farther ; the latter causes the process of emigration to renew itself, and it increases in intensity.

"*Annotation.*—The therapeutic complexion which I
give this chapter may be an example to the student, how
directly the results of pathological histology may also
be applied to the practical treatment of the physician."
pp. 107–108.

The reader will observe how little support Prof.
Montgomery will obtain from Rindfleisch in this controversy, and one is not a little surprised that a gentleman of so much sagacity and penetration as Prof. Montgomery possesses should fall into such an error.

. Now let us see whether I have placed my friend "in a
false position." Prof. Montgomery's own words are,
" In the commencement of a case of inflammatory disease, if the patient is not too young, or too old, or too
feeble for antiphlogistics, we bleed, purge, give vera-

trum, or aconite etc." According to this rule very
few, cases would be bled at all. "The other anti-
phlogistics, as mercury, opium, tartar emetic, veratrum viride, aconite, cold, etc., we use with extreme
caution, and on the earliest indication for their use,
promptly administering tonics and nutrients." It
is very evident that by the above we are to understand Prof. Montgomery to mean that we must bleed
every case of inflammation "that is not too young, too
old, or too feeble." This is the rule he lays down, and
that we are to resort to tonics and nutrients only after
we have reduced the patient, and he begins to show the
effects of our treatment on his vital powers. If by
these measures Prof. Montgomery does not carry "the
issue of the malady on the point of his lancet," then
no language can convey such an idea. If Prof. Montgomery does not mean what he says, the fault is not
mine. And I believe that every intelligent man on
reading all the papers that have come from my learned
friend's erudite and fertile pen during the progress of
this controversy, will come to the conclusion that I
have in no wise misrepresented him.

Prof. Montgomery says that all the great systematic
writers on medicine sustain his view of the question.
Let us see how far they, in a general sense, speak of
blood-letting as a therapeutic measure ; but they nevertheless hedge it around with a far more abundant caution than does my distinguished friend. As systematic
writers, they say that blood-letting is a remedy for inflammation, but even Watson would reflect a thousand
times before he resorted to it once, in fact, it is evident
they practically regard it as a loved memory of the past
only. Prof. Montgomery, in attempting to grapple

with my facts and arguments adduced from the writings of many distinguished men in opposition to him, claims that their experience was derived mainly, if not wholly, from the poor, miserable devils that infest European hospitals, and claims that the hostility the phlebotomy system has encountered, arose from its ill effects upon such subjects. Right here is where Prof. Montgomery is in error again.

The annals of the profession for thirty years show that hostility to the antiphlogistic or blood-letting system of treating inflammations first commenced with men who were engaged in large private practice among the well-to-do classes. The murderous results that the antiphlogistic treatment produced on these classes of well-to-do people brought it into odium. The large mortality of pneumonia, bronchitis, and other inflammatory affections among the better classes, was brought under statistical notice by Pfeufer, of Heidelberg, in an able paper, somewhere about 1844. In comparing with hospital practice the results of private practice, the difference was but little, indeed. We all recollect the able manner in which Sharpter handled this question, and what an effect it had upon Brodie, Gull, B. Jones, W. F. Mackenzie, Hilton, Sky, Stokes, and other distinguished men. These men, it must be remembered, were long in private practice before they went into hospitals. The most remarkable feature in this overhauling of a long petted system of practice, was the remarkable change that came over the French school under the leadership of Louis. This great man was among the first to arrive at the conclusion that the antiphlogistic treatment of disease was a great mistake. He, too, found that the reduction of inflammatory products were in no way effected by phlebotomy, and Gull, in one of his first papers, showed that there was no reliance to be placed upon it. About this time Trosseau was becoming prominent in Paris as a clinical lecturer. He never lost an opportunity of impressing on the minds of his hearers, that if blood-letting at times did good, there was more certainty of its doing harm than otherwise. The investigations and studies of the German school, in the natural history of disease, as well as in pathology, soon brought all the facts within the limits of comparatively clear demonstration that blood-letting as a therapeutic agent, had so few merits that it could safely be abandoned in practice. With this view Niemeyer concurred as well as others of the German school.

Prof. Montgomery endeavors to draw an argument from the numerical mortality attending pneumonia during the prevalence of the restorative treatment. It seems to me that Prof. Montgomery has severely forgotten the past history of our profession. Any man of ordinary attainments can easily satisfy himself that the mortality attending pneumonia and other pulmonary diseases has been gradually growing less during the last twenty years. During the antiphlogistic regime the mortality of pneumonia was near 70 per cent. In fact, thirty years ago it was fully that. The mixed treatment, which Prof. Montgomery so much lauds, had its day as well. With it the mortality was somewhat reduced, though it was still large. Thirty years ago, if a physician lost only 40 per cent. of his cases of pneumonia, he was considered to be a very fortunate practitioner. To-day the man who loses 15 per cent. of his cases of ordinary pneumonia, is regarded as a very indifferent practitioner, indeed.

What the learned professor says relating to pneumonia and its mortality in this city, I shall not dwell long upon. Every painstaking physician knows that pneumonia, bronchitis. and other pectoral affections are very prevalent among children and infants. The common sense view of mortality reports, show a high mortality among subjects under 15 years of age. We find among these a pretty high share of pneumonia and other pulmonary affections, but the disease is mostly of the catarrhal kind, and every well-informed physician knows that there is a marked difference between the gravity of this kind of pneumonia and that known as "croupous." I believe that I can with safety affirm that 95 per cent. of croupous pneumonia will recover without any very active treatment. In fact, I think that the antiphlogistic treatment, no matter how cautiously carried out, would both increase the mortality and lengthen the duration of the disease. I am confident the best minds of the profession will sustain me in this statement. On the other hand, no sane man would dream of treating a case of catarrhal pneumonia with phlebotomy, mercury, or tartar emetic. These cases from the very outset, need not only a restorative treatment but careful stimulation to carry them through. The robust adult is seldom attacked with catarrhal pneumonia, while the feeble infants, children and many aged people suffer from it almost exclusively. Let Prof. Montgomery draw a moral from the above facts.

The effort now being made in certain quarters to revive the bleeding system of treatment is meeting with more and more opposition every day from clinical facts and figures. Sebert, of Berlin, has shown that 246 cases of pneumonia were treated in 1870 with the loss

of less than 6 per cent., the treatment was quinine, carbonate of ammonia, veratrum viride, wine, nutrients, and
occasional blisters.   Dr. Watters, of Liverpool, England, gives an account of fifty-nine cases of acute pneumonia, treated on the restorative principles, with a loss
of but two cases.   Dr. Parton, of Indianapolis, Indiana, reports ninety-six cases of pneumonia treated with
carbonate of ammonia, nutrients, good nursing, with a
loss of two.   Dr. Witherspoon, of Bruceville, Indiana,
reports seventy-two cases treated in the same way with
a loss of two, and Dr. Stevens, of Russellville, Indiana,
reports thirty-five cases treated the same way with
one death.   These facts are reported in *Butler's Half-
yearly Compendium* for 1871.   But Prof. Montgomery
insists that sthenic cases of acute pneumonia, when not
intercurrent with another disease, "when it occurs in
young, robust subjects, when not epidemic, when the
pulse is hard and quick, the respiration hurried and
labored, and the bodily temperature high in the beginning of the disease, a free venesection will certainly do
good." Head of Confucius! I would guarantee that
one thousand such cases of the type above mentioned,
could be successfully treated without the loss of a single drop of blood, or the use of tartar emetic or calomel, and with a mortality ranging from 3 to 5 per cent.
Every experienced physician knows that these sthenic
cases of croupous pneumonia seldom die when carefully
treated on the restorative plan.   A mortality of 10 per
cent. of such cases as Prof. Montgomery instances
would show bad treatment, or gross carelessness in private practice.   Dr. Parks' opinion that in this disease
the liver is always implicated, is worth but little in a
clinical point of view.   The fact is, the most of the

autopsies from which Parks derives such opinions are from subjects that have died from intercurrent disease, or have had bad treatment tending to derange the functions of the liver. We all are aware that the class of cases known in this country as "bilious pneumonia," are of a typhoid type. We are also aware that the yellow color of the skin often suddenly comes on just before resolution of the inflamed lung, and gradually subsides with absorption of the exudation. These are clinical facts, and these cases do much better when well fed and properly nursed, than when calomel, antimony and other barbarous treatments are inflicted upon them.

Prof. Montgomery advises the advocates of the restorative treatment to "consult old authorities, and see the enormous extent to which venesection and purgation was carried without *any fatal* consequences, the very cautious, moderate and discriminating use of these measures recommended in my plea, will be looked upon as abundantly conservative." This sounds a good deal as hetrodox, as there is a lack of consistence in the position assumed. If there is no danger in this method of treatment, why caution against it? But I venture to say that Prof. Montgomery is too good a physician to adopt the system of practice he recommends, however well he may think it looks in the pages of a medical journal.

The experience of observant physicians has not directly led them to infer "that if sthenic cases of acute inflammations are allowed to go on, without the controlling and ameliorating influence of bleeding and evacuants, a far more dangerous form of prostration and debility will ensue, or perhaps irremedial structural lesions take place." This was once the theory, and the

practice was thoroughly in accordance therewith, and
the death rate was exactly proportioned. Chambers
very aptly remarks, that we can in a measure, tell the
character of the treatment by the mortuary. It is well
also to recollect that many writers say that the type of
diseases has changed from sthenic to asthenic, while
others affirm that there is no change of type, only a
change of thinking and observing for the better. This
latter view is more in harmony with the truth.

Before concluding this paper I wish to say a word
upon what Prof. Montgomery calls a " mixed system "
of treatment, viz : half depletory and half restorative.
Prof. Montgomery seems to forget that when the antiphlogistic system was seriously attacked, and its baneful influence exposed, there was a kind of compromise
entered into so as to afford a " mixed system." It is
well known to posted men that this mixed system did
not mend the matter much. Even Dr. Allison was
forced to admit that the loss of blood was likely to do
immense damage even when the patient was well fed,
so much so that he at last acknowledged it a two-edged .
sword that was as likely to be wrong as right. It is a
fact well attested, that these so-called sthenic cases are
as ready to take on asthenic conditions and end fatally
as any others ; hence it has been fully acknowledged that
we have no guide by which to be directed in using it.
Prof. Montgomery is too sagacious a thinker not to see
the force of this argument, and the facts attending it.'

The case cited by Prof. Montgomery is of no value
to him in this controversy. He does not claim that he
had a case of inflammation of the brain or its membranes. Farther, it is now well known to all physiologists, that " we cannot, in fact, lessen to any considera-

ble extent the quantity of blood within the cranium by arteriotomy or venesection ; and that when by profuse hemorrhage, destructive to life, we do succeed in draining the vessels within the cranium of any sensible portion of red blood, there is commonly found an equivalent to this spoilation in the increased circulation or effusion of serum serving to maintain the plentitude of the cranium." It is well known that these perturbations of the nervous system pass without the aid of active treatment. The most that can be made from Prof. Montgomery's reasonings is what one may naturally draw, a *post hoc proctor hoc* argument.

In closing this paper I assure Prof. Montgomery of my high esteem and respect for his distinguished talents as an able physician, and an excellent observer. He has the misfortune of being on the wrong side of the question ; he has nevertheless handled his part of this controversy with remarkable ability. Were our positions reversed, it is doubtful whether I could have sustained my side so long. *Magna est veritas et prevalibat.*

802 Washington Avenue.

REMARKS ON THE USE OF THE HYPODERMIC SYRINGE.

By R. W. ERWIN, M. D., Athens, Ohio.

Every one who has had occasion to use this instrument, has no doubt discovered that its employment in a certain proportion of cases requires care, to prevent

alarm to patients or their friends.   A means so potent
for good, as the hypodermic syringe, ought not from
carelessness, or want of knowledge, or skill in its use,
to pass into neglect.   Experience warrants me in making the following observations.   As a whole, they are
not new; but to those who are beginning, or who have
little acquaintance with this form of medication, they
will prove valuable.   First, it is best never to use the
syringe for the injection of morphia in cases of children.
The rapidity of its absorption, and the fact that this
class of patients do not bear preparations of opium
well, is sufficient evidence against it.   Strychnia and
certain other articles, are not open to the same objection—want of toleration.   To the children's class is
to be added hysterical women, in the use of atropia.
Much of it will cause a change of doctors, *nolentes
volentes*.   In instances where the toleration of morphine
has not been tested, the dose ought not to exceed one-
sixth of a grain.   From that quantity, even, I have seen
alarming results.   One case* in particular comes to my
mind, in which strong contraction of the pupils, marked
dyspnœa and delirium ensued in five minutes.   There
was no disease of the circulatory or respiratory organs
to account for the trouble in respiration.   Nothing except intestinal colic, which the injection was designed
to relieve, existed.

Such cases are rare, but that every one will meet
them is probable.   It is very easy, in case the first dose
does not relieve, to repeat it, but it is not an easy thing
when overdone to undo it.   Two-thirds the interval for

---

* In this person, a very prominent minister, opiates invariably cause distress
in the stomach.   He assures me that violent colic will almost immediately follow
a dose of paregoric.

repeating the dose by the stomach, when pain is severe, is sufficient; if relief is not obtained, the injection can then be given again with safety. The same rule will govern the necessity of the repetition as governs internal administration. The difference in time is due to the fact, that often the quantity of liquid in the stomach being considerable, and the organ inactive, medicine may lie an hour or two before entering the circulation. However, unless the pain is very intense, and has undergone very little abatement, an hour is as short an interval as is prudent in untried cases. Persons accustomed to take $\frac{1}{2}$ gr. to $\frac{1}{3}$ gr. internally, provided the solution is not too concentrated, will bear with impunity from $\frac{1}{8}$ to $\frac{1}{4}$ gr. hypodermically. On one occasion I injected a quarter of a grain of morphine of a strength of 5 grs. to the drachm. In less than two minutes my patient, a strong young man, had his pupils dilated to their utmost, was very palid, and had a quick and frequent pulse—purely the result of fright, from rapid absorption. No harm was done, except to prejudice him against that form of medicine. In this instance it was not thrown into a blood-vessel, a thing easily prevented by carrying the point well through into the cellular tissue, and then holding it up in loose fold, while the injection is slowly made. Three minims thrown into the cellular tissue, if no hemorrhage occurs in it, will be absorbed or carried into the circulation in from two to five minutes. In all cases where morphine is not used habitually, the strength of the solution should not exceed $\frac{1}{4}$ gr. to twelve or fifteen minims of water. One grain to a drachm of water is an excellent formula. Ten minims of it equals $\frac{1}{6}$ gr. It will insure gradual absorption, and freedom from

41

alarming effects. Next, the solution should be neutral. Acid ought not to be employed with morphine or atropine preparations; it only increases the smarting and danger of inflammation. Strychnine is not as soluble, and where a concentrated solution is required, acid will be necessary. Even here if the salt is employed, and the water heated, the quantity will be inconsiderable. One grain of the sulphate of strychnine to the ounce of water, dissolved by the aid of heat, is a good formula for hypodermic purposes, and secures a neutral preparation. Ten minims of it equals $\frac{1}{12}$ gr. of the alkaloid. Usually the seat of pain should govern the place of insertion. The effect is more prompt, and the popular idea, that medication directed to the seat of trouble is best, is complied with.

In affections of the viscera of the chest, abdomen and pelvis, the abdominal regions are to be selected as being less painful, and less liable to tenderness afterward. This is true in a marked degree. The needle ought never to be entered in parts that have to the patient the sensation of numbness or coldness. There is less vitality in them, and hence more risk of making a sore.

The only abscesses or ulcers I ever saw following the use of morphine, was in the case of a pregnant woman. She had been suffering from severe neuralgia in front and outer part of thighs, induced by the fœtal pressure. There was numbness in the part. One injection was made beyond the affected portion, and two in it. The first gave no trouble, while the others produced two ugly corroding ulcers difficult to heal.

Many dislike the syringe from the pain and shock its introduction causes. I have seen the needle thrust into the skin with as much force as the combattant would sabre his victim. Of course such a thing would produce dread from the shock. It should be done gently. The integument and fascia, after being pinched off into a fold, are to be entered by gradually carrying the point of the needle through them—when fairly through, the fluid should be as slowly discharged, in order to allow the cellular structure to receive it without being torn. The pinching diminishes the sensibility, and unless there is hyperæsthesia, the injection will cause very little suffering. The ease with which the needle enters depends somewhat upon the shape of the point. Two or three kinds are manufactured: First, a flat or spear-shaped point; a three edged point, and a rounded one. The latter is most to be condemned as being painful. The first is most easy of introduction, but is likely to be followed often by bleeding, yet I think it is to be commended. The next thing is a step on a graduated piston-rod to insure against accidents in haste, or when operating in feeble light. Any one who has tried this arrangement will not desire a change.

A few words in reference to extempore preparations of morphine will conclude this paper. There is no use in carrying an elaborate apparatus for its production. A drachm vial which can be carried in a pocket case, and morphine powders put up by weight, is all that is necessary. The syringe will answer for a graduated measure. In the absence of the vial, I have taken a clean tablespoon, and dissolved the morphine in it, by first drawing the water into the syringe, and then throwing it upon the morphine. All that is necessary aside from the syringe, is to carry carefully weighed powders

of morphine, which is the best for safe internal administration.

Since writing the foregoing, I notice in the October
number, *Boston Journal of Chemisty*, an article by Dr.
Ephraim Cutter, Woburn, Mass., in which he describes
a new form of hypodermic syringe, and also mentions
some things that receive attention in this article.   It is
what I would call, from the description of the inventor,
telescopic hypodermic syringe   The cylinder is like a
small test tube being closed at the distal end.   At the
open end a hollow graduated piston-rod enters.   Upon
the proximal end of the rod is screwed the needle, which
is made of alumina alloy to prevent rusting.   Instead
of pushing in the piston to discharge the liquid, the
cylinder is pushed over it, and the solution passes
through the piston into the needle, from which it is
discharged.   To close it, the needle is unscrewed and
put into the hollow of the piston-rod, and it in turn is
pushed into the cylinder.   The advantages claimed for
it, are, its portability and diminished liability to get out
of order, from drying of the leather on the piston-rod.

REST, ITS THERAPEUTICAL VALUE, AND MODE OF APPLICATION IN CERTAIN DISEASES OF THE CHEST.

By Eugene C. Gehrung. Denver, Colorado

Simultaneously with the progress of rational medicine,
has the therapeutical application of rest been brought
into prominent and honorable notice.   Several so-

called exhaustive treatises, have been written on this subject, but still the field is not entirely gone over, and it is to be hoped that this contribution is only one of the many which the subject in question shall suggest. Although the means I advocate in this paper, have been used' long ago in traumatic affections of the chest; yet in the pathological affections of the same part they have—so far as my information goes—remained entirely unnoticed. The diseases for which I would propose therapeutical application of rest, are, pneumonitis, pleuritis, pleuro-pneumonitis, and possibly bronchitis. It remains then to describe its method of application, which consists in *bandaging* the chest to such an extent, that thoracic breathing is almost prevented, and abdominal breathing substituted in its place. The compression of the chest-walls is to be made with a broad bandage with rollers, or with any other contrivance that may have the same ultimate effect. For the double purpose of equally distributing the pressure of the bandage, and protecting the parts from the effects of sudden changes of temperature, previous to placing the bandage, I cover the chest with a thick layer of cotton batting.

The results of these simple operations are remarkable. Not only can the pain in the above enumerated affections be thus controlled at will, but likewise all the other symptoms may be made to rapidly disappear. Indeed the patient will recover in so short a time, that we may almost doubt the correctness of our diagnosis. By the employment of this method, all the usual complications and sequelæ may be likewise avoided. No pleural exudations, no pulmonary consolidations, etc., the too frequent after-effects of these diseases. Neither will abortions occur if the patient happens to be a pregnant female. Such at least have been the favorable results obtained in the cases I have treated in this way. To be fully successful, it is necessary to commence the treatment at the very onset. I fully believe that any failure which may occur with this treatment in the hands of other practitioners will result from its too late application ; but even then much good of a palliative kind will result. The bandage acts, in these cases, on the principle of a splint applied in inflammatory affections of the joint. It is, of course, inadmissible in these organs to produce complete rest ; but, nevertheless, the partial rest obtained in this way appears to be all that is required in arriving at the above quoted beneficial results. The walls of the chest encased in this manner are so doubled in their strength and firmness, and the patient, provided with such firmly resisting support, depends no longer on the former yielding and elastic chest surroundings, to resist the succussions caused by the cough ; the mental as well as the physical relief is instantaneous. The patient, who previously was obliged to consider each respiration lest it should cause him pain, is now relieved of all care. In fact, he cannot, even if he would, draw a deep breath, for the bandage does not allow of it.

In the few cases where I have had an opportunity of making thermometric observations, this mode of treatment succeeded far better in permanently reducing the temperature, and the pulse as well, than the administration of cardiac sedatives. The noted reductions of temperature were a fall of from 4° to 6° F. I will give the following case in illustration :

Case ——, the patient a young married lady at the

sixth month of pregnancy, showed all the signs of a pleuro-pneumonitis, such as the rusty colored sputa, pleural friction sounds, pleuritic pain, râles, etc.; the pulse was 140; the temperature 105° F. I wrapped her chest thickly in cotton batting, gave a cardiac sedative and anodyne, and succeeded satisfactorily in reducing the pulse, and, to a certain extent, moderated the temperature and alleviated the pain. But so soon as the effects of the medicines disappeared, the symptoms returned with violence, and her condition was as bad as before. Then I applied the bandage as described, and ceased giving any more medicine. To my great satisfaction the patient declared herself *at once* free from pain, and altogether comfortable. The fever flush disappeared rapidly, and when I applied the thermometer it registered a fall of 4° in the temperature, the pulse beating about 100. In this condition, with orders to take no medicine whatsoever, I left her. In the night I was called again, the patient having become much worse. Upon inquiry I found that, feeling uncomfortable, she had the bandage removed about eight hours before. I ordered it immediately re-applied, prescribing at the same time a placebo, and when I returned the next day I found her up and well, and reporting also that she felt the motions of the fœtus, the absence of which motions, during her illness, had depressed her extremely. She has since been delivered of a healthy child.

To mention more cases would simply be to repeat the same successful results as in the above, either in the experience of others reported to me, or that occurring in my own practice. It should also be here stated that, even in chronic cases, this treatment is an adjunct to whatever other means may be used.

Hospital Reports.

CITY HOSPITAL.

By T. F. Prewitt, M. D., Resident Physician.

A case of gunshot wound in the head—the patient surviving for eleven months, with the bullet in the brain.

Chas. Burklin, æt. 32, confectioner, was admitted to the City Hospital, March 9, 1872, with a gun-shot wound of the head, inflicted by himself, having first attempted to kill his wife by shooting her. The wound, made by a small pistol ball on the day before, was located a little to the left of the median of the forehead, and about an inch and a half above the supraorbital ridge. The patient had been a hard drinker, and had suffered with delirium tremens during the past winter, and had been drinking prior to and at the time of the attempt upon his life. At the time of his admission, he was suffering with great irritability of the stomach, nausea, and vomiting. He was rather morose, seemed indisposed to talk, and not altogether rational. His answers to questions, however, were always relevant, both upon admission and afterwards. The general disturbance was so disproportioned to the apparently serious character of the wound, that some doubt was entered at first whether the bullet had really entered the cranium. By the introduction of a probe, however, to the depth of half an inch, the bony circumference of the track through the skull could be readily traced. No further attempts at probing were made.—I would state here that Dr. A. Hammer, who saw him immediately after the injury, has since informed me that he passed a probe to the depth of *six inches*, into the cavity of the cranium, the instrument passing in without the slightest force, and apparently meeting no resistance.—The irritability of the stomach was attributed at the time, partly to the brain lesion, and partly to the condition of the stomach induced by drinking. He was therefore ordered sul. morp. gr. ¼ with chloral at night, to procure sleep, and ward off if possible an attack of delirium tremens. In this we succeeded, the patient at no time showing any marked delirium, though it was evident his mind was not just right. He did not seem to appreciate his position, expressed frequently a wish to go home, manifested no anxiety about his own fate, though when told that his wound might, and probably would prove fatal, he expressed a hope that it would kill him quick. He asked repeatedly about his wife, manifested a good deal of anxiety about her condition, said that he did not know why he had shot her, that he must have been crazy, and at one time when insisting upon being permitted to go home, and upon being told that he would be thrown into prison if released from the hospital, he said they could not hurt him for it—referring to the shooting of his wife—that he was crazy when he did it.

March 11th (two days after admission).—Patient sleeps well; bowels regular; pulse 80; temperature 100¼; stomach not so irritable.

12th.—Slept pretty well last night. Stomach less irritable.

13th.—No pain in head, but complains of being giddy; no longer throws up his food; has some appetite. Pulse 72; temperature 100° F.

For several days the condition of the patient varied but little, the pulse ranging from 72 to 80 and the temperature standing at 99°.

20th.—Pulse 80; temperature 99¼°. During the day the patient had a chill. The wound was somewhat inflamed, and eyelid of left eye puffed up.

21st.—Patient passed a restless night. Has some fever; pulse 100; temperature 103°. Appetite failing, and general condition not so good; wound inflamed, closed and fluctuating. On opening it with a probe, a bloody pus was discharged.

22nd.—Condition better; pulse 88; temperature 99°.

23rd.—Pulse 80; temperature 99°.

April 16.—Patient has gradually improved up to this time; is now convalescent; pulse and temperature normal. Reopened wound which had been closed for a day or two, and fluctuated a little, with the discharge of a watery and bloody pus. Is somewhat nervous, but has a good appetite.

April 19.—The patient was discharged greatly improved, with the external wound closed, his general health pretty good, and no marked impairment of intellect.

Burklin was now remanded to jail for trial, was subsequently

convicted of assault with intent to kill his wife, and sentenced
to the penitentiary.

For the following notes of his case while in that institution,
as also for the notes of the *post-mortem*, I am indebted to Dr. R.
E. Young, Physician to the penitentiary.

CONTINUED HISTORY.

By R. E. YOUNG, M. D., of Jefferson City Hospital

Saw Charles Burklin **Jan.** 23rd, 1878. He had then been an
inmate of the hospital since January 6th, 1878. Admitted by
the Physician.

Diagnosis.—Intermittent fever for which he was treated up to
time I first saw him.

On examination he presented the following signs and symptoms: pain in the head in the region of the external wound,
which was about ¼ an inch to the left of the median line, and
1¼ inches above the supraorbital ridge of the left half of the
frontal bone; he also complained of great heaviness of the
head.

His skin was moist, but abnormally cool; feet and hands
much colder than rest of the body; pulse frequent and feeble;
tongue slightly furred and tremulous when protruded. His
bowels were in a soluble condition, and discharged their contents generally twice a day, but he was not conscious of the
motions. His urine had a natural color, and was normal in
quantity, and contained neither albumen nor sugar, its specific
gravity was generally 120. The urine was also involuntarily
discharged, but did not dribble away, being discharged at intervals as in health. His temperature was at this time 97 in
the axilla; his appetite generally poor; appearance listless,
when aroused there was a slight stare about the look. There
was little or no change in the above signs and symptoms until
Jan. 28th, when he was attacked with erysipelas of the œdematous variety. His skin now became dry and hot; temp. 101° F.
to 108° F.; pulse 130 and feeble. The inflammation began at
the external wound, and extended backwards including the left
ear. This inflammation yielded readily to treatment, lasting
only six days.

Feb. 4.—Burklin sunk into a semi-comatose condition, from
which it was difficult to arouse him. When aroused, his con-

versation was of a incoherent nature. His answers were generally in monosyllables, and frequently these did not appertain
to the questions asked. His memory of passing events from
the time I first saw him was very vague, but he had an acute
remembrance of the events that occurred between the time he
shot himself, and the time he was admitted to the prison, at this
place (this fact was learned from a fellow prisoner who was in
jail with him, and nursed him while sick in this hospital).
Nothing further occurred in Burklin's history from his recovery
from erysipelas, except that he grew more listless, and it was
more difficult to arouse him from that semi-comatose condition
into which he had sunk. He gradually wasted away, taking
little food, and it was with the greatest difficulty he could be
induced to take food at all. There was no perceptible change
in his temperature or pulse, as recorded previous to attack of
erysipelas, until about 24 hours before his death. His temperature now sunk to 96° F. in axilla, and his pulse grew so frequent and feeble, that it could not be counted.

Feb. 13, 7.20 P. M.—Burklin died of æsthenia.

The *post-mortem* was made on the morning of February 14th.
On removing the calvanium the dura mater was found to be
unusually adherent to the inner table of the frontal bone,
around the margin of the wound. The brain was removed
from the cavity of the cranium intact. Upon the under surface
of the anterior left lobe of the cerebrum was a large sac apparently filled with pus. The sac extended in width from the
longitudinal fissure, to the outer and under border of the left
anterior lobe of the cerebrum. The anterior border of the sac
was a few lines posteriorly to the anterior border of the left
lobe, and extending backwards nearly to the fissure of Silvius.
In front of this sac, and incysted, lay a small leaden bullet,
with some small fragments of bone. That portion of the brain
lying in front of the sac, was adherent to the dura mater. (This
fact was observed by my student, and also by one of the
prisoners, present at the *post-mortem*.) The sac on its under
surface, was not formed by the dura mater, nor was it attached
in any way to it. The ventricles had no communication with
the sac. There was a straw-colored liquid in the left ventricle
and also in the subarachnoid space at the base of the brain.
No other lesions were observed. When the sac was opened,
about 6 oz. of pus was discharged.

Proceedings.

ST. LOUIS MEDICAL SOCIETY.

St. Louis, Oct. 4th, 1873.

Dr. T. F. Rumbold exhibited instruments of his invention for treating diseases of the throat, nose and ear. See October number of this Journal for particulars.

Dr. Clayton Keith read a paper on yellow fever, its history, differential diagnosis from pernicious malarial fever, etc. He stated that the first recorded case occurred in 1647, in the West India Islands. With few exceptions it had been confined to cities on the coast of the Atlantic, Mediterranean, and Gulf of Mexico. It had not appeared on the Pacific coast. The cause he believed more or something in addition to malaria.

Dr. Edgar spoke of the derangement of the spleen, in marsh fevers, and that it *contra-indicated mercurials*; which he feared received too little attention by the profession generally. That, while quinine was doubtless the best antiperiodic we know of, a *cold saturate of the bark* was more valuable in preventing relapses of intermittents. Haydon's saturates he had found reliable in preventing relapses.

Dr. Hughs remarked that the appearance of frost is the signal for the departure of yellow fever.

Yellow fever is certainly not a disease of the same grade as bilious fever, and it has symptoms *sui generis*, which all observers have noticed as distinguishing it symptomatically from every other disease.

Whatever may be the diversity of cadaveric signs, the symptoms of the living, or, perhaps quite as often of the dying patient, are not to be mistaken.

The vomit is so characteristic—decomposed blood—that the Spaniards at once found an appropriate name for the disease in this striking symptom.

The face, as it does in almost every other grave disorder (and this is emphatically a grave disorder in every sense of that term), when the physician is seeking for a sign, here mirrors the disease.

Its expression has been found peculiar and characteristic by all writers, and the color of the eye and face (bloodshot and yellow) have never failed to attract attention.

Yellow fever is certainly something more than the miasmatic fevers we are accustomed to see, because of its peculiar symptoms, because of its tendency to seldom re-attack the same person, because of its seeming to require animal decomposition combined with vegetable decay under certain definite degrees of heat prolonged, eighty degrees, and certain latitude not higher than about thirty-six degrees north for its propagation; whereas the miasmata, as we call them, prevail almost everywhere where there exists marshes and vegetable decomposition alone.

It also disappears while the miasmata continue in force, tarrying often through the fall, winter and spring, until a return of about eighty degrees of temperature, and yellow fever comes again, or postpones its return for many seasons.

Perhaps yellow fever is a specific disease engrafted upon a typho-malarial empoisoning of the blood, due to telluric emanations, the result of vegetable and animal decomposition combined.

This view is in harmony with all the facts as they have heretofore existed and as they exist now down the river.

But what is miasm? Neither the microscope nor chemistry have revealed it. We have thus far touched not, tasted not, handled not this conjectural source of so many morbific influences by any of the aids which science has given to medical investigation.

Miasm is malaria, and malaria is bad air. This is all we know. The distinguishing characteristic of that malaria which produces our autumnal fevers, and which you suppose to emanate from vegetable decomposition, is unknown to us.

Malaria is one of the hypothetical facts of medical science.

We are familiar with it in its effects.

Its specific nature and what is the chemical difference between the malaria of vegetable and animal decay remain to be proven.

Discussion in regard to the miasmatic origin of a disease before we had determined the specific nature of miasm, will be comparatively fruitless.

We know "only this and nothing more."

When yellow fever prevails, something is the matter with the atmosphere. Whether it be a condition brought about by the decomposition of vegetable or animal matter, or both combined, or whether infinitesimal animalculæ are the messengers of propagation, or whether all these play a part, aided by prolonged heat, we cannot certainly tell.

But none of the facts condemn us if we call yellow fever a specific disease, engrafted upon a typho-malarial state of system. The question then remains open as to whether its specific nature is due to the admixture of animal exhalations or animalculæ.

Dr. Coles read a paper on infinitesimal divisions in the system — being a criticism upon certain experiments of homeopathic writers, and pointed out their fallacy.

Dr. Hurt said he had read the proceedings of a homeopathic society in Paris, in which the potentation of infinitesimal doses was admitted to be a fallacy, so that the homeopaths are not a unit on this subject, and do not limit themselves to the theory laid down by their founder.

Dr. Hodgen drew a diagram on the blackboard to illustrate a case of paralysis. The patient first experienced a partial paralysis of the left eye, then of the muscles of the left side of the face and mouth, extending to the breast, arms and legs. He showed the origin of the disease in the brain.

Dr. Hodgen also described another case of paralysis—origin, a small abcess of the brain.

Dr. Bryson made remarks on paralysis and nervous diseases.

Dr. Kennard spoke of a case of cerebro-spinal meningitis, some symptoms of which were similar to those in the case spoken of by Dr. Hodgen.

Adjourned.

St. Louis, Oct. 11th, 1873.

Dr. H. A. Buck made the following observations:

If reports are correct, important changes in the epidemics of cholera and yellow fever have occurred this year in the Mississippi valley. Heretofore in this country, yellow fever has prevailed in epidemic form almost exclusively in the cities on the Atlantic or Gulf, and principal river towns near the coast. This year they have left their former haunts for towns in the interior. This change naturally excites inquiry as to the cause.

May it be due to the sanitary regulations adopted in our large cities, but sadly neglected by the smaller towns? From this or other cause it would appear that our large cities are becoming more healthy than the small cities and towns.

There still exists diversity of opinion as to the etiology of yellow fever and its mode of communication; the latter we believe similar to that of Asiatic cholera in some respects, like cholera it may be transmitted in textile fabrics, but not like it from the dejections from the body, hence not so much as cholera through the medium of drinking water. Yellow fever has failed to be communicated by taking the *black vomit* into the stomach.

Persons leaving a place infected with yellow fever for one free from such influence have taken the disease with them, but failed to extend it in the new locality, showing, as we think, pretty conclusively that there must be *special local causes* favoring the production of the disease, otherwise it may not prove communicable. When or where yellow fever first appeared is not recorded, whether in Europe, Asia, Africa or America.

We believe yellow fever to be a *specific disease*, but often complicated by some form of malarial fever, leading some physicians to consider it a pernicious fever of the malarial family. It seldom strays from the belt included by 40° N. and 20° S. latitude, differing in this respect from other fevers. The diagnosis of mild cases is often obscure. The most characteristic features are: "flush of the forehead and glare of the eyes," pain in the back and limbs, *continued fever*, tenderness over the epigastrium. Where convalescence takes place without yellowing the skin, or black vomit, unless the disease was epidemic, its true character might not be suspected.

The epidemic this year seems of the most malignant type, at least in *Memphis* and *Shreveport*.

The supportative treatment seems to have been the most successful. Louis and Trousseau made numerous post mortems, and compared the appearance or color of the liver to that of butter, mustard, or coffee, attributing the yellowness to fat cells in the liver. Until we know more of the *etiology* and *pathology* of the disease we should move in the treatment, like a ship without a compass in a dark night, let the "anchor drag" and feel our way until light appears.

St. Louis, Oct. 18th, 1873.

The Society met at the usual time and place. Dr. Newman presented a gall bladder impacted with gall stones, several of which had escaped through the walls of the sac, causing the death of the patient.

Dr. Gregory related a case of injury of the knee-joint with a rusty hatchet, penetrating the cavity of the joint, through which wound the synovial fluid gradually escaped, inducing inflammation of the joint on the third day, when he was called and applied a plaster-of-Paris splint, securing perfect immobility of the joint, at the same time the inflamed joint was left free from pressure and accessible for treatment, the case promised well so far.

Dr. Hodgen presented a simple appliance to pass liquids in and out of the stomach, consisting of a rubber tube three or four feet long, attached to a smooth elastic rubber bougie eighteen or twenty inches long, to pass into the stomach after being filled with water, on the principle of the syphon. By depressing the free end below the stomach, its liquid contents would flow out, when the action could be reversed by placing the free end into a vessel filled with water and elevating the same above the end in the stomach. In this way the stomach could be emptied and washed out without resorting to the stomach pump so often not at hand or out of order, on account of its valves. The tube recommended being free from valves or other complication, and of trifling cost compared with a stomach pump, favored its universal adoption.

Dr. G. Sumrall gave an interesting account of the disease which was epidemic at Pilot Knob during the past summer, describing the symptoms and treatment of one hundred cases or more treated by himself, with the results—most of the mortality he thought due to bad nursing.

On motion the regular order of business was suspended and an invitation extended to Dr. Montgomery to address the Society, (he having just returned from a visit to Europe,) which was accepted, and the Doctor gave an interesting and graphic description of many magnates in the profession abroad. He mentioned that histology and etiology were the favorite studies in the Berlin and Vienna schools, somewhat to the neglect of *therapeutics* as the Doctor thought.

On motion the Society adjourned.

Reviews and Bibliographical Notices.

THINKERS AND THINKING. By John Darby. Philadelphia: J. B. Lippincott & Co. 1873.

He must be a thinker of no mean capacity himself, whose common-place book is worth publishing. It does not appear that the author of this work is distinguished in philosophy. The book certainly contains many things that are good, and some that are new; but to use Lessing's criticism, *the good things are not new; the new things are not good.* Apparently a good history of philosophy, and an encyclopædia would furnish the bulk of the work. The comments are weak and sentimental; the style stilted and pedantic—method it has none. An instance of the writer's feeble imagination and sentimentalism may be found on p. 240, in the picture of Emerson and Holmes.

On the whole, it is a second-hand book of fourth-rate ability; and if it has any *raison d'être,* in these times when sensible men can only afford leisure for choice reading, we fail to discern it.

L.

AN ESSAY ON THE PRINCIPLES OF MENTAL HYGIENE. By D. A. Gorton, M. D. Philadelphia: J. B. Lippincott & Co. 1873.

[For Sale by the St. Louis Book & News Co.]

Here is an author who believes in moral as well as medical practice; who believes that the mind is to be medicined as well as the body. He is convinced "that man's great want is more religion;" and he sets forth in vigorous phrase his thoughts on this subject.

But his "religion" is by no means the staple of the popular creeds, his prime article is evidently a belief in right-mindedness. "The bane of hygeine (he says p. 10) like that of religion is superstition." "True religion is not in the market, cannot be bought and sold, bartered for, nor begged with prayer. It is distilled in the human mind by slow and silent processes, and is in truth as truly an evolution in humanity as passion or reason." p. 129. "Belief is strongest where reason is weakest." p. 150. "The faith that was and is so potent on the life and

habits of the unlettered savage and barbarian, the church is
still holding out to a civilization that has long since turned its
back upon her, and which, instead of leading as she used to do,
and ought always to do, is dragging heavily in the rear." p.
158. Referring to Mr. Mayhew's assertion that the great need
of the London poor was the " word of God," says our author
" this is giving pearls for food ; baptism for baths ; piety for
pure air; the light of revelation for the light of heaven." p. 87.
He believes in fastings, but " thinks they are chiefly good for
gouty people, or those having enlarged livers, or troubled with
spinal irritation." p. 60. There is much more, however, in this
book than the above quotations would indicate. It is full of practical suggestions on the power of medicinal agents ; on keeping the equilibrium between corporeal and mental exercise ; on
the influence of knowledge in diminishing crime ; on the
fallacy of chemical analysis in determining the effect and value of
foods; and on the requisitions of marriage. Moreover, although
the book is written in a style which will recommend it to
the general reader of average intelligence, he seeks to inculcate
a more scrupulous integrity, a higher sense of honor in the
members of his own profession. " Faith, hope, charity, honor,
honesty, virtue—mental hygiene comprehends the nurture of
these ennobling graces." p. x.

Then he says that " the climate of the whole Atlantic coast
is particularly irritating and unfavorable to long life and good
morals." (p. 24.) We, of course, have another reason for being
content with our continental residence ; we are afraid, however,
that our maritime brethren will not heartily endorse the
generalization.   L.

S. Zickel's Deutsch-Americanisches Hand-Lexikon des
   Allgemeinen Wissens. In zwei Bänden Gross-Quarto. Voll-
   ständig in circa 60 Heften *a* 15 cents. NewYork : S. Zickel,
   No. 19 Day street. 1873.

We have received two Nos. (24 & 25) of the above work, and
from these specimen numbers we have reason to believe the
work when complete will be very valuable. It is in three-column
pages ; two volumes of nearly a thousand pages. It contains
geographical names with description of towns, water courses,
etc., etc., and also proper names of distinguished persons.

The numbers appear semi-monthly. The statistics are quite full, one small item from which we quote : Emigration 1871, by way of Bremen : from Germany, 45,674, Austria, 8,828 , other states, 6,514 ; by way of Hamburgh: from Germany, 80,260, Austria, 1,172, other states, 10,792 ; total by the two parts, 102,740, in 295 ships. The average per year for 1869-70-71 was over 106,000.

We think the work would have been far preferable published in Roman letters, much easier for the scholar, and none the less valuable for any. G.

BOOKS AND PAMPHLETS RECEIVED.

PRACTICAL HYGIENE, A Manual intended especially for medical officers of the army, and for civil medical officers of health. By Edmond A. Parks, M. D., F. R. S., etc., etc. Fourth edition. Philadelphia : Lindsay & Blakiston. For sale by the St. Louis Book & News Co. Price $6.

A TREATISE ON MENTAL PHILOSOPHY. By N. Christensen, St. Louis.

THINKERS AND THINKING. By J. E. Garretson, M. D. Author of Odd Hours of a Physician, etc. Philadelphia: J. B. Lippincott & Co. For sale by the St. Louis Book & News Co.

CHEMISTRY : INORGANIC AND ORGANIC, With experiments. By Charles London Bloxam, Prof. of Chemistry in King's College, London, etc., etc. With 295 illustrations. From the Second and Revised English Edition. Philadelphia : Henry C. Lea. For sale by the St. Louis Book & News Co.

MEDICAL JURISPRUDENCE. By Alfred Swaine Taylor, M. D., F. R. S. Seventh American Edition. Revised from the author's latest notes, and edited with additional notes and references. By John J. Reese, M. D. With illustrations on wood. Philadelphia: Henry C. Lea. 1873. For sale by the St. Louis Book & News Co.

MENTAL HYGIENE, An Essay on the Principles of. By D. A. Gordon, M. D. Philadelphia: J. B. Lippincott & Co. 1873. For sale by Gray, Baker & Co.

LECTURES ON CLINICAL MEDICINE. By A. Trousseau, late Prof. of Clinical Medicine in the Faculty of Medicine, Paris, etc., etc. Translated from the Third Revised and Enlarged Edition. By Sir John Rose Cormack, M. D., F. R. S., and P. Victor Bazire, M. D. Complete in two volumes. Philadelphia: Lindsay & Blakiston. 1873. For sale by the St. Louis Book and News Co.

TRANSACTIONS OF THE MEDICAL SOCIETY OF THE STATE OF PENNSYLVANIA, 1873.

TRANSACTIONS OF THE MEDICAL SOCIETY OF CALIFORNIA, FOR THE YEARS 1872 AND 1873.

TRANSACTIONS OF THE MEDICAL SOCIETY OF MINNESOTA.

A TREATISE ON THE PNEUMATIC ASPIRATION OF MORBID FLUIDS. By George Dieulafoy. Philadelphia: J. B. Lippincott & Co. 1873. For sale by Gray, Baker & Co., St. Louis.

PHYSIOLOGY, Text Book—General, Special, and Practical. By John Hughes Bennett, M. D., F. R. S. E. With twenty-one photo-lithographic plates. Philadelphia: J. B. Lippincott & Co. 1873. For sale by Gray, Baker & Co., St. Louis.

MIDWIFERY, A Manual of, including the Pathology of Pregnancy and the Puerperal state. By Dr. Karl Schroeder. From the Third German Edition. Translated into English by Charles H. Carter, B. A., M. D., B. S., London. With twenty-six engravings on wood. New York: D. Appleton & Co. 1873. For sale by Gray, Baker & Co., St. Louis.

PERITYPHLITIS. By William T. Bull, M. D. A Thesis to which the first prize was awarded by the Faculty of the College of Physicians and Surgeons. New York: D. Appleton & Co., 557 Broadway.

LONG ISLAND COLLEGE HOSPITAL, Brooklyn, New York. Annual Announcement and Circular. Session 1873-74.

CHANGES IN TEMPERATURE AND PULSE IN YELLOW FEVER. By Joseph Jones, M. D., Prof. of Chemistry, etc., University of Louisiana.

VISITING LIST, Physician's, for 1874—twenty-third year of its publication. Philadelphia: Lindsay & Blakiston. For sale by the St. Louis Book & News Co.

PRACTICAL CHEMISTRY, An Introduction to, including Analysis. By John E. Bowman, F. C. S. Edited by C. M. Bloxam, F. C. S. Sixth American, from the Sixth Revised English Edition. Philadelphia: Henry C. Lea. 1873. For sale by the St. Louis Book & News Co.

MEDICAL DIAGNOSIS, The Student's Guide to. By Samuel Fenwick, M. D., F. R. C. S. From the Third Revised and Enlarged English Edition, with eighty-four wood cuts. Philadelphia: Henry C. Lea. 1873. For sale by the St. Louis Book & News Co.

LECTURES ON DISEASES AND INJURIES OF THE EAR, at St. George's Hospital. By W. B. Dalby, F. R. C. S. With twenty-one illustrations. M. B. Cantab. Philadelphia: Lindsay & Blakiston. For sale by Gray, Baker & Co.

HIP-JOINT DISEASE, Mechanical Treatment of. By Charles Fayette Taylor, M. D. New York: Wm. Wood & Co. 1873. For sale by Gray, Baker & Co., St. Louis.

LECTURES ON THE FEMALE PERINEUM AND VESICO-VAGINAL FISTULA. By D. Hays Agnew, M. D. With numerous illustrations. Philadelphia: Lindsay & Blakiston. 1873.

NEW CATALOGUE OF TEXT-BOOKS AND MANUALS. By Lindsay & Blakiston, Philadelphia: For Gratuitous Distribution.

DISEASES OF THE EYE. A Treatise. By Soelberg Wells, F.JR. C. S. Second American, from the Third English Edition, with Additions. Illustrated with 248 engravings on wood, and six colored plates. Together with selections from the test types of Prof. F. Jaeger and Dr. H. Snellen. 8vo. pp. 836. Philadelphia: Henry C. Lea. For sale by the St. Louis Book & News Co.

REPORT OF THE DISEASES OF INDIANA, for the year 1872. With a brief outline of the Medical Topography and Climatology of

Different Localities. By George Sutton, M. D., of Aurora, Indiana. Indianapolis Sentinel Company, printers. 1878.

SCRIBNER'S ILLUSTRATED MAGAZINE, For Boys and Girls. November, Vol. I, No. 1. Conducted by Mary Mapes Dodge. The present is a good time to subscribe for this monthly, particularly valuable for the young folks. New York : Scribner & Co.

MEDICAL JURISPRUDENCE, Principles and Practice of. By Alfred Swaine Taylor, M. D., F. R. S. Second Edition, in two volumes. 8vo. pp. 724 and 672. Philadelphia : Henry C. Lea. 1878. For sale by the St. Louis Book & News Co.

Our Medical Schools

Commenced their regular term of Lectures on October 13th, with *larger classes* (we are informed) than had matriculated at that time in former years. *The Missouri School* occupy their new edifice, a neat substantial structure, with all the modern appointments for the comfort of students, and convenience of teachers, situated on the southeast corner of Christy Avenue and 23d street, adjoining St. John's Hospital. The changes in the Faculty are Dr. E. Montgomery, elected to the chair of Materia Medica and Therapeutics; Dr. C. E. Michel, Chair of Histology and Diseases of the Eye and Ear; and Dr. H Tuholske to the chair of Anatomy.

The St. Louis School occupy, as formerly, at the corner of Seventh and Myrtle streets.

The vacancy in the chair of *Physiology and Medical Jurisprudence*, occasioned by the death of Prof. J. W. Clemens, has been filled by the appointment of Dr. Gustavus Baumgarten, formerly editor of this JOURNAL; his devotion to science, and critical scholarship, give assurance of success in this field of labor.

As the close of the year approaches our subscribers who have not remitted their subscriptions for the present year will excuse us for reminding them of the fact, and requesting them to do so at their earliest convenience.

Meteorological Observations.

METEOROLOGICAL OBSERVATIONS AT ST. LOUIS, MO.

BY A. WISLIZENUS, M. D.

The following observations of daily temperature in St. Louis are made with a MAXIMUM and MINIMUM thermometer (of Green, N. Y.). The daily minimum occurs generally in the night, the maximum about 3 P. M. The monthly mean of the daily minima and maxima, added and divided by 2, gives a quite reliable mean of the monthly temperature.

THERMOMETER FAHRENHEIT.

SEPTEMBER, 1873.

Day of Month.	Minimum.	Maximum.	Day of Month.	Minimum.	Maximum.
1	77.0	92.0	18	65.0	89.0
2	70.0	84.0	19	45.5	65.5
3	72.5	88.5	20	47.0	67.5
4	66.5	84.0	21	48.5	74.5
5	66.0	85.0	22	53.5	60.0
6	59.0	77.0	23	50.5	71.5
7	60.0	77.0	24	53.5	64.5
8	53.0	76.5	25	48.0	70.0
9	53.5	80.5	26	64.0	86.0
10	59.0	86.5	27	67.0	88.5
11	62.5	91.0	28	69.0	75.0
12	67.0	79.0	29	53.0	62.0
13	52.0	64.0	30	44.5	65.0
14	45.0	67.0	31		
15	51.5	82.0			
16	57.0	79.5	Means	58.1	76.7
17	62.0	89.0	Monthly Mean 67.4		

Quantity of rain : 2.46 inches.

Mortality Report.

FROM SEPT. 20th, 1873, TO OCT. 25th, 1873, INCLUS.

	DATE	White. Males.	White. Females.	Col'd. Males.	Col'd. Females.	Under 5 yrs.	5 to 10	10 to 20.	20 to 30.	30 to 40.	40 to 50.	50 to 60.	60 to 70.	70 to 80.	80 to 90.	90 to 100.	TOTAL.
Saturday	27	77	66	2	2	75	3	4	12	12	11	14	9	6	1	...	147
"	4	90	52	4	3	75	9	11	15	14	10	7	5	1	2	...	149
"	11	74	55	4	2	61	5	8	14	17	9	11	6	3	1	...	135
"	18	77	43			62	4	7	8	12	14	6	4	2	1	...	120
"	25	74	41		2	52	4	5	10	18	10	8	4	5	1	...	112
Total,		392	257	10	9	325	25	35	59	73	54	46	28	17	6		663

Abortion......... 2
Atelectasis .. 2
Abscess of Liver. 5
Accident 4
Anemia 3
Asphyxia........... 5
Atrophia 1
Bronchitis........12
Cancer............. 7
Colitis . 1
Chill, conges ... 5
Cholera Morbus 13
" Infantum..24
Conges. of Bowels 5
" Brain ...18
" Lungs 5
Consumption.......61
Convulsions 36
Croup............11
Debility 8

Diarrhœa 26
Diphtheria........12
Disease Hip Joint . 1
Dropsy 10
Drowned 6
Dysentery. 32
Eclampsia 4
Encephalitis........ 1
Enteritis.... 21
Enteralgia 1
Entero-colitis. 3
Fever, congestive 13
" intermittent .. 5
" gastric 1
" puerperalis. 8
" remittent 19
" typhoid 31
" continued .. 1
Gastritis............ 3
Hemorrhage........ 6

Hernia 1
Hydrocephalus. ... 7
Icterus Gravis .. 1
Inanition 5
Inflammat'n Brain 3
" Bowels. 2
" Throat. 1
Intussusception 1
Jaundice............ 2
Laryngitis.......... 2
Lockjaw........... 4
Marasmus 43
Meningitis 18
Mening.cereb-spin 2
Œdema of Lung .. 2
Old Age........... 1
Paralysis........ 2
Pyemia............ 1
Pleuritis............ 3
Pneumonia........27

Phebiatis 1
Phemphigus........ 1
Premature Birth ... 6
Rheumatism........ 1
Rupture Urethra.... 1
Scarlatina 2
Scald 2
Scrofula............ 2
Small Pox. 12
Shot Wound....... 1
Softening of Brain.. 1
Suicide............ 3
Summer complaint 8
Tabes Mesenterica.. 1
Teething...... 22
Ulcerat of bowels 2
Uremia....... .. 2

Total........663
Stillborn...........46

Long Island College Hospital,

BROOKLYN, NEW YORK.

THE REGULAR COURSE OF LECTURES,

In the Long Island College Hospital, will commence on the fourth day of March, 1874, and end the last week in June following.

FEES.—Matriculation, $5.00. Professors' Tickets, $100.00. Demonstrator's fee, $5 00. Graduation fee, $25.00. Hospital Ticket gratuitous.

SAMUEL G. ARMOR, M. D., Dean,

1y—sept

Brooklyn, New York.

THE SAINT LOUIS

Medical and Surgical Journal.

DECEMBER, 1873.

Translation.

PRINCIPLES OF TREATMENT FOR CROUPOSE PNEUMONIA.

By PROF. TH. JÜRGENSEN, of Kiel.

(*Volkmann's Clinical Lectures.—Translated from the German by Dr. Henry Kirchner, St. Louis, Mo.*)

[Continued from page 546.]

Quinine when administered in proper time and quantity, diminishes the temperature for at least twelve hours. The minimum, 1.5° to 2.5° less than the temperature of the beginning, takes place from five to seven hours after taking the remedy. The falling off and rising again take place in a pretty straight line, as I have shown by measurement, every five minutes.

On the manner of giving the quinine, depends a great deal. In moderately severe cases I give it, to grown persons, after the following formula :—

Quiniæ sulphatis   -   ʒss.
Acid. hydro clorici q. s. ad solut.
Aq. destillat.   -   -   ʒiss.

To be taken at once in the evening between 6 and 8 o'clock. To children to the fifth year, I give about ¼ grain for

43

each year, after that age 7½ to 15 grains, according
to circumstances. These normal doses may be increased without detriment. You can give, in intense
febrile conditions, to a vigorous adult, 75 grains; to a
child under a year old, 15 grains, always in one dose.
I have used both quantities frequently; slowly increasing my doses have I gathered my experience; never saw
disadvantage, and I am positively of the opinion that
even those boundaries for·quinine are not in the least the
most extreme. I know many will doubt the propriety
of such large doses. With facts only fools quarrel.
He, whose aim is to cure the sick at the bedside, does
not act from tradition, but knows what he wants and
never hesitates a moment to act accordingly. I only
caution against one thing: You are not advised to
give a pneumonic, who has at any time a temperature of
41°C. which, after an insufficient abstraction of heat,
quickly rises again, 5 grammes (75 grains) of quinine
at one dose. This is allowable only when repeated,
thorough, cold baths reduce the temperature for only a
short time, and smaller doses of quinine have no effect.
Even then, I first try three or four grammes (45 to 60
grains). And again, I emphasize that the heart be the
determining ·point for the physician. Whoever carefully notices the pulse goes sure, and who does not,
easily stumbles.

In my cases I have never observed detrimental effects of quinine on the heart. With the temperature the
pulse diminishes, but at the same time remains full and
strong, or gets better than it was before. The subjective inconveniences are not much greater with large
doses, than with smaller ones—they disappear quickly.
Frequently emesis occurs shortly after taking the quin-

ine.   If it occurs one-half to three quarters of an hour
after taking the quinine, the dose need not be renewed,
as the resorption in the suggested form is speedily accomplished ; only when *periculum in mora* you must not
hesitate, but rather give too much than too little.

But frequently the stomach rejects it after the lapse
of some minutes ; you can frustrate this by letting the
patient bend over as soon as the quinine is taken, and
open his mouth to allow the generally profuse sali-
vation to run off. Often small pieces of ice, swallowed as
soon as sickness of the stomach occurs, prevent emesis.
But should it occur in spite of this, I give, one-quarter
to one-half hour later, another, and eventually the third
dose—generally the second dose is not thrown off.   If
we should not succeed, what may sometimes happen, to
give quinine *per orem*, we may give it in injection—with
this we nearly always succeed—the resorption from the
rectum is, as it appears, as vigorous as from the stomach.
If you have to employ quinine by injection you must instruct the apothecary not to be too liberal with the acid,
and take three or four fold more of water for its solution,
than stated before.   In too much irritation of the rectal
mucous membrane the unwelcome dose will be thrown
off.   A bland vehicle and a few drops of tr. opii are
with very few exceptions sufficient to effect a tolerance
of the intestine.   In order to get the whole effect of
the single dose, quinine must not be given daily, but a
lapse of time of forty-eight hours must intervene between two doses, therefore it has to be given every other
evening.   By forced doses we also succeed in lowering
the temperature for twenty-four hours.   But it is never
so decided as in the first named instance. I should think
that such properties would suffice to bring the high

rank of quinine as an antipyretic to acknowledgment everywhere. And yet there are often enough heard doubting, or even negative voices. Most frequently absolutely too small or broken doses were used. The form also has to be considered. If you give a person with fever, quinine in powder for a long time, without giving him an acid lemonade, you must not wonder when, now and then, the effect is altogether *not* experienced, or dyspeptic disturbance ensue. The same objection holds in dispensing quinine in pills. Subcutaneous injections of quinine I have given up, as they frequently create abscesses. The diet of pneumonics is conditioned by the position that one assumes in the question of principle: should the physician allow fever patients to eat? With me the question is decided for some time. The assumption that feeding causes an increase in temperature, and therefore should be interdicted, because you must not pour oil into the fire, appears to me untenable, even if proof were brought by those gentlemen, who hitherto did not bring it, that the supposed increase in temperature really does take place. But even if it was so, I would nourish my patients. For the nutriments brought into the organism save a greater loss to the tissues and give compensation for the losses already sustained. Would you rather buy wood or burn your chairs, when compelled, in a temperature sufficiently cold, to keep your room warm? It is a fact sustained by experience, that fever patients who are not starved get well much sooner, and why appears to me transparent enough.

It depends upon finding the proper form of nutriment. This is found much easier when by proper treatment you prevent the patient from being exposed to

a continued high temperature; you can in such case impose much more upon his digestive organs. I am convinced that you can contribute to keep his appetite
awake by having his mouth and teeth cleansed several
times a day. I hold it to be very proper to add not too
little salt to every meal. Leaving its high significance
as nourishment out of question, it has a tendency
to cleanse his mouth, and at the same time improve
his appetite. If the patients are willing to take it,
I allow them some scraped beef lightly broiled, several times a day, with bread and butter; in small portions that are taken, say one hour after the bath, for
three or four times daily, is the best manner. I never
compel patients to this nourishment. In somewhat
severe cases, *I demand* that there be taken one to two
tablespoonsful of good *bouillon*, with one or two eggs,
per day; also in the course of the day (determinable
for each case) a certain quantity of milk diluted with
one to three parts water, always to be added not too
small a quantity of salt.

I consider it a *sine qua non* that a pneumonic gets a
quantity of wine, varying according to his age and custom of living; for us the 8 per cent. Bordeaux is the
most convenient. For the adult, about one-half to one
bottle daily. Whatever is not used before and after
the bath can be taken *ad libitum*, mixed with water, in
the course of the day. I also allow good beer. It is
sure that by alcoholic drinks the heat of the body is
rather diminished than increased; more than probable,
alcohol is a direct guardian of the tissues. The formerly existing prejudice in this direction has been shown
to have no foundation, especially by *Bouvier* and *Binz*.

There are two objects to be mentioned yet at this

point, that are of importance during the increase of debility of the heart—neither the pain from which a pneumonic suffers, nor the sleeplessness should be left unsubdued. That continued pain diminishes the resistance of the patient is a fact. Here in addition, the pain from the inflamed pleura `hinders respiration. I always found·it to the purpose to make local subcutaneous injections of morphia. The dose may be a small one, from 1 to 1½ centigrammes ($\frac{1}{6}$ to $\frac{1}{8}$ gr.) will suffice. The often very harrassing cough has to be viewed from the same standpoint. If the pain is very severe, the demand to subdue it is the same as that of inducing sleep. Sleeplessness must not be suffered in pneumonia. Every one of us, I suppose, has had his strength tested by a sleepless night. The weakly are more affected by such a loss of rest than the stronger. Every pneumonic becomes weak by his disease, no matter how his constitution may have been before. The loss of sleep will bear upon him worse than on the healthy. The malaise caused by loss of sleep is for me a weighty cause for therapeutic interference. This sleeplessness often disappears as soon as an antipyretic treatment is instituted, without further trouble. Should this not be the case, then I employ the somnifera in decided doses. In children, the antipyresis, in very few exceptions, is sufficient to bring on sleep; a circumstance that saves the physician a great deal of embarrassment. There are cases where the sole therapeutic aim should be to effect sleep. There are those, where a condition exists that manifests itself by continued delirium, accompanied by muscular twitchings, sometimes even maniacal outbursts, with complete sleeplessness. Sometimes in only incomplete antipyresis, a full dose of quinine suffices, that by many will be taken as a direct hypnotic. To this category belongs the pneumonia of drunkards, that, without producing the "school shaped" picture of delirium tremens, are distinguished by the accompanying delirium, and finally the delirium tremens itself, originating with the pneumonia.

No matter what may be the cause, a continually increasing work is always imposed, (frequently from the beginning,) upon the weak heart (drunkard), by a continued muscular action. Soon enough will the pulse tell the inability of the heart to master this task. Sleep, and with it a reduction of this muscular work is the sole remedy. I have produced sleep in such cases by very large doses of the proper preparation: lately mostly by chloral hydrate, 5 to 8 grammes, (75 to 120 grains) for the single dose, whenever smaller ones fail.

Never forget in fever patients to give a sufficient quantity of properly diluted muriatic acid, to prevent a decomposition of the chloral hydrate in the stomach, the surface of which may not re-act acid enough, or even be alkaline. In giving this or any other remedy of the kind you must not forget the energetic stimulation of the heart. Without this, a thorough-going medication is not allowed. With it, you need not hesitate to transgress the exclamation point* of the pharmacopœia, whenever a necessity exists to create sleep.

Allow me to remark, that in severe acute diseases, I do not like the darkened sick-rooms. If you place the bed in such a position that the daylight does not strike

---

* The German laws demand an exclamation point from the physician when he wishes to transgress the usual doses.—K.

the patient's eyes, it will be sufficient. It appears to me that a patient fares best when exposed to light.

We have now arrived at the second part of our proposition. It runs: *Conquering the already existing debility of the heart.* For the cases that you treat from the beginning, and in whom your prophylactic endeavors have been insufficient, mark the rule—: *the sooner you notice the coming of debility of the heart, the easier it is to bring your patient over it.* The reason for this is evident. Debility of the heart muscles produces a slowness in the circulation. Slowness of circulation causes a disturbance in the nutrition of all the organs. The longer it lasts, the deeper are the alterations called forth by the same. If even the normal rapidity of the blood is reestablished after a while by the strengthening of the activity of the heart, it yet requires some time, equivalent to the disturbance, to repair the damage. And this damage is most apparent in those parts that require most blood—these are the laboring muscles: heart and respiratories. On this circumstance I lay a great deal of stress, and direct my attention to the first symptoms that indicate a reduction in the activity of the heart. I believe that the success I enjoy at the bedside is not a little due to this attention. Besides the quality of the pulse, the relation between its frequency and that of respiration ; finally the approaching cyanosis has to be watched. The temperature shows no constant difference in the initiatory stage of collapse.

It is often only transient ; for I suppose that these light and lightest disturbances that are found upon close examination in every single case, are caused only by a spreading of the local affection. This the thermometer does not always show. It rests with the physician,

whether he is to interfere here. In a robust patient I
do not do it before all appearances are somewhat more
definite. But I know that you can act sooner without
harm.

The picture of outspoken collapse with its most
prominent symptom, œdema of the lungs, is so characteristic, that its outlines will be indelibly impressed
upon any one who has seen it once. That here is
the beginning of the end will be clear to the dullest
mind. Collapse of high grade surely leads to death
when the physician renders no help. What is to be
tried here, has to accomplish much. But what is to be
tried? Here the separating point of views is of the
most telling significance. The importance of the thing
requires the closest consideration. Hitherto I have
spoken of debility of the heart, but have not mentioned
how its consequences manifest themselves. That in
pneumonia the right ventricle in the first instance is over-
taxed, has been mentioned before. If the heart cannot
accomplish its work, the disturbance created thereby
shows itself here first. So then by the diminished work
of the right ventricle, a stagnation is produced in the
pulmonary circulation, the left ventricle becomes empty
as a consequence; in higher degrees an accumulation of
the blood in the veins of the general circulation takes
place, on account of the difficult passage through the
never-sufficiently emptied right ventricle, and on account of the insufficient *vis a tergo*. In the more developed condition of insufficiency of the heart, œdema of
the lungs may ensue. In lethal cases this is never wanting. The much-discussed cerebral œdema called forth
by insufficient circulation of the vena cava superior,
may develop in exceptional cases as a variety. The

symptoms described generally as cerebral œdema may, with equal justice, be considered as those that a lasting fever calls forth with impeded exchange of gases—an insufficient blood respiration. Similar symptoms are produced just as seldom as in pneumonia, in all severe febrile diseases.

The *emptying of the left ventricle* is always, and under all circumstances, a very considerable disadvantage; the laboring muscles, heart and respiratories do not receive in consequence a sufficient quantity of blood. By this their ability to work is most effectively disturbed. It is therefore more to the purpose to put the term, *insufficiency of the heart*, in place of œdema of the lungs, as a cause of death in pneumonia. This is something more than a mere alteration of the name. In speaking of œdema of the lungs you easily come to the conclusion that it only is a purely mechanical exclusion of air from the blood, caused by the serum poured into the alveoli, that hereby the exhalation of carbonic acid is difficult, and so the carbonic acid retained in the blood causes death. That a filling up of the alveoli of the lung with a fluid interferes with the exchange of gases, is sure. But with this circumstance comes into consideration that the retardation of the circulation preceding the œdema caused by the debility of the heart, retards the interchange of matter in the tissues; a retention takes place in them of all products of oxydation. It is preferable, therefore, to choose your name from the cause and not from the effect, and this cause is insufficiency of the heart.

Within the last ten years an opinion has been propagated that deviates from the one on which we base our views. *Niemeyer* speaks so definitely of an œdema

of the lungs produced by collateral fluxion in pneumonia, that the reader, not very familiar with the matter, is
seduced into the belief that this was the usual occurrence. The proof of the opinion reads something like
this: The occlusion caused by the pneumonic exudation within the distribution of the pulmonary artery,
calls forth a fluxion (an increased and accelerated flow)
towards the parts not filled by exudation. The blood-
pressure acts upon capillaries in the lungs, that are not
like those of other organs imbedded in more or less resistant tissue, but are to the larger part of their walls
almost naked or entirely so, so that they are unable to
resist an increased pressure of the blood. These capillaries are first expanded and afterwards allow their contents to transude.*

A consequence of the view used by Niemeyer thera-
peutically is: that an increase in the heart's action induces an increase in the accumulation of fluid in the
alveoli. That this deduction is not to the point is
easily proven.

1. If these coarse mechanical conditions took place,
why don't you always find collateral œdema, as soon as
the disease befalls a robust individual? Why do we
find œdema in the weakly and not observe it in the
strong?

2. In emphysema of the lungs, spoken of in Niemeyer's, work exactly from this point—with the wasting
of capillaries is constantly connected hypertrophy of
the right ventricle; an increase of the living power is
therefore created by the heart in every contraction, and
consequently an increase of pressure in the capillaries

* Niemeyer even goes farther than that; he allows that increased action of
the heart alone creates hyperæmia and œdema in the lungs.

of the lung over-filled by "collateral fluxion." Œdema of the lungs does not appear as long as the right ventricle remains hypertrophic, but only when it undergoes fatty degeneration.

How does this agree with Niemeyer's views above?

3. You never find an increase in the sounds over the right ventricle during the existence of lung affected with œdema. (Thierfelder.)

4. I have seen in all, something like a thousand cases of pneumonia. Among these is one, in whom, forty-eight hours after invasion of the disease, œdema of the lungs was noticeable. In all the rest, later. This one was treated with stimulants in the most lavish and persevering manner, and he recovered.

I cannot give positive figures, but I believe I can rely on my memory, having had an eye on these circumstances for years. Very definitely I remember two cases of pneumo-thorax, when, a few hours after its invasion, paralysis of the heart appeared with œdema of the lungs. Even here, where the collapse of a whole lung created the most welcome opportunity for a "collateral active œdema"—it disappeared after the administration of the most active stimulation, *coup sur coup.* The experience of one is always only a drop in the sea. But how many physicians see œdema of the lungs during the period when the local alterations establish themselves? How many of us notice œdema of the lungs together with increased heart's action in pneumonia? I believe I can now drop the subject without further inquiry.

If even the impossibility of œdema of the lungs originating in this wise cannot be demonstrated theoretically, yet experience teaches its occurrence to be rare indeed.

If it does occur, there is possibly existing with the physical cause, also a physiological one—want of resistance in the vessels, as in those disposed to phtisis, in drunkards, etc. If those purely mechanical conditions brought forward by Niemeyer, were indeed the predisposing ones, then œdema of the lungs ought to occur necessarily at the beginning of pneumonia. But have we to do with a *passive* œdema caused by the inability of the right ventricle to overcome the resistance created in the lung circulation—what is to be done then?

The school teaches that a lessening of the general mass of the blood causes a lessening of the heart's labor, the mass to be propelled will be less. At the same time the amount of fluid transuded into the alveoli is re-absorbed by the tissues. Venesection diminishes the work of the heart and allows the œdema to vanish by resorption. Venesection therefore is fully indicated in passive œdema of the lungs. Experience teaches that indeed the threatening condition disappears after venesection, sometimes very quickly, so that there are few remedies that can boast of such eminent efficacy.

And yet: Is this remedy the most rational, or are there still others that might produce the same result? If venesection was an indifferent thing, any discussion would be unnecessary. But it is the contrary. How does it generally work when we venesect in pneumonia on account of existing œdema? After the lapse of twenty-four hours, and sometimes much earlier, the condition is the same as before venesection. You take the lancet again—and the symptoms of œdema vanish again. But if the crisis, the natural decision, does not set in very soon thereafter, the patient will perish by a third or fourth necessary venesection. You

will have to be satisfied therefore in your mind the first
time you open a vein, that the operation is justified
only in order to gain time for the appearance of the
spontaneous end of the disease, and I would myself in
the given case not hesitate to open a vein if *I saw no
possibility to succeed in any other way*—in order to gain
time.   But can't we succeed in a less dangerous way to
obtain the same results?   If we could stimulate the
heart and stimulate so long until the impediment in the
lung circulation was overcome, the task would be accomplished.   Experience will have to decide on the
question, whether a tiring out would not follow the increased activity, so that the same consequences were
created for the heart as by venesection.

Let us look at the principle of both methods.   Every
laboring muscle wants oxygen in proportion to the
amount of labor it has to perform.   *Ceteris paribus,* the
quantity of oxygen carried into the muscles, is dependent upon the quantity of red blood corpuscles.   These,
of course, venesection diminishes.   Less oxygen is
therefore taken into the blood after venesection.   When
the demand exceeds the quantity contained in the blood,
it is only compensated by an acceleration of the circulation.   For, as the number of red blood corpuscles
may be considered as a constant quantity for the time
under consideration, there only remains the possibility,
that in the given time, the extent of contact between
the blood and the air in the lungs for the taking in of
oxygen, and at the same time between the blood and the
tissues for the giving off of carbonic·acid has to be increased.   Another thing to be taken into consideration
is, that a lessening of the burden, which venesection
caused in the first instance to the heart, is of very short

·duration, as the volume of the blood is very soon re-
plenished by resorption from the tissues. That means,
·expressed in one sentence :—

*Heart and respiratory muscles must labor harder after
venesection than before, when the same quantity of oxygen
is to be carried into the tissues.*

The requirement of oxygen for the body will only
be diminished by venesection, when a considerable
lowering of temperature takes place in consequence,
and then only as long as such low temperature lasts.
As a rule the requirement of oxygen will remain the
same, or is increased after venesection, therefore, the
only transient improvement caused by abstraction of
blood is readily understood. Only the diminishing of
the requirement of oxygen—the crisis—disposes to a
lessening of the inner muscular labor.

Venesection therefore is a very doubtful friend in
need. Comparable to the usurer, who is ready to lend
money upon security, in order to take finally everything the debtor owns. For the moment, the loan
helps him out of the ʼscrape, but if there is no cutting
down of expenses, the catastrophy will only be a question of time.

I have to point to a contradiction, although an apparent one. How does it come, when the above deduction is correct, that immediately after venesection, heart
and respiratories work better and stronger than before ?
This occurs, because for the moment the right ventricle
is eased of its burden, so that it is able to drive more
blood into the left one. And if the left ventricle re-
·ceives more blood after venesection than before, the
heart and respiratory muscles receive with the increase
· of blood also an increase of oxygen.

Entirely different are stimulants. Here the heart is stimulated to increased labor, but by the remedy itself is put into a condition to accomplish the work. Each stronger contraction brings more blood into the left ventricle from the over-filled right one; carries with it more oxygen and helps to get rid of the dross of oxydation; is of value, therefore, in the first instance to the heart. The blood quantity is intact; it only is necessary to call forth a stronger exertion for a short time, to get out of the momentary dilemma. Under these circumstances, stimulants are not only the whip but also the oats for the heart. For it brings oxygen to the heart, without which, no muscular labor is possible. How the decision will be after this theoretical reasoning cannot be uncertain.

If the last named way is the right one, of course you will choose it. Experience has taught that it is so. We indeed succeed by discriminate and bold employment of stimulants to keep pneumonics alive for three or four days after debility of the heart ensued; mostly we can keep them even longer.

In the lighter degrees of debility of the heart, a full dose of strong wine suffices in the majority of cases, say, 150 grammes (about 8 ounces) of port, madeira, sherry, etc., to make them disappear. The quantity of the single dose, of course, has to vary according to the individuality of the patient, especially according to how he is used to stimulants. If these lighter attacks follow each other frequently, I order an emulsion of camphor, 3 grammes to 200 water (45 grains, to about 10 ounces), a tablespoonful every two hours. If the condition continues without momentarily assuming a threatening character, I order one tablespoonful of strong wine every hour or half hour alternately with the emulsion of camphor. Sudden collapse of considerable intensity is very appropriately treated with musk, 5 to 15 centigrammes (⅜ to 2 grains) per dose, with one or several tablespoonfuls of champagne. You can give this quantity every ten minutes or every half hour until the patient takes a turn for the better. Musk, like champagne, acts quickly; camphor slower, but its effect lasts longer. In severe cases, with frequent intercurrent attacks of debility of the heart, I give after the musk, champagne and camphor for a longer period in order to hold on to the gained advantage. Almost quicker than musk with champagne, acts hot grog—one to two parts cognac or rum, or if nothing else is to be had, whisky, to one part water or one part strong coffee or tea. I give of this one or several tablespoonfuls every ten minutes. Sometimes you see wonders from it. But here too, the effect is not lasting, you have to continue in order to keep its effect alive.

To make definite rules for the employment of stimulants would be useless. You must set up a principle according to which you will employ them at the bedside, and on quiet observation you will soon learn to go sure.

If you notice the first symptoms early, it will enable you to do away with the "heavy artillery." But if it has to be ordered to the front, make it a rule that a maximum boundary for stimulants must not exist, that when the weaker are inefficient, you must employ the stronger and increase the dose if necessary. Perseverance only leads to glory; whoever is timid, when it is necessary to act otherwise, belongs elsewhere, and not at the sick-bed.

44

The adherents of venesection have arrived at the point that they employ stimulants after venesection. That within certain boundaries some results may be obtained in this way is sure. But do not hesitate to make the whole step forward, relinquish venesection and combat œdema of the lungs from the beginning with stimulants. The first trial will not be the last one. Should the patient be bathed, when symptoms of debility of the heart are established? Theoretically, the answer is, the bath transiently increases the labor of the heart, but it diminishes on the whole its labor. If the heart can bear the transiently increased labor, you may bathe; in the opposite case, not. Practically, the thing is this: If you have to contend against the deepest collapse, you can, with sufficient care in the choice of stimulants and the temperature of the bath, treat most of your patients by direct abstraction of heat. All can bear large doses of quinine. Taught by experience, I have gone a little farther. Whoever is well-acquainted with the treatment of pneumonia according to the principle herein laid down, and by a low per cent. of mortality, will always go ahead more daringly, than one who has to gather his experience first. Never forget: the most dangerous enemy to the heart is an excessive temperature, and that is brought down by the bath surely and quickly.

To one circumstance I wish to direct your attention. Not very seldom, collapse appears in weakened patients at the time of crisis, or even several days thereafter. Usually it disappears very soon spontaneously, but sometimes becomes dangerous. I believe you will notice this collapse less often when you allow for five or six days after the disappearance of the fever a light wine. You must always prepare the family or the attendants for such a possibility, and make your arrangements *before hand*, because prompt action is here of the greatest importance. A *short* re-convalescence of our patients we aim to obtain by sufficient nourishment, especially albuminous substances, and a sufficient quantity of beer or wine, and endeavor to reduce it to the narrowest limits. Preparations of iron we use with predilection. You know the form in which we use the metal on dyspeptics :

R Ferr. hydrogen. reduct. 8 grm. (120 grains.)
  Extr. chinæ reg. frigide purat. 2 grm. (30 grs.)
  F. l. a. pilul. No. 100, c. pulv. cinnamon.
3 times daily 3 pills, 10 minutes after meals.

You begin with one pill and increase gradually, when a high degree of dyspepsia exists.

When resorption exists I can not pressingly enough recommend ol. terebinth. I give 6 times daily, every time 12 drops in milk or capsules, of an increase in the dose I have seen no advantage, although you can go far beyond this, without harm. When you give with each dose a sufficient quantity of milk, say 3 to 5 ounces, you will have no gastric disturbances.

The views here demonstrated have that preference from the beginning, that they render clear the whole doctrine of pneumonia from a unitary standpoint, and at the same time discuss the measures to be taken. But in therapeutic affairs success is the sole judge, and any deduction, as enticing as it may sound, is worthless, unless it is based upon experience at the sick-bed. I know that my views were not born at the desk, but are gathered in the sick-room—that my theory is derived from practice.

But, by their fruits ye shall know them; and so in conclusion, I will not show any statistics, but a simple enumeration of the last 200 cases, treated at the Polyclinic according to the principles which I have delineated as the guiding ones. There is no selection, but case after case in chronological succession, taken from our protocols. *Statistics in pneumonia that are to be of value*, must be *death statistics*, I believe.

If you have not the control over thousands, there is too much room for accident. Examine the list carefully, and I am convinced that you say with me that the treatment has accomplished what possibly could be expected. I hold that all cases should be counted that died with the clinical diagnosis "pneumonia," and were ratified by the anatomical knife. This excludes all arbitrariness. If I take 400 cases that were treated before I could carry out my principles against 400 other cases, it shows the mortality reduced to one-half; but this reduction is still too small for me. My death statistics may speak for me.

Of the 200 treated according to the foregoing, *nine were under one year old*, no death; under five years old, sixty-three, of whom *two died;* from six to ten years old, thirty-eight; *two deaths.* From ten to twenty, sixteen and no death; from twenty to thirty, thirteen and no death; from thirty to forty, fourteen and *two* deaths; from forty to fifty, fifteen, of whom *eight* died; from fifty to sixty, *fourteen*, and *two* deaths; from sixty to seventy, *ten*, of whom *four died;* from seventy to ninety, *seven*, and *four* deaths; at ninety three, *one.*—Males, 114; females, 86. Total, 200, of which number, twenty-four died. Many incidents attending the fatal cases, cf interest as explanatory of that result, we are compelled to omit.

Gentlemen, the several cases will be in your memory yet, when you stood hesitating at the bedside, where a severe pneumonia threatened the life of your patient, and where you found that your apparently useless interference brought the sufferer out of danger. I need not tell you that my treatment is not an heroic one. You formed your judgment at the bedside, and this sufficiently satisfies me that it is a correct one. Allow me to direct your attention to the cardinal point: *Pneumonia is no disease after a specific pattern, and you are never to fashion your treatment after a pattern.*

Original Communications.

DO THE MANIFESTATIONS OF VENEREAL DISEASE DIFFER IN THE MALE AND THE FEMALE.

By Thomas Kennard, M. D., St. Louis,

[Continued from page 590.]

In the article which I had the honor of reading before this Society at our last meeting, I stated that I did not believe that it was possible for any one to decide, positively and truthfully, that any initial venereal lesion would not be followed by constitutional symptoms, because it lacked the characteristic induration, either of the sore, or of the inguinal glands, or both; and that the different forms of syphilitic infection varied so much, and that the induration was often so slight, or so completely wanting, that the majority of observers were frequently in danger of mistaking the true form of the disease for the chancroid, or soft sore: and hence we found so many cases of constitutional syphilis following the non-indurated sore. I pointed out the fact, that induration was the exception, and not the rule in females; and therefore in many cases it was impracticable to distinguish the infecting from the non-infecting primary lesion in women.

I also contended that the infecting chancre might commence, either as an abrasion, a pustule or a simple crack in the mucous membrane, and its appearance differed in no particular from lesions formed by accident, and consequently excited no alarm or suspicion, even in the mind of the patient, as to the origin of the lesion, and that this was especially likely to occur, because there is always a period of incubation in true chancres, and that these primary lesions healed or were lost sight of, before the disease manifested itself.

I unhesitatingly conceded that the young or dualistic school had done much to clear up the inextricable confusion that formerly prevailed, in regard to the doctrines of syphilis, and that the distinctions drawn by them between the chancre and the chancroid, as a general rule, were true, and answered all clinical purposes most admirably, but that they would not hold good in every instance, for like every other disease, syphilis varied somewhat, under varying circumstances. I confessed that I was a dualist, so far as the truthfulness of that doctrine applied as a general but not as a universal rule. I am also a unicist, in believing that there is but one true syphilitic virus—and that one attack of constitutional disease protects against a second in the same individual, but not in the sense that there is but one venereal virus, or but one mode of manifesting the true syphilitic virus. I do not accept induration as an infallible test of the nature of any and every venereal lesion, but believe, that anto-inoculability or non anto-inoculability of any venereal sore is a much better guide to a correct diagnosis, as proven by the experiments of M. Clero, M. Rollet, M. Fournier, and others, to say nothing of the clinical experience of every surgeon, which is, that hard sores never duplicate themselves on the same individual, and that chancroids are always liable to do so.

I now desire to record my views in regard to the prevalence

and curability of the disease, its prognosis, the modes of contagion between adults, and its communicability to the offspring.

The most momentous questions to any one suffering from venereal disease are: Is it true syphilis that I have? Will it infect my blood? and if so, can I be radically cured? Such questions are universally asked us, and we should endeavor to be able to answer them promptly, honestly and correctly. It has been the fashion so long, to consider this disease as absolutely incurable in the great majority of cases, that it has inspired the unprofessional with a holy horror of it, and has induced many experienced surgeons to believe, that it could not be thoroughly eradicated from the system, and a few, that its baneful effects might be transmitted even to the third and fourth generations. The study of syphilis has been prosecuted so sedulously, however, within the last twenty years, and its natural history been so thoroughly examined into, that it no longer causes either the patient or the experienced physician any very great anxiety, except in rare and malignant cases. Syphilis is not near so common a disease, as the majority of people believe, nor is it near so persistent, if left to the efforts of nature, or resistant to treatment, as most authors tell us. If it were so, how few healthy children would now be borne, after four centuries of active propagation. That it is not so, is proven by the very small number of cases of hereditary syphilis that we meet with, compared with the number of cases of syphilis that we treat every year, and the very small proportion of deaths that are recorded annually in our large cities, from that disease. The general healthy appearance of our people in every walk of life, proves that the blood of but few of them is contaminated by this virus; and the bills of mortality show how seldom the direct cause of death is attributed to syphilis. In New York we find that the—

* Number of deaths during 1866, was 21,206, of which 44 were from syphilis.

"	"	"	1867,	"	23,443,	"	76	"	"
"	"	"	1868,	"	24,889,	"	77	"	"
"	"	"	1869,	"	25,167,	"	77	"	"
"	"	"	1870,	"	27,175,	"	106	'	"
"	"	"	1871,	"	26,976,	"	142	"	"

* F. R. Sturgis, M. D., *American Journal of Medical Science*, July, 1872.

and in Philadelphia, the—

Number of deaths during 1860, was 11,568, of which 9 were from syphilis.								
"	"	"	1861,	"	14,468,	"	9	" "
"	"	"	1862,	"	15,097,	"	21	" "
"	"	"	1863,	"	15,788,	"	28	" "
"	"	"	1864,	"	17,582,	"	25	" "
"	"	"	1865,	"	17,169,	"	30	" "
"	"	"	1866,	"	16,802,	"	22	" "
"	"	"	1867,	"	13,983,	"	25	" "
"	"	"	1868,	"	14,698,	"	43	" "
"	"	"	1869,	"	14,786,	"	21	" "
"	"	"	1870,	"	16,750,	"	28	' "
"	"	"	1871,	"	16,993,	"	19	'

In our own city, St. Louis, we have found, from a critical examination of the reports of the Board of Health, that there were during the—

Year ending Dec. 31st, 1867, 6,538 deaths with 8 from syphilis.					
"	"	1868, 5,193	"	17	"
"	"	1869, 5,884	"	5	"
"	"	1870, 6,676	"	30	"
"	"	1871, 5,265	"	9	"
"	"	1872, 8,047	"	9	"

It is true that the indirect cause of death is often believed to be some syphilitic taint in the blood, when the certificate assigns it to some more acute malady, but if it be justly attributable to that disease, the syphilitic cachexia should be easily enough diagnosticated. The truth is, that it is no longer such an all prevailing, unmanageable and inexterminable disease, as some persons would have us believe, but in the great majority of cases, is just as curable under proper treatment as any other troublesome malady. It is evidently becoming much milder and more manageable under our improved methods of treatment, and in St. Louis (more especially since the enforcement of the social evil law), we do not meet with many aggravated cases of venereal disease of any kind, either in public or private practice, and if the system of registration, inspection, introspection, segregation and prompt and efficient treatment was properly carried out, we might almost stamp out syphilis from our midst.

The ordinary duration of constitutional syphilis engrafted upon a robust constitution is two years, but this period may be greatly shortened and mitigated by judicious treatment, or very much prolonged by mismanagement. I am thoroughly convinced from experience, that in many instances its external manifestations may be obviated entirely by prompt mercurial treatment of the disease, when convinced by the initial lesion that constitutional infection has occurred.

We may, too, with a reasonable degree of accuracy, prognosticate the mildness or severity of the primary; from the long or short period of incubation; from the early or late appearance of the eruptions; from the uniformity or irregularity of the intervals between the different kinds of eruption, for a great degree of correspondence is found to exist in all of these particulars. In very many cases we have only a few of the milder forms· of eruption, and the poison seems to have been eliminated before progressing to the ulcerative stage; in others we may have severe attacks of several forms of eruption, either separately or following each other so rapidly, as to become mixed on the same patient; in others again, we may have some of the special organs involved, or the joints and superficial bones affected; and yet I believe that the majority of all these cases are readily amenable to treatment, and can be thoroughly and radically cured. Certainly I have seen a number of cases of obstinate psoriasis rupia, and ulcerations, and a necrosis of the bone entirely cured. When the vital organs—the brain. the spinal cord, the lungs, the liver, the kidneys and the arteries become involved—the one or more, the case becomes far more serious, but even then, some constitutions are strong enough to bring about recovery, either partial or complete. Age, strength of constitution and the mode of living has much to do with the course of syphilis. Infants and old people are destroyed by it far oftener than the young and middle-aged. The former, because they are imperfect beings, sprung from a poisoned source, and consequently have their vital organs diseased before they are brought into the world, and often die in their mother's womb; the latter, because the natural debility consequent upon old age is greatly increased by the depressing effect of the syphilitic virus, and the system is not able to eliminate it. Hence, we find that the great majority of deaths from syphilis occur in children under five years of age, and over ninety per cent. of that number die before they reach one year. Hereditary syphilis may originate either where both parents are suffering from constitutional disease at the time when fecundation occurred, in which case it would be almost impossible for the fœtus to escape, or where the mother alone is syphilitic and either furnishes a diseased ovum in the first place, or contaminates it by furnishing it the nutritive elements which nourish the child in utero; or the father may be the only one syphilized, and may communicate the disease directly through his poisoned semen, or, what is much more common, by communicating the disease to the mother before, at the time of, or very soon after impregnation. The child may also contract syphilis by becoming inoculated from a syphilitic mother during labor, or from vaccination or nursing. The majority of authors deny that the syphilitic disease can be communicated directly to the fœtus through the semen of the father, and especially when the mother remains pure, and although I am free to admit that such cases are very rare exceptions, I am still thoroughly convinced that they do occasionally occur, as in the case which I reported to this Society a few years since, and which was published in the Sixth Volume of the *Medical Archives*, and attracted much attention among specialists in this department. This very striking case has been commented on at great length, and criticized in the *New York Medical Journal* by Dr. Frederick R. Sturgis, the partner of Dr. Bumstead, in an able article on the Etiology of Hereditary Syphilis. In this report I stated that it was an instance of the transmission of syphilis by a diseased father, while the non-syphilized mother remained uninfected, proving that the poison reached the child only through the impure semen of the father. That the disease is communicated to the fœtus through the mother at the time of impregnation, or in the early stages of its existence, in the great majority of cases, is very well proven and generally acquiesced in, but still I am not convinced that wherever the child is diseased, the mother is also, and wherever the mother remains healthy, the child cannot be infected. The mother however, although generally the immediate cause of the disease in her child, is nine times out of ten the innocent one, for she has been infected by her husband, and thus ignorantly and unintentionally poisons the fruit of her womb. There can be no doubt of the greater degree of virtue among married and child-bearing women than among men, and hence the origin of the great majority of cases of hereditary syphilis can be traced back directly to the father, although it is generally imparted to the fœtus in utero through the mother. The inherited disease will, as a rule, be more or less severe in the child, in proportion to the virulence of the disease in the parent communicating the same and the length of time that has intervened since syphilitic symptoms manifested themselves in either or both parents. It may be ˆtransmitted at any stage of the constitutional disease, from six months to twenty years, or more, after the infection of the parents, and often when the disease is latent in them. It is not generally believed or satisfactorily determined that the hereditary disease may be transmitted to the third and fourth generations (though some authorities are inclined to credit the statement that it may descend through several generations), nor can I see any good reasons for such belief. Neither has it been determined whether an adult who has suffered from hereditary syphilis, is from that fact more or less exempt from receiving the disease anew in his own system. It is however very probable that to a certain extent he is protected.

In the adult, beyond doubt, the most common mode of communicating venereal disease in its primary form, is sexual intercourse, either natural or unnatural, and infection occurs either mediately or immediately. Either directly from a diseased to a healthy person, the usual mode, or the two parties copulating, may be both healthy, and yet the prostitute may retain in her vagina gonorrhœal, or chancroidal pus, or the poison of syphilis received from a previous connection with a diseased man, and thus without being infected herself, may communicate it to the second man, or *vice versa*, the man to the woman. Most authors of the present day admit the possibility of this mode of mediate contagion. Both men and women from want of cleanliness, may serve as a vehicle for contagion in this manner, as has been demonstrated beyond peradventure. It may be communicated in this manner, also by dirty, infected clothing, and by neglect in cleansing catheters and other surgical instruments.

No one denies that syphilis is generally communicated by direct inoculation from the indurated chancre; very few doubt that the early secondary lesions will also frequently serve as vehicles for the transmission of the virus, whilst only a limited number contend that the later secondary and tertiary sores possess the power of propagating the disease. The mucous patch, perhaps, communicates syphilis more readily than any other secondary lesion, and it is claimed that it will impart the disease by simple contact with any crack or fissure, as the primary ulcer does. Its extensive prevalence and location has, however, I think´more to do with its infecting powers than its form or peculiar nature, as it most commonly is found around the nipple at the entrance to the vagina, and in the mouth. Other secondary lesions will also communicate the disease to the non-infected. One of the most common methods of communicating secondary disease is by suckling, when it may originate either from the nurse or the nurseling, more commonly from the latter. Sometimes very many children are infected from their nurses, and *vice versa*, producing real epidemics in foundling hospitals and lying-in asylums.

Vaccination from virus obtained from a syphilitic child, is also sometimes a fruitful source of contagion, and has caused epidemics among children, accompanied by great mortality. Several alarming outbreaks of this kind have been recorded by authorities that were considered reliable. Lancereaux has collected nineteen observations of syphilis being propagated by vaccination. They include 851 individuals, vaccinated from syphilitic children; 258 of them were inoculated with syphilis, the rest escaped. The most remarkable outbreak of syphilis by vaccination of late years, is that which occurred at Rivalta, near Aqui, in Piedmont, in 1861.

Dr. Pacchiotti, of Turin, who was employed by the Italian government to report on the attack, has published an account of it. The facts are briefly these. "In May, 1861, an apparently healthy child, named Chiabrera, was vaccinated at Rivalta, with lymph sent from Aqui for the purpose. Ten days after this vaccination (June 7th), 46 healthy children were vaccinated at one sitting from this child. Again, on the 12th of June, 17 other healthy children were vaccinated from one of the 46. Thirty-nine of the 46 received syphilis with the vaccine disease, and 7 of the second series of 17, making a total of 46 out of 63 children, in a mountain village, simultaneously inoculated with syphilis. Some months elapsed before the vaccination was suspected to be the source of the children's bad health. By the 7th of October, when attention was drawn to this spreading disease, six of the 46 syphilized children had died without receiving any treatment, 14 were recovering, and three were in a precarious condition. * * * In addition to the children, twenty women suckling them were inoculated with syphilis from the children. Through the mothers the disease had reached some of the husbands, and even the elder children of the different families." (Berkeley Hill, page 64.) Now, a rigid inquiry into the case of the child Chiabrera, convinced Pacchiotti that the disease was communicated to it by a nursing woman, afterwards proven to be syphilitic, and not through the vaccine lymph, because the vaccine disease ran a regular course in Chiabrera, and the mother and father were perfectly healthy until sometime after the disease appeared in the child, whereas in all the other infected children the vaccine ran a very irregular course, and showed from the beginning that some poison had been introduced by the vaccination.

I mention this fact in conformation of what I have contended for on two previous occasions, years ago, when this subject was under discussion in this Society, viz : that syphilis is not communicated by syphilitic poison in the lymph, but by syphilitic blood intimately mixed with the vaccine lymph, or in other words, that vaccine lymph, *per se*, does not contain the syphilitic virus. That this is the way that syphilis is communicated by vaccination, I do not for one moment doubt. We know by positive experiments that secondary syphilis may be communicated by the blood, by the inoculation of a healthy person with the blood of a syphilitic person, as has been proven in many instances, by Pellizari, of Florence, Gibert, of Paris, Waller, of Prague, Lindwurm, of Munich, and many others, whose experiments were conducted in public, and the effects attested by numerous witnesses. This is the only rational explanation, too, in those cases where the foetus in utero is infected entirely through the mother. Syphilis has never been known however to be communicated through the blood of patients suffering from tertiary syphilis, by means of inoculation, although the experiment has been repeatedly tried. It is also believed by some authors, that the disease may be communicable through the milk, the saliva, etc.; but this question is still *sub judice*, and not likely to be positively determined, as the secretions, except the semen, are very likely to become mixed with the virus from syphilitic ulcerations or eruptions, and in that way to always render our experiments unsatisfactory, and liable to contradiction.

I am not as yet convinced that the disease may be imparted to a healthy person, by the natural or artificial mode of inoculation of the vaginal discharge of a syphilitic woman, or one who has had syphilis, but at the time has no local manifestation of the disease whatever. Drs. Morgan, Hammond, Carmichael and others, have, however, adduced many proofs of the truth of this doctrine, both by experimental inoculation, and from the records of their clinical experience, which we can only contradict, as the dualistic believers do, by deciding that all conclusions that do not prove the truth of their law, are drawn from wrong premises, and attributable to ignorance and inexactitude of observations.

TREATMENT OF PUERPERAL CONVULSIONS.

By Ulysses L. Huyette, M. D., Rolla, Mo.

In this paper, it is our desire to lay before the reader what seems to us to be the true course in the treatment of puerperal convulsions. We are satisfied that the most frequent condition under which this affection is met, is anæmia. That the opposite state will favor its occurrence, we doubt not, but that it is by far the less common, we hesitate not to assert, and it is of convulsions attended with the former condition we propose now particularly to speak. It is a well-established fact, that a want of vascular supply to the brain and spinal cord predisposes to convulsive action. The nervous centers evince the want of healthy blood by a morbid irritability, a sensitive, excitable state. This is the state of the pregnant anæmic female, her nervous system wrought up to its greatest tension, and the excitement of labor suffices to destroy the balance and produce spasm. Many modern females pass through pregnancy amid much suffering and discomfort, and as the weary days and months go by, their powers fail, the hue of health has left the cheek, and pale, bloodless and enfeebled, they enter the parturient work. A physiological, normal function is transformed into a pathological condition. Thus, many of our patients arrive at the close of gestation, and the system, when called upon to pass through the ordeal of labor (which requires all the nerve-force of a healthy organism,) is unfitted for the task. The result then too often is, that when labor has progressed to a certain extent, the nerve-centers fail to respond in a normal way, and convulsions occur. Instead of regular motor action, which is the response of a healthy state, we behold spasmodic irregular muscular contractions. Thus we perceive the chief source of this disorder is in the nervous centers, and the parturients are merely the exciting causes.

There is another feature to which we ask attention, viz : that convulsions *per se* are periodic, being characterized by paroxysms and intervals. This must be evident to all, and it is to this point we wish to call attention, for it has much to do with the treatment.

What are the indications in the case we have described ?

1st. To restore, if possible, the circulation in the nervous centers. (This want of vascularity may be due, either to anæmia, in which case the general supply is deficient, or to congestion when there is an abnormal distribution of blood in the brain. It is of small account which of the two conditions exists, for the remedy will be the same.)

2d. To take advantage of the periodicity of the affection.

3d. To remove the exciting cause by promoting speedy delivery.

The first two indications are fulfilled by the use of sulphate of quinia. It should be administered in large doses during the intervals of muscular contractions, the object should be to bring about the constitutional effects of the drug as speedily as possible. If the case is such that it cannot be administered by the mouth, it can be used subcutaneously.* From the use of quinia we have had most satisfactory results in the treatment of this class of diseases. It should be borne in mind that the work

*[Or what is better, by enema.]

should be done promptly, hence the importance of large doses of the remedy. The *modus operandi* must be manifest to all, it increases the cerebral circulation, thus giving rise to a condition the opposite of the one upon which this disease depends. We hear a great deal said about speedy delivery, and we rested long under the delusion that the first object should be to evacuate the uterus of its contents, but experience teaches us that in a great number of cases this affords no relief, the convulsive action continuing as strong after as before the operation. We insist that the first object should be to allay the morbid state of the nervous system, and restore, if possible, the functions to harmony. If the case be such to preclude the use of quinia, the patient having sunken to the condition when time is not allowed to obtain its effects, chloroform will alone afford a chance for life. It should be administered to complete anæsthesia, and the patient kept profoundly under its influence until the probabilities of a return of the convulsions cease to be apparent, especially should the patient be profoundly asleep when the placenta is delivered, for this is a period when many succumb, an event which might often be prevented were the patient allowed to remain longer under the influence of the anæsthetic. More danger exists, and we dare say more deaths follow a too early suspension than from excessive use of chloroform. In one case that I recall, I kept the patient completely under the influence for twelve hours, and notwithstanding (before I saw her) she had writhed in convulsions at varying intervals from five in the morning until seven in the evening, the whole process of delivery having been completed with no consciousness on her part whatever. She awoke from her chloroformic sleep refreshed, asked when her baby was born, and had a happy convalescence. But it is to the use of quinia we wish to allude. Doubtless, many such cases might be prevented by resorting to this remedy prior to labor, when the patient is anæmic, nervous, and predisposed to convulsions. By way of recapitulation, we say our grounds for the use of quinia are:

1st. Because it is an anti-periodic, convulsions being strictly periodic.

2d. It restores the supply of blood to the head, the want of which is proven to be a potent cause of this affection.

3d. It should be used in large doses so that the constitutional effects may be quickly obtained, and when, during the intervals the patient is unable to swallow, it should be given subcutaneously.

With these hints we leave the subject.

That quiniæ as an anti-periodic might be useful in epilepsy as a preventative, we doubt not, and we are sanguine that it will prove an efficient agent in all cases of convulsions due to want of vascularity of the nerve-centers. It is even questionable whether it is contra-indicated in plethora, for in all cases, contraction of the cerebral capillaries accompanies convulsions; hence, might we not reasonably expect from the action of this remedy upon the great sympathetic system, a dilatation of the vessels of the brain.

WHAT I THINK—PROFESSIONAL JOURNALISM.

By CHARLES LEONIDAS CARTER, M. D., Holden, Mo.

For nearly a score of years I have been in the habit of writing for the medical press, and yet, I have never written an article on the phenomena and details of a special disease. No man ever made a medical philosopher by studying the details of special cases. The professional ermine becomes only those who apply to underlying truths, and philosophic principles for correct diagnosis, prognosis, and therapeutics, and for correct deductions of every kind. While the geologist reasons inductively, from the effect back to the cause, the pathologist should reason, in the main, deductively, from cause up to effect.

After this prelude, I think it is obvious that if we reason more from first principles, though "case doctors" do croak "*theorists*" at us, we should have but little difficulty in comprehending special cases.

Now, without writing an article on syphilis, yellow fever, or cholera, I desire to notice in brief review some views of these maladies presented in the last JOURNAL. Also the discussion on

45

the more general, and therefore more important question of antiphlogistic therapeutics. All those who presented the views referred to, possess high literary and professional attainments, and are worthy of being heard whether they are right or wrong.

Dr. Thomas Kennard on the duality of syphilis and its differential manifestations in the male and female, has, I think, shown himself a fair controversialist and an able writer. The idea, too prevalent among practitioners, that syphilis is of two kinds—that chancres are infecting, or non-infecting, or, to use their corresponding synonyms, hard and soft, is a fateful fallacy.

Without going over all the grounds, so well-traversed by Dr. Kennard, it is a fair deduction from impartial observation, and as well from the ever varying susceptibility of the human organism to this, and to every morbific element, that this virus will produce in one person a soft, and in another a hard chancre, and that either form is inoculable, and that either may be followed by secondary and tertiary syphilis. I regard it as an important fact, not generally known in the profession, that soft chancre is more common in females than males, and that they often impart the disease from mere erosions.

Dr. Buck, speaking in the Society of the etiology of yellow fever and its similitude to cholera, said: "both diseases may be transmitted in textile fabrics, and that cholera may be communicated, by the dejections and effluvia from the body." This is true beyond question, and in this, the doctor guided by reason and independent thought, ignores the "rut" and takes his position in the advance line of professional thinkers.

But he thinks yellow fever cannot be communicated by dejections, and presumptively, too, not from effluvia arising from the body. In this I think he errs. I hope he will give this subject more thought, then apply impartial observation. All malignant forms of disease are communicable from one person to another, either by inoculation or by infection. I presented this view in my Treatise on Pathology, and I am fully satisfied it is a fact to which the profession must come, and the sooner the better. Of course there are various degrees of activity among contagions, and the negative proves nothing, or it would prove that small-pox is not contagious.

On this subject, Dr. Chas. H. Hughs, whom I remember as one of my brightest class-mates in 1857-8, remarked that "yellow fever is certainly not a disease of the same grade as bilious fever." In this I concur, but I would add, it has the same prime element, though in a much more intense degree, and in its character malignant, from which arise its symptoms *sui generis*.

Next comes the question of antiphlogistic therapeutics, affirmed by Dr. Montgomery and negatived by Dr. Adolphus. Each is an able exponent of his position. If the discussion had taken place in the days of Armstrong and Rush, the decision would have been for the affirmative; but as the members of the profession of to-day are the umpires, the verdict is overwhelmingly for the negative. The world moves.

It is a wonderment that some intellectual and erudite medical men yet adhere with tenacity to the old depletory system; even now, when science is yielding her choicest blessings, and the light of physiology and pathology is glowing on our altars, and exposing to view retrospectively, frightful errors, and prospectively, lighting our way and guiding our feet to new mines of knowledge, potential in elevating our profession, and rich in blessings to our race.

Believing that, with all his known merits, Prof. Montgomery is on the wrong side of the question at issue, I would suggest that there are hope and comfort in the adage "*quid docet discit*," for certainly those who teach may learn.

Having made this article an ark of varieties, if you will allow the antiphrasis, I desire to record my views on another subject, and that is *professional journalism*. For seventeen years I have been a subscriber and occasional contributor to this JOURNAL, and I think it is as good as any of them, but the journals are all filled up too much with "squibs" from case doctors, giving the details of cases that are supposed to be *wonderful*; they do not instruct nor interest, but bore those who study and comprehend general principles.

Again, all importance is attached to the *medicines*, especially by those doctors and journals of the "salad" variety. It should be known that the great fountain of knowledge which elevates the doctor above the snob, is accessible only through anatomy, physiology and pathology, and the collateral sciences.

The inscription written on the pyramid thousands of years ago, "Man, know thyself!" is an injunction too little heeded.

We are to study man physically, and mentally. We are to study the varied conformations of the brain, the temperament and the texture; and thus bring to view the mind, the motives and the actions.

Few who embark in physic have, or ever get to have, any considerable knowledge of the natural sciences. An uncultivated mind thrust in professional science is like a "squaw patch" in a dense forest. All around is darkness, and the intruding man is regaled in his musings by the chirp of the katydid, and the croak of the owl; while the tined lightning cuts mystic gambols on the dark portentious cloud.

Our journals should give wider scope to the collateral sciences. I say, clear away the brush over the line, and let in the sunshine of reason. Give us more room. Give us more resources to breathe, to see and to think. Give us more elevated and thorough conceptions of man, of God, and of this stupendous universe.

Correspondence.

Editors of St. Louis Medical and Surgical Journal:

In your November number I notice another article from Dr. Adolphus, criticizing my paper on the "Antiphlogistic Treatment," but as it is but a re-iteration of the doctor's former criticisms, I judge it unnecessary for me to reply at this time, as I believe, I fully, fairly and candidly answered all the doctor's objections in my article, published in the *St. Louis Medical Archives*, in December, 1872.

As I understand the "*Archives*" has ceased publication, I would ask you Messrs. Editors, to copy my paper of December last in some future number of your Journal, as defining my position on the treatment of inflammatory disease; and as a reply to Dr. Adolphus, and all others who are infatuated with the belief in alcoholic stimulants, and a universal system of stuffing, and on the other hand, to those who believe in the " rose water system," or expectancy in therapeutics.

Respectfully yours,

EDWARD MONTGOMERY, M. D.

1316 Olive Street, Nov., 1873.

Proceedings.

SPRINGFIELD, MO., MEDICAL SOCIETY.

SPRINGFIELD, June 6, 1873.

Dr. J. E. Tefft read a paper on " The Possibility and Probability of the Communication of Constitutional Diseases by Vaccination," in which the following conclusions are enunciated:

1. No constitutional or general disease is communicable by vaccination, except those in which the blood will communicate it by inoculation.

2. Scrofula, tuberculosis, carcinoma, the essential fevers, and the contagious exanthemata, not being under any circumstances communicable by inoculation of blood, cannot be communicated through the medium of vaccine lymph.

3. The blood of a syphilitic patient is inoculable in direct proportion to the activity and virulence of the disease, and if the disease is not so active, developed and aggressive, as to be easily detected by simple inspection, the blood is not inoculable at all.

4. That so-called latent syphilis cannot be communicable by inoculation of blood, for the simple reason that, if the blood of the subject is in such a state as to communicate the disease to another person, it would *a fortiori* infect his own tissues, or, in other words, it would not be latent.

5. It follows from the above that there is no fear of the com-

munication of syphilis by vaccination, if the vaccinifer has no visible symptoms of disease.

6. There is no fear of communicating skin diseases if reasonable care is used in selecting the virus.

7. The doctrine that vaccine lymph is a specific product, capable of producing the specific disease vaccinia, and that alone, is probably true.

8. Neither lymph nor the dried crust should be used for the purpose of vaccination without a careful examination of the subject from which it is taken.

9. Vaccine virus should be collected only by medical men, and the greatest care should be used.

10. The possibility and probability of communicating diseases by vaccination has been much over-stated, and is not such as to furnish any argument against the practice.

LINTON DISTRICT MEDICAL SOCIETY.

The semi-annual session of this Society was held at Montgomery City, Mo., Nov. 4th, 1873, and continued in session two days. The meeting was called to order at 2 o'clock, p. m., by the president, Dr. S. N. Russell.

The Committee on Credentials reported the following named physicians present: Drs. S. N. Russell, T. P. Rothwell, Wesley Humphrey, W. H. Lee, and Pinckney French, Mexico; Dr. A. W. McAlister, Columbia; Dr. W. E. Evans, Rocheport; Dr. W. W. MacFarlane, Fulton; Drs. W. B. Adams and Thos. Hill, Danville; Dr. James M. Foreman, Jonesburg; Dr. J. A. Matthews, Ashley; Dr. W. F. Humphreys, Concord; Dr. Isaac Moore, Portage des Sioux; Dr. W. T. Maupin, Columbia; Drs. S. T. Buck and A. T. Barnett, Wellsville; Drs. J. R. Bodine and Walter Caldwell, Montgomery City; Dr. H. H. Middelkamp, Warrenton; Dr. John Snethen, Americus; Dr. Thos. Peery, Wellsville; Dr. Virgil A. Willis, Price's Branch; Dr. J. C. Goodrich, Wentzville, (honorary member.)

Committee on Medical Education made an able report, which was adopted.

Committee on Publication made a verbal report, which was adopted.

Five scientific papers were read and discussed. Also a report on the Medical Department of the State University was presented and adopted.

We regret the want of space for the report entire. The following concluding paragraphs will be read with interest:

"This together with the disinterestedness of the faculty, being paid by the State, the nine months' session of the college, and the superior advantages offered the students in having access to every other department of the University, must commend the institution to medical men and medical aspirants, favorably at least.

"After a thorough investigation of the subject, your committee are of opinion that in the building up and sustaining of schools, enforcing so rigid a discipline, and of such high standard of education, lies the only solution of the perplexing question of medical education. Medical diplomas have been made merchandise of all over our country. Would you stop this terrible bartering with the lives of your fellow-men, then encourage and sustain only schools of a higher order, such as the Medical Department of the State University proposes to be.

"All of which is respectfully submitted by your committee.
J. W. LANIUS.
WM. H. LEE."

On motion of Dr. H. H. Middelkamp, the report was unanimously adopted, and on motion, the committee, with the Secretary added thereto, were instructed to present the report to the consideration of the Board of Curators of the State University at their next meeting.

The following members were appointed to furnish and read papers at the next meeting on the subjects named:

1. Connection of Diseases of the generating organs to Insanity. Dr. W. W. McFarlane, of Fulton.

2. Jaundice: its Pathology, Diagnosis and Treatment. Dr. T. P. Rothwell, of Mexico.

3. Typhoid Fever. Dr. W. T. Lenoir, of Columbia.

4. Croup. Dr. W. B. Adams, of Danville.

5. Best appliance for the Treatment of Fracture of Clavicle. Dr. W. G. Elliott, of Rocheport.

6. Best appliance for Treatment of Fracture of or near Ankle

Joint with or without Dislocation. Dr. W. E. Evans, of Rocheport.

7. Therapeutical Actions of Gelseminum. Dr. Moore, of Portage de Sioux.

8. Comparative Dangers of Ether and Chloroform as Anæsthetics. Dr. W. F. Humphreys, of Concord.

9. Diseases peculiar to Females. Dr. V. A. Willis, of Price's Branch.

10. Post partum Flooding. Dr. J. M. Foreman, of Jonesburg.

Louisiana was selected as the next place of meeting.

Dr. J. A. Mathews, of Ashley, was appointed chairman of committee on arrangements.

A public meeting was held at 7 o'clock, at which time addresses were delivered by Drs. Russell, Middelkamp, McAlister and Rothwell. A vote of thanks was tendered the citizens, Prof. Kurtz and the physicians of Montgomery City for hospitalities received at their hands by the visiting members of the society. Col. D. P. Dyer delivered a very interesting speech and said he was glad the society had concluded to hold their next meeting at Louisiana. He wanted all the members to bring their wives, and promised them a hearty welcome from the citizens of old Pike. The Society then adjourned to meet at Louisiana on the first Tuesday in April, 1874.

H. H. MIDDELKAMP, *Secretary.*

Reviews and Bibliographical Notices.

SEX IN EDUCATION; OR A FAIR CHANCE FOR THE GIRLS. By Edward H. Clarke, M. D. Boston: J. R. Osgood & Co., 1873.

[For sale by Gray, Baker & Co.]

Henry Ward Beecher is reported as saying that "exaggeration is a good thing; it helps you see an object better."

We think the general verdict will be, that both in tone and statement there is somewhat of over-emphasis in this book.

The stress that is laid upon the *evils* which our author forcibly describes, is perhaps not too great—they are confessedly most common and most grave ; but the *cause* of those evils we suspect, is too complex to be included under any single term. Certainly after carefully reading this book, we are not convinced that all, or the principal part of the female disease and debility of our times is to be charged against our system of popular education.

If we run our eye over the catalogue or shelves of our libraries of medicine, we are struck with the immense number of treatises, great and small, that have been written on " *The Diseases of Women.*" And if we notice the date of these works we shall find that some of the profoundest and most comprehensive were authorities long before there was any martinetism in our public schools to complain of—whether in St. Louis or Boston. And if we consider the question of authorship we shall also find that England, France and Germany, not to specify smaller nationalities, have contributed very largely to the burdening of the aforesaid shelves ;—showing that the foreign practitioner found no lack of cases at home to arrest his attention. We simply mention these facts because, in reading such a work as this of Dr. Clarke, they are likely to be lost sight of, as we are resistlessly borne on by his trenchant English into the black and fathomless sea of our own present distress.

"I once saw (says Dr. Clarke, p. 178-9) in the streets of Coblentz, a woman and a donkey yoked to the same cart while, a man, with a whip in his hand, drove the team. * * * A German girl yoked with a donkey and dragging a cart is an exhibition of monstrous muscular and aborted brain development. *An American girl yoked with a dictionary and dragging a catamenia, is an exhibition of monstrous brain and aborted ovarian development.*"

The last sentence of this quotation which we have given in italics, might have been made the motto of the book. "The law of periodicity," "the rhythmical action," which characterizes the female organization, is made the pivot about which every argument turns. And especially between the ages of fourteen and twenty he urges the strictest attention to this royal demand of womanhood. Now Dr. Clarke deserves the gratitude of the community for calling attention to this matter in a book which may be suitably and profitably read by every intelligent parent, and should be read by every teacher and employer of girls. It suggests a care, and delicacy of treatment too seldom observed, whether in home, or shop, or school. No thoughtful person versed in the elements of physiology, can doubt that, for want of the proper recognition of this tidal movement and function of woman, and especially while still reaching upward to maturity, health is sacrificed and lives are lost.

But why brain-work should be singled out from all other work as the chief offence against nature; why the girl seeking an education is held up as the one pity-compelling and melancholy example whose privileges instead of being extended, should be limited even to the taking away of "even what she has,"—this is not so plain. In spite of this book, the subject we think, remains open for discussion and for difference of opinion.

Of course, some admissions are made which show a wider outlook. Incidentally something like the following drops in : "We live in the zone of perpetual pie and dough-nut; and our girls revel in those unassimilable abominations." "The gifted authoress of *The Gates Ajar* has blown her trumpet with no uncertain sound, in explanation and advocacy of a new clothes philosophy, which her sisters will do well to heed rather than to ridicule." He approves, as seen among the Germans, their "open-air, oxygen-surrounding, blood-making, health-giving, innocent recreation : not gas, furnaces, low necks, spinal trails, the civilized representatives of caudal appendages, and late hours." Here also is an admirable passage : "Girls, young ladies, to use the polite phrase, who are about leaving or have left school for society, dissipation, or self-culture, rarely permit any of nature's periodical demands to interfere with their morning calls, or evening promenades, or midnight dancing, or sober study. Even the home draws the sacred mantle of modesty so closely over the reproductive function as not only to cover but to smother it. Sisters imitate brothers in persistent work at all times. Female clerks in stores strive to emulate the males by unremitting labor, seeking to develop feminine force by masculine methods. Female operatives of all sorts, in factories and elsewhere, labor in the same way, and when the day is done, are as likely to dance half the night, regardless

of any pressure upon them of a peculiar function, as their
fashionable sisters in the polite world. All unite in pushing
the hateful thing out of sight and out of mind : and all are
punished by similar weakness, degeneration and disease."

But, especially impressed with the idea that brain-work is
most fatal, and that the opening of the doors of Harvard University to young women would be the consummation of our
national wickedness, our author says: " the scope of this paper
does not permit the discussion of these other causes of female
weaknesses." He contemplates therefore the number of brain-
cells necessarily used up by the girl who " studies Latin for an
hour," and the " aching heads" which "signalize the advance of
neuralgia, tubercle, and disease:" and from his clinical notes he
selects cases of girl-patients who were proficient in " Latin,
chemistry, philosophy, geography, grammar, arithmetic, music,
French, German, and the whole extraordinary catalogue of an
American young lady's school curriculum." And against co-
education he inveighs—so far as it is " identical education—" as
a " crime before God and humanity, that physiology protests
against, and that experience weeps over."

Dr. Clarke, however, gives the impression that all our higher
institutions for the education of girls exclusively, fail,—perhaps even more signally than our mixed schools—because in all
their methods they conform to a boy's standard and organization, and are adapted to a boy's wants and regimen. His own
experience justifies the inference " that the ratio of invalidism
among female-college graduates is greater than even among
the graduates of our common, high, and normal schools."
Appropriate co-education he has no objection to. " Isolation is
more likely to breed pruriency, than commingling to provoke
indulgence." He has no sympathy with conventual instruction,
although that system seems to us to be free enough from all
charge of being conformed to a boy's regimen. With us, at
any rate, it is no copy of the public school curriculum or drill.

To close with, this book refers us to foreigners for healthy
mothers and children, and rather vaguely to European methods
of education as giving us better models to follow.

Now, there are natural reasons, aside from political ones, why
some provinces or nations remarkable for their fecundity pour
their surplus population with unceasing flow into the United

States. Our greatest increase is from Ireland and Germany. These nations are fertile at home, and for the present remain fertile here. But what ethnologist would think of attributing this fact to their respective systems of education? We find female sterility prevalent in certain districts of France, in Egypt, in Persia. Barrenness has been lamented in Syria and Palestine ever since Abraham's time. What had their systems of education to do with it? Nothing certainly in the sense in which an education refers to the study of Juvenal or geography, to chemistry, or co-education. So, while we ought to insist not less strongly than Dr. Clarke does, that no clearly understood law of a girl's nature should be broken or ignored, in the school-room *or anywhere else,* we are not ready to lay the chief burden of American female sterility upon the cause of popular education. The severe requirements of the "high pressure principle" which was introduced into public schools twenty years ago, have nearly everywhere fallen into disrepute, if they are not absolutely null and void.

Of co-education, only the other day the principal of the Mary Institute, one of the largest and very best collegiate schools for girls in the West, and a man not ignorant of physiology, said to us, "I have always believed in the co-education of the sexes, and I believe so still." And in the St. Louis High School the methods of which he, himself, as former principal, did much to perfect, we shall see a "double-sexed" school which we are persuaded will stand the test of comparison with any other, whether judged by thorough mental training, physical health or respectable morals. And, if we mistake not, Prof. Harris, City Superintendent of the schools of St. Louis, can show from actual statistics, that the headaches and absences from the public schools on account of sickness, belong by no means to those who rank highest in their class recitations, or spend the greatest number of hours in study. Girls from fourteen to eighteen years of age, though weighted with the catamenial function, are more mature in mind, and, as a rule, get their lessons more easily and in much less time, than boys of the same age. And now-a-days, neuralgia, hysteria, menorrhagia, dysmenorrhœa are complaints of the least educated women, and the tuberculous Irish are crowding into our hospitals.

How many a time in journeying through the agricultural districts of our Western States, have we found the young or middle-aged woman of the house, feeble in health, or utterly disabled. " Can you keep us to-night ?" " I would," says the robust farmer, "but my wife is sick." And upon inquiry, in a startling number of cases, we find the husband, now in the prime of his strength, with his second or even third wife. Here is something to start our melancholiest thoughts. And no man who has lived outside of Boston, would think of attributing this condition of things to school education.

Finally, one word on the economy of the higher education for girls, for which we wish to put in a plea.

To give young women "a fair chance" at Harvard, Dr. Clarke says, "an additional endowment of from one to two millions of dollars is necessary." This he evidently feels will remain the perpetual bar to their admission. We confess we have not much faith in the experiment of grafting into the stock of any ancient university, the scion of female education. But that the higher, the collegiate education, if you please, of girls, is already one of the most important questions of the age, and is destined to become even more absorbing, is everywhere indicated.

Instruction in all our schools, whether we look at primary grades, or to high schools and seminaries, is more and more entrusted to the hands of women. Less and less do well educated men look to teaching as a profession. The compensation does not warrant it; and the expenses of our system of education we may safely predict, will not suffer any material increase of salaries. Moreover, the teaching of youth is a vocation which, after fair trial, all admit a woman is fitted to pursue; it is honorable, it is self-supporting, and as wages now are, the same outlay will secure more culture, tact, talent, and executive ability in a female teacher, than in a male.

This fact being established, then, that the deliberate action or choice of the American people is, that the instruction of its youth shall be chiefly given into the charge of female teachers, there is no advantage of mental discipline and culture from which they should be ultimately excluded. By this position, as in some sense controlling the future destinies of the republic, they should somehow or somewhere have access to the best opportunities of the higher education. They should have all the

breadth of culture and thoroughness of training which they
are capable of receiving. No class, not even the members of
the learned professions, as they are called, more need the broad-
ening influence of university life, with its recitations, libraries
and lectures; with its contact with the best minds in the varied
departments of literature, natural history and science. So
much at any rate is requisite, if our schools and seminaries are
to advance with the advancing knowledge of our day; if they
are to respond fitly to the fresh demands of a nation that is
ever raising the ideal of intelligence and power.

Our verdict then, in brief, of Dr Clarke's timely book is,
that it has the merits and the demerits of an exaggeration. It
will be much more widely read, than if its tone were more
judicial It will call attention to an often overlooked, neglected
or despised theme, to a function of sex, which in every occupation should have due recognition. If as Mr. Greg says,
"error is necessary to float and vivify truth," we are of
opinion that this work will not fail in the requisite amount.
The danger is, that the cause of the evils that affect society,
being too narrowly stated, there is aroused in quarters where
there is no occasion for it, a mysterious dread of all intellectual
efforts, a fanatical fear and superstitious distrust of any valuable system of education whatever.   J. C. L.

THE MECHANISM OF THE OSSICLES OF THE EAR, AND MEMBRANA
TYMPANI. By H. Helmholtz, Prof. of Physiology in the University of Berlin, Prussia. Translated from the German with
the author's permission, by Albert H. Buck, and Normand
Smith, of New York. With twelve illustrations. 8vo., pp.
69. New York: Wm. Wood & Co., 27 Great Jones st. 1873.

This essay of sixty-nine pages, first appeared in *Pflüger's
archive für Physiologie,* in 1869. In it the subject is considered in
its anatomical, physiological, and mathematical bearings; and
from the ability of the author, as also from the method of the
experiments, the production must be regarded as of the highest
authority. It is divided into eight sections. Our author (as did
B. Riemann), proposes as the chief task of aural mechanics, to
explain how the apparatus of the middle ear can transmit from
the air to the fluid of the labyrinth such extraordinarily fine
shades of vibration—as we know it actually does—the excur-
sions of the stirrup in the fainter tones being too small to be

detected "even with the highest powers of our modern microscopes." He does not believe the statement, " that it is the task
of the apparatus of the middle ear to transmit to the fluid of the
labyrinth the changes in atmospheric pressure at every movement of time, with perfect accuracy and constant relative
strength," because the facts do not warrant such a conclusion.
"Accuracy in perception requires only that every tone of a
given pitch should cause the same sensation, both in kind and
intensity, every time that it is reproduced." p. 8.

Sec. 2. *Anatomy of the Membrana Tympani.* * * * " The
plane that passes through the groove in which the membrana
tympani is inserted is inclined at an angle of 55° to the axis of
the external auditory canal. * * * The membrana tympani
is not stretched out flat in the ring to which it is attached, but
its centre or navel is strongly drawn inward by the handle of
the hammer, with which it is united; for this reason the membrana has the shape of a funnel whose point or end corresponds
to the tip of the handle of the hammer, and whose meridian
lines are convexed toward the hollow of the funnel."

Fig. 2 shows the form of the membrane, "a point of great
importance in the mechanics of the conduction of sound," as
taken in a cast with stearine. By this it is shown very clearly
" that the radii drawn on the surface of the membrana tympani
are convexed outward toward the external auditory canal. At
the same time it can be seen that as a result of this drawing in
of the navel, the upper half of the membrane is made to lie in
almost the same direction as the upper wall of the canal, while
the lower half stands almost at a right angle with the axis of this
canal. * * * This perpendicular portion of the membrana
tympani, which is situated, as a rule, just below the tip of the
manubrium, reflects back through the external auditory passage the light that is thrown upon it, and thus gives rise to
the triangular 'bright spot.'" p. 20.

" The membrana tympani consists essentially of a peculiar
tendinous membrane, which, although only one-twentieth of a
millimetre ($\frac{1}{500}$ in.) thick is yet comparatively very strong.
Externally it is clothed with a thin continuation of the skin of
the external auditory canal, internally by a thin continuation
of the mucous membrane of the middle ear. Taken together,
these layers have a thickness of 0.1 mm. ($\frac{1}{250}$ in.) * * *

The middle and strong layer of the membrana tympani is fibrous, and consists partly of radiating, partly of circular fibres. The radiating fibres lie on the outer side, the circular on the inner of the layer. * * * In the centre of the membrane the circular fibres form a very thin layer which gradually increases in thickness towards the periphery; at the extreme periphery, however, they disappear altogether (according to Gerlach), or at least (according to J. Gruber) form a very much thinner layer than in the centre. * * * The tendinous fibres of these layers are very dense and unyielding; they lie close to one another, and offer great resistance to any distending force. Through their great power of elastic resistance they differ materially from the very much more yielding yellow elastic tissue. * * * This peculiarity of construction of the membrana tympani is a very important element in the mechanical working of this membrane. * * * It is not to be considered as an elastic, yielding membrane, but as an almost inextensible one." pp. 20-22.

Sec. 7. *Mechanism of the Membrana Tympani.* "The membrana tympani is to be considered as a tense membrane, which, however differs essentially from those which have been hitherto studied in acoustics, in fact, that it is curved. Its tension is modified by the handle of the hammer which draws it inward, and . which is itself retained in this position by means of ligaments of attachment, and by the elasticity of the tensor tympani. If the radial fibres of the membrana tympani were not united by transverse ones, they would be stretched in a straight line, * * hence, we conclude that the radial fibres are drawn toward one another by circular fibres, and that the latter are also made tense at the same time. * * In the concussions which sound produces, the pressure of the air acts sometimes upon the convex, sometimes upon the concave surface of the membrana tympani, according as this pressure is alternately greater or less in the meatus than in the cavity of the tympanum; in every case the pressure of the air acts perpendicularly upon the membrane, also perpendicularly upon the curve formed by the radial fibres, which curve it at one time increases and at another diminishes."

The bones singly and in combination have been thoroughly examined, and their action, individual and combined, carefully observed. The essay closes with a "*Mathematical appendix, having particular reference to the mechanism of curved membranes.*" The translation has been very fairly done. G.

WÖHLER'S OUTLINES OF ORGANIC CHEMISTRY. By Rudolph Fittig, Ph. D., etc. Professor of Chemistry in the University of Tübingen. Translated from the Eighth German Edition, with additions, by Ira Remsen, M. D., Ph. D., Professor of Chemistry and Physic in Williams College, Massachusetts. Philadelphia: Henry C. Lea, 1878. 12mo. pp. xxxii, 518.

This little book, upon the "chemistry of the compounds of carbon," is in no wise, a complete text-book upon organic chemistry, but is rather a descriptive catalogue of organic bodies, arranged methodically upon the basis of their known constitution and relation to each other. It is, therefore, but a chapter of the great unwritten hand-book of modern chemistry, and one which can only be read by the light of the chapters which necessarily come before it upon chemical physics and philosophy, and elementary chemistry. As a guide to systematic instruction in organic chemistry, as to a student following the courses of a German University, the book is admirably constructed, as its eight successively revised editions attest. A *treatise* on organic chemistry it is not, and does not pretend to be.

The translator and editor has prefixed to the book a chapter of fourteen pages on the "constitution of chemical compounds" in order to aid the beginner in his attempt to comprehend certain terms, upon which he would otherwise, perhaps, stumble at the very outset of his study, and to render his entrance into the apparently labyrinthic structure somewhat less dark and indefinite." To the average *American* beginner in organic chemistry, a much fuller introductory chapter, or, still better, a reference to a few of the best introductory books, would be useful and welcome. J. G.

LECTURES ON DISEASES AND INJURIES OF THE EAR. Delivered at St. George's Hospital. By W. B. Dalby, F. R. C. S., M. B. Cantab., Aural Surgeon to the Hospital. With twenty-one illustrations. Philadelphia: Lindsay & Blakiston.

As reprinted from the London edition is a neat 12mo. vol. of 225 pp. The author has accomplished what he started out for in

46

this little work—"to describe as shortly and clearly as possible the pathology and symptoms of diseases of the Ear, and in directing attention to the treatment of these affections, to place before the reader the general results to be expected from remedial measures." The book does not appear as claiming to be an exhaustive treatise, neither will Mr. Dalby obtain a title to much originality. He has effected all that he probably designed, and has given to the profession a work which will admirably meet the wants of those who seek only for practical information, and are not concerned about the minutiæ which appertain to scientific study. We are in need at this time of all that may be said upon such a subject, to the importance of which the whole profession has become now fully awakened.

Mr. Dalby justly condemns the practice of those who are in the habit of treating diseases of the ear (or diseases of the eye for that matter, or diseases of the lungs), neither having made the essential preparations in study, nor having appliances. We see every day the fruits of this injudicious labor; and to those who would perform as simple an operation as the removal of inspissated cerumen from the external auditory meatus seems to be, he addresses this epigrammatic proposition:—"you know that it is an unvarying rule in surgery, that before a patient be cut for stone, while he is on the operating table, the presence of the stones should be unquestionably demonstrated."

The treatment as laid down for, what the author is pleased to call, "purulent catarrh of tympanum," is liable to criticism. And this leads us further to say, that Mr. Dalby's nomenclature is very objectionable, and we regard it an unfortunate feature in his little book. This should not detract, however, from what real worth it possesses, and we commend it to any who are interested in the subject of diseases and injuries of the ear. S.

THE DISEASES OF THE PROSTATE: THEIR PATHOLOGY AND TREATMENT, comprising the Jacksonian Prize Essay, for the year 1860. By Sir Henry Thompson, F. R. C. S., etc. Fourth Edition, xiii plates, pp. 355, 8vo. Philadelphia: Henry C. Lea. 1873.

The First edition of "Thompson on The Enlarged Prostate" was issued in November, 1857. In 1861 the Jacksonian, prize for the previous year, by the council of the Royal College of Surgeons of England, was awarded to the author for an essay on "The Healthy and Morbid Anatomy of the Prostate Gland." In September, 1861, the *first edition* and the prize essay were incorporated in a *second edition*, under the new title, viz: "The Diseases of the Prostate: their Pathology and treatment." In 1868, a *third edition* was issued, with such addition and changes as seemed to be called for. The *fourth edition*—the present—came forth in July of the present year; and of it the author says, "In preparing a new edition of this work, I have found it necessary to make several additions. At the same time I have compressed the existing material, so much as to reduce somewhat the size of the volume, at the same time, as I hope, to increase its utility." This work has been so long before the profession, and the author so well known, as to require but a brief notice from us at this time. The above history of it will show its origin and progress.

On the use of injections to dissolve phosphatic deposits, he remarks, page 846, "I have used the acetate of lead very largely in connection with phosphatic deposits, and I have arrived at the following conclusions. First, that the maximum strength that most patients can bear without suffering irritation afterwards, is a solution of one grain to three ounces of distilled water. Secondly, that it suffices to prevent accumulation of the product, and has often checked the formation of phosphatic calculi, in those who had previously been habitually subject to them. Thirdly, that in some cases, notwithstanding its daily use, phosphates still form, and cohere to form calculus. Lastly, that in some instances, it is inferior in efficacy to a solution of hydrochloric acid. The last-named is a more powerful solvent of the triple phosphate than either the nitric or the phosphoric acids. The strength to be used may vary from one minim to two and a half minims to the ounce of water. Consequently this acid and the acetate of lead are the two agents which I mainly rely upon for the purpose in question."

The same paragraph closes this as the former edition; and this contains nine pages less. The work stands among the highest on the subject. I wonder if the author still thinks Prof. S. D. Gross, of Philadelphia, is "Dr. Gross, of Louisville.".

The appearance and finish of the book are improved by passing through the Philadelphia house.   H. Z. G.

A TREATISE ON THE DISEASES OF THE EYE. By J. Soelberg Wells, F. R. C. S., Doctor of Medicine of the University of Edinburg; Professor of Ophthalmology in King's College, London; Ophthalmic Surgeon to King's College Hospital; and Surgeon to the Royal London Ophthalmic Hospital, Moorfields. *Second American,* from the *third English edition, with additions.* Illustrated with two hundred and forty-eight engravings on wood, and six colored plates, together with the selections from the test types of Prof. E. Jæger and Dr. H. Snellen. Philadelphia: Henry C. Lea, 1873. 8vo., pp. 836.

The first English edition of Wells on Diseases of the Eye was published in December, 1868; the second in May, 1870; and the third quite recently. It has been translated into French and German, and the volume before us is the *second* American from the last English, "a portion of the sheets" however, "had already been printed" before the new English edition appeared, hence, for that portion, the additions are put in the appendix.

We will now pass on to mention some of these additions.

Mode of Examining the Field of Vision, page 26.—The instrument proposed is by Mr. Brudenell Carter, and is a modification and simplification of Förster's Perimeter. The description is taken from the *Lancet,* July 6, 1872.

Treatment of Chronic Granulations by sulphate of quinine, as recommended by Mr. Bader. "About as much as would go on the point of a pen-knife is to be applied, twice daily, with a camel's hair brush to the inside of the lower lid." He uses it in cases accompanied by pannus.

Treatment of Symblepheron, page 99.—The operation is ingenious and is best understood by the description accompanied by the illustration.

Phlyctenular Corneitis.—Page 112. * * * * "In the treatment of herpes corneæ accompanying catarrh of the respiratory organs, the insufflation of calomel generally greatly relieves the pain by causing rupture of the minute vesicles. Atropine and a bandage should also be applied. In the form accompanying herpes zoster, injections of morphia and electricity are often very serviceable in alleviating the sufferings of the patient."

Treatment of Ulcers of the Cornea.—In obstinate and chronic ulceration of the cornea with slight or no corneal vascularization, and in which there is a lax condition of the conjunctiva in the retro-tarsal fold, "Dr. Hosh strongly advises the application of pure nitrate of silver to the retro-tarsal fold." It should be applied with a finely pointed crayon, to a narrow rim of the fold, and immediately washed off with a solution of salt and water, and not re-applied till the eschar is entirely removed.

Indolent Hypopyon Ulcer.—Page 188. "Operative interference is, however, only indicated in the more advanced and graver cases, when the ulcer is considerable in extent, its bottom and edges infiltrated with pus, and the hypopyon large. In such cases either a large iridectomy, or Sæmisch's operation should be performed; on the whole, I have found the former the more successful proceeding of the two." In mild cases, a compress bandage, atropine and warm fomentations will suffice. Sustaining and tonic treatment should be adopted, the patients generally being in a depressed state of health. Prof. Horner prefers iridectomy in the more severe cases, and he does not operate at all in mild cases.

Treatment of Conical Cornea.—Page 152. Three methods have been introduced for the treatment of conical cornea. Mr. Bader excises an elliptical piece of the apex of the cone; and uses Gräfe's cataract knife in the operation. Mr. Critchett uses a double-bladed knife by which a small elliptical piece (both sides of which are exactly equal and sharply defined) of the cornea will be excised.

Mr. Bowman employs a drill, operating somewhat on the plan of a trephine, and excising a circular portion of the cone, not entirely, however, through the cornea, but leaving the membrane of Decemet, and puncturing it with a needle. Mr. Bowman speaks highly of this method. Our author, however, concludes as follows: "At present it must be admitted that all these more modern methods are still upon their trial and nothing decisive can as yet be said as to their relative advantages or disadvantages." He thinks the simplest and easiest is Gräfe's method—that of forming a central ulcer. "Should a central leucoma be left, an iridectomy would improve the sight, and tattooing the opacity would improve the appearance."

The various other changes and improvements in the use of the ophthalmoscope; in the operation for cataract; in the discovery and measurement of astigmatism; the various methods of treating diseases of the lachrymal apparatus. On the last subject the American editor adds: "Dr. Williams, of Boston, advocates the use of flexible probes with bulbous extremities, of the size of Bowman's series, but slender for one-third of the distance from the bulb to the flat disk in the middle. They are of alloyed silver, and have an elastic flexibility without being able to bend upon themselves in encountering obstructions. Dr. Williams has found in practice that these probes adapt themselves to the sinuosities of the passages, and can be introduced with more facility and less pain, and are less likely to take a wrong passage than Bowman's probes, which, if not bent so as precisely to correspond with the direction of the duct in each particular individual, often lacerate the mucous lining of the passages, giving rise to pain and hemorrhage, and retarding cure by causing local inflammation."

The work is thoroughly practical; up to the latest advances of the science; and is the one which we have recommended as a text-book from the time the first edition was issued. The additions made to the American edition are quite numerous and have been selected by one competent to judge of their value.

The work is gotten up in excellent style.

CHEMISTRY: INORGANIC AND ORGANIC, WITH EXPERIMENTS. By Charles Loudon Bloxam, Prof. of Chemistry in King's College, London; in the Royal Military Academy, Woolwich; and in the Department of Artillery Studies, Woolwich. With two hundred and ninety-five illustrations From the second revised English edition. Philadelphia: Henry C. Lea. 1878. 8vo. pp. 700.

It is now six years since the first edition of Bloxam's Chemistry was published; and, as the author remarks in the preface to the present (second) edition, "the adoption of the atomic system of notation has become so general among English chemists, that I have felt obliged to employ it in the present edition." Under this system, hydrogen being the unit, he has thought best to study it first, and whilst oxygen is a diatomic element he "found it absolutely necessary to assign to it (oxygen) the second place." While acknowledging the beauty and value of the new system, yet he sees "the necessity of propounding the difficult hypothesis of the finite divisibility of matter at the commencement of a study, which has been recommended to the student as strictly experimental;" and while accordingly the combining weight of hydrogen in water must be represented as 2, the perplexing and unnecessary inquiry being suggested to the mind of the pupil, why it is set down as 1 in the lists of combining weights.

This new system is being adopted; and new nomenclature also (in part), by the last edition of the U. S. Pharmacopœia, A few examples will illustrate the change: water, HO (old system); H_2O, (new system.) Old system: nitrate of potash, KO, NO_5; nitrate of soda, NaO, NO_5.

CHEMICAL NAME.	COMMON NAME.	ADDITIVE FORMULA.	SUBSTITUTIVE FORMULA.
Nitrate of Potash.	Nitre, Saltpetre.....	K_2O, N_2O_5	K_2O_3
Nitrate of Soda...	Peruvian Saltpetre.	$Na_2O \ N_2O_5$	$NaNO_3$
Nitrate of Silver.	Lunar Caustic.......	Ag_2O, K_2O_5	$AgNO_2$

In the above table which may be taken as a representative of the formation of salts—either carbonates or sulphates,—the nitrates are represented by two formulæ: the *substitutive* representing each salt as derived from one or more molecules of HNO_3 (nitric acid, p. 168), by the *substitution* of the metals (in this case potassium and sodium), for the hydrogen; the *additive* formula shows the oxides—potassa and soda—combined with anhydrous nitric acid N_2O_5.

It will be observed that the salts are regarded as combinations of the acid with the particular metal, and not with its oxide. Hence in the U. S. Pharmacopœia we have now potasii citras for the old potassæ citras, calcii carbonas præcipitata for calcis carbonas præcipitata.

The index is especially convenient, having the chemical formulæ attached, as for example, potash, 293, is written in the index, "potash, K_2O, 293." From this the student can ascertain at a glance the formulæ of the substance sought, and having it so frequently before his eye, it becomes familiar.

The work is from the highest authority, and a valuable text-book.

The typography is in the usual excellent style of Mr. Henry C. Lea.

PHARMACEUTICAL LEXICON. A Dictionary of Pharmaceutical Science, containing a concise explanation of the various subjects and terms of Pharmacy, with appropriate selections from the Collateral Sciences. Designed as a Guide for the Pharmaceutist, Druggist, Physician, etc. By. H. V. Sweringen, Member of the American Pharmaceutical Association, etc. Philadelphia: Lindsay and Blakiston. 1873, pp. 576 8vo.

The contents of the volume before us, in addition to the Lexcon proper, may be stated as on the title-page: Formulæ for Officinal, Empirical, and Diatetic Preparations; Selections from the Prescriptions of the most eminent physicians of Europe and America; an alphabetical list of Diseases and their Definitions; An account of the various modes in use for the Preservation of Dead Bodies for interment or dissection; table of signs and abbreviations, weights and measures, doses, antidotes to poisons, etc., etc., and as an item of curiosity, a few leaves from a Dispensatory published in the seventeenth century.

Part First.—The Lexicon comprises 428 pages, giving the various articles of the materia medica, pharmaceutical preparations, etc., etc., with brief descriptions of each; indeed, all the elementary substances are included. There is no division of the words into syllables, nor marks of accent. This we think an omission which should not have been made. While it is not a matter of special importance, yet a uniformity of pronunciation is highly desirable.

The list of *Select Prescriptions* comprising 42 pages including those for hypodermic use, contains many very valuable combinations, approved by our most eminent practitioners. It is not sufficient, in the practice of medicine, to know the general, or the special, action of a given drug, or even the indication for its administration, it is convenient and sometimes very important to give it in such form, and so combined as to act most kindly and efficiently.

In this list are to be found prescriptions to meet almost every shade of difference in indication. Especially at this time, when so much is being done to improve the preparations for agreeable administration, we cannot afford to be indifferent on this subject.

The directions for the preservation of dead bodies is very full, giving the methods used in most of the largest hospitals and colleges in England.

The work is very convenient for reference, and is such as we can cordially commend. It is gotten up in the usual good style of Lindsay and Blakiston. G.

ON THE TREATMENT OF DISEASES OF THE SKIN, with an analysis of eleven thousand consecutive cases. By Dr. McCall Anderson, Prof. of Practice of Medicine in Anderson's University, Physician to the Cutaneous wards of the University Hospital, etc., Glasgow. Philadelphia: Henry C. Lea, 1873. 8vo. pp. 84.

The work before us is divided into two parts: First, *analysis of the eleven thousand cases;* second, *the therapeutics of diseases of the skin.* The classification, the author tells us, is a modification of that adopted many years ago by Dr. A. B. Buchanan, of Glasgow, and its aim is to serve a clinical purpose. Ten thousand of the cases were in hospital, and one thousand in private practice, and are divided into " two great classes namely: (*a*.) functional; and (*b*.) organic. The organic we divide into two great classes.

" 1. Those defined by uniform causes.

" 2. Those not defined by uniform causes.

" The diseases defined by uniform causes are arranged under four heads, namely : 1, parasitic affections; 2, syphilitic affections; 8, strumous affections; 4, eruptive fevers. The diseases not defined by uniform causes comprise all affections of the skin not included in any of the preceding groups, and are arranged pathologically under three heads, namely: 1, inflammations; 2, new formations; 8, hæmorrhages." We are compelled to say that judging from the diseases put down among the *functional* affections, and those among the organic, the classification is not very clear.

" With regard to affections due to vegetable parasites, which were 656 in number, there is much difference of opinion, and consequently much variety in their classification. Thus, Wilson holds that there are no such diseases—the plant-like structures met with in ring-worm, etc., being, in his opinion, mere degenerations of the structure of which the skin is composed. Others, while admitting the class of vegetable parasitic affections, hold that they are all due to one and the same parasite ; while my own opinion, as fully explained elsewhere, and as indicated in the present statistics, is that, regarded from a

clinical point of view, there are four fungous growths, productive of four distinct affections, which under no circumstances are transmutable." The *first* of these, *tinea favosa* is due
to the presence of *achorion Schönleinii,* and occurs generally
among the lowest classes. There were 160 cases of it. *Second,*
ring-worm, or *tinea tricophytina* (due to the presence of *tricophy-
ton*) was met with 178 times. *Third, tinea versicolor,* that brown
patchy eruption which occurs upon the trunk of the body (due
to the presence of the *microsporon furfur*), was met with 120
times. The *fourth* and last, *tinea decalvans* (due to the *microsporon Audouini*) occurred 197 times. * * * It is quite evident
that all persons are not equally under the influence of vegetable parasites, a certain soil, as in the case of the higher plants,
being necessary in order to their growth; and debilitated and
strumous persons seem especially liable to be attacked. Hence
constitutional treatment to improve the general health."

He regards "tinea circinata, tinea tonsurans, and tinea sycosis, as mere varieties of ring-worm, the first affecting non-hairy
parts, the second the head, the third the other hairy parts of
the body, especially the beard."

In some cases local treatment alone proved sufficient, and
"consisted of parasiticides, such as the perchloride of mercury
(two to four grains to the ounce), the hyposulphite of soda (half
a drachm to a drachm, to the ounce), and sulphurous acid. * *
Where hairy parts were involved it was generally found necessary to extract the hair in addition to using the parasiticides,
with a view of removing along with the roots, the fungous
matter which lay embedded in the follicles and beyond the reach
of the remedy—especially so in tinea favosa and tinea sycosis.
In obstinate cases of tinea tonsurans and tinea decalvans strong
local applications—including blistering—were employed successfully."

The parasitic affections, dependent upon an animal, are "included in two forms of disease—scabies and phtheiriasis."
While for the former, sulphur is the common remedy, he very,
much prefers "sponging the whole body, night and morning,
with a solution of chlorate of lime as recommended by Dr.
Christison, or annointing it every night—for three successive
nights, with an ointment of styrax: liquid styrax, one ounce;

lard, two ounces: melt and strain." And for the latter, ointment of staphisagria and lotions of perchloride of mercury.

In that troublesome affection, acne vulgaris, which so frequently makes its appearance about the period of puberty, and in females often becomes aggravated at the menstrual period, he says, "a very elegant formula for a stimulating lotion was recommended to me by Dr. Buckley, of New York, and which is as follows:—sulphate of zinc and sulphuret of potassium, of each one drachm; rose water, four ounces: shake the bottle; cover the parts affected with pieces of lint dipped in the lotion, which are to be removed when the lint is dry. To be used night and morning."

PART SECOND. *Therapeutics of Diseases of the Skin.*—"My remarks are intended to be suggestive only, and I must leave the filling in of the picture to the subsequent experience of the reader." As hints or suggestions, the author's remarks are quite judicious in reference to the treatment of cutaneous affections.

Of *local treatment* he says, "it is *especially applicable to eruptions dependent upon local cause.* * * Frequently, however, as in cases of eczema, an eruption is called forth by a local cause, which would have failed in producing such a result, had there not been some constitutional derangement. Such cases require a mixed treatment."

Of *poultices* he says, "the most soothing poultices with which I am acquainted are made with cold water and potato starch."

Soothing ointments.—He speaks in the highest terms of the benzoated oxide of zinc ointment, brought prominently before the profession by Wilson, "and which is much improved by the addition of two drachms of spirit of camphor to each ounce of the ointment, being thus rendered softer and at the same time more cooling."

Soothing lotions :—(a) Solution of subacetate of lead, one drachm; glycerine, four drachms; distilled water, six ounces. (b) Dilute hydrocyanic acid, two drachms; bicarbonate of soda, one drachm; glycerine, four drachms; rose water, five ounce and a half."

The impermeable dressing—vulcanized India-rubber and vulcanized India-rubber cloth—is highly spoken of for some cases of eczema and psoriasis, especially when affecting the hands.

The work contains a large amount of information for so small a volume, and is especially valuable with reference to treatment. The author speaks of that which he has seen and knows. G.

THE PHYSICIAN'S VISITING LIST FOR 1874. Twenty-third year of its publication. Philadelphia: Lindsay and Blakiston.

[For Sale by the St. Louis Book & News Co.]

If there is a practicing physician in the land who has not used this aid to accuracy (in keeping accounts with patients) and punctuality in meeting professional engagements, he will find the purchase of a copy the best investment of *a dollar and a half* he ever made.

VOLTAIRE'S definition of a physician is: "An unfortunate gentleman expected every day to perform a miracle, namely— to reconcile health with intemperance."—*Boston Med. and Surg. Journal.*

ELIXIRS AND FLUID EXTRACTS.—We are much pleased with the samples found on our table from the accomplished Pharmacist, Herbert Primm, corner Washington Avenue and Fourteenth street.

These preparations, (Ferrated Elixir of Gentian, Fluid Ext. of Valerian, Elixir Phosphate of Iron, Quinine and Strychnine, Elixir Calisaya, Iron and Strychnia, Elixir Valerianate of Ammonia, Elixir Pepsin, Bismuth and Strychnia, etc.,) are made by Mr. Primm expressly for his dispensing trade, which enterprise is to be commended in him, or other dispensing Pharmaceutists for their own benefit, as well as for the public who patronize them.

A FRIENDLY WORD "fitly spoken," *i. e.*, at the right time and place, by our friends, might soon double the JOURNAL'S field of usefulness.

ORIGINAL material designed for the present number has been crowded out by Book Reviews of unusual interest.

Meteorological Observations.

METEOROLOGICAL OBSERVATIONS AT ST. LOUIS, MO.
By A. Wislizenus, M. D.

The following observations of daily temperature in St Louis are made with a MAXIMUM and MINIMUM thermometer (of Green, N. Y.). The daily minimum occurs generally in the night, the maximum about 3 P M. The monthly mean of the daily minima and maxima, added and divided by 2, gives a quite reliable mean of the monthly temperature.

THERMOMETER FAHRENHEIT.
OCTOBER, 1873.

Day of Month.	Minimum.	Maximum.	Day of Month.	Minimum.	Maximum.
1	45.5	66.5	18	48.5	60.5
2	49.0	72.0	19	37.5	54.0
3	57.0	75.0	20	37.0	55.0
4	56.5	70.0	21	34.0	60.0
5	56.0	73 0	22	47.0	66.5
6	36.5	52.5	23	32.5	44.5
7	36.0	60 0	24	30.5	54.5
8	41.5	70 0	25	36.0	59.5
9	48.0	78.5	26	46.0	53.0
10	54.5	81.0	27	32.5	50.0
11	63.0	74.5	28	26.5	38.0
12	45.0	64.5	29	23.5	43.0
13	43.5	73.0	30	36.0	59.0
14	51.5	79.0	31	26.0	40.0
15	52.0	78.0			
16	61.0	70.5	Means	43.6	62.8
17	62.0	72.5	Monthly Mean 53.2		

Quantity of rain : 2.77 inches.

Mortality Report.

FROM NOV. 1st, 1873, TO NOV. 22nd, 1873, INCLUS.

White,	Males,...... 235.	Females, ... 167.	Total, ... 402.
Colored,	Males ...... 11.	Females,...... 4.	Total, ... 15.

Total,.. 417.

AGES.

Under 5 years......147	30 to 40............ 50	70 to 80........... 16
5 to 10............ 14	40 to 50............ 47	80 to 90........... 7
10 to 20............ 24	50 to 60 31	90 to 100........... 3
20 to 30............ 40	60 to 70............ 28	

Abscess of Liver 2	Croup............12	Hydrocephalus...... 1	Pneumonia..........22
Accident 5	Cystitis 1	Hepatitis............ 1	Pleuritis. 4
Anemia 2	Debility 12	Hydrothorax....... 1	Peritonitis 5
Atrophia 1	Diarrhœa 6	Inanition 3	Phlebitis 2
Atelectasis.... 2	Diphtheria........ 2	Inflammat'n Bowels 3	Rheum. of Heart 1
Albuminuria 1	Dropsy............ 5	" Lungs.. 3	Scarlatina 3
Ascites . . . 1	Dysentery 10	Jaundice 1	Scald. 1
Asthma............ 5	Dentition 3	Laryngitis 2	Small Pox..........13
Apoplexy........ 5	Eclampsia 2	Lockjaw.......... 7	Syphilis 3
Angina Pectoris.... 1	Enteritis............ 8	Marasmus 20	Spinal Disease...... 1
Bronchitis 5	Empyema 2	Measles 2	Softening of Brain.. 1
Bright's Disease . . 2	Fever, congestive 2	Murder 2	Scirrhus 1
Cancer.. 3	" remittent. 3	Meningitis 9	Ulcerat of bowels . 2
Cholera Morbus . 1	" typhoid . 15	Mening. cereb-spin.. 6	Uremia... 1
" Infantum . 7	Gastritis 3	Morbus coxarius . 1	
Cirrhosis of Liver 3	Hypertrophy 1	Metritis 1	Total........417
Concussion Brain.. 2	Heart Disease 1	Metro Peritonitis 2	
Conges. of Bowels... 1	" Valv. " 3	Œdema of Lung.... 1	Stillborn............39
" Brain . 5	Hernia Umbilical... 1	Old Age............ 8	
" Lungs.. 3	Hæmoptysis........ 1	Paralysis.......... 3	
Consumption........44	Hemorrhage........ 6	Poison............ 1	
Convulsions 22	" Lungs.. 1	Premature Birth.... 6	

Lightning Source UK Ltd.
Milton Keynes UK
UKHW020624120219
337137UK00005B/538/P